Chronic Pain Epidemiology

Chronic Pain Epidemiology
From Aetiology to Public Health

Edited by

Peter Croft

Fiona M. Blyth

Danielle van der Windt

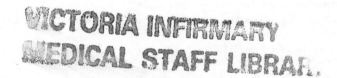

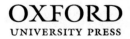

OXFORD
UNIVERSITY PRESS

OXFORD

UNIVERSITY PRESS

Great Clarendon Street, Oxford OX2 6DP

Oxford University Press is a department of the University of Oxford.
It furthers the University's objective of excellence in research, scholarship,
and education by publishing worldwide in

Oxford New York

Auckland Cape Town Dar es Salaam Hong Kong Karachi
Kuala Lumpur Madrid Melbourne Mexico City Nairobi
New Delhi Shanghai Taipei Toronto

With offices in

Argentina Austria Brazil Chile Czech Republic France Greece
Guatemala Hungary Italy Japan Poland Portugal Singapore
South Korea Switzerland Thailand Turkey Ukraine Vietnam

Oxford is a registered trade mark of Oxford University Press
in the UK and in certain other countries

Published in the United States
by Oxford University Press Inc., New York

British Library Cataloguing in Publication Data
Data available

Library of Congress Cataloging in Publication Data
Data available

Typeset in Minion by Glyph International, Bangalore, India
Printed in Great Britain
on acid-free paper by
the MPG Books Group, Bodmin and King's Lynn

ISBN 978–0–19–923576–6

10 9 8 7 6 5 4 3 2 1

Oxford University Press makes no representation, express or implied, that the drug dosages in this book
are correct. Readers must therefore always check the product information and clinical procedures with
the most up-to-date published product information and data sheets provided by the manufacturers and
the most recent codes of conduct and safety regulations. The authors and the publishers do not accept
responsibility or legal liability for any errors in the text or for the misuse or misapplication of material
in this work. Except where otherwise stated, drug dosages and recommendations are for the non-pregnant
adult who is not breastfeeding.

Preface

In this book we consider the idea that chronic pain is a condition in itself, which can be studied in populations and assessed as a public health problem, using concepts and ideas from classical epidemiology.

The book does not attempt to cover the epidemiology of all painful conditions. We have selected some individual conditions as examples, together with chapters on general topics and methodological issues. Our aim is to provide a framework and basis for thinking about chronic pain in populations and about the potential for its prevention in public health terms.

The book owes much to the ideas of the late Geoffrey Rose, who first introduced the idea of sick populations in a lecture at the North Staffordshire Medical Institute, Stoke-on-Trent, UK, subsequently published as an article in the *British Medical Journal* (Rose, 1981).

Rose, G. 1981: Strategy of prevention: lessons from cardiovascular disease. *BMJ* **282**, 1847–51.

Contents

Contributors

Fiona M. Blyth,
Head, Pain Epidemiology Unit,
University of Sydney Pain Management
Research Institute at Royal North Shore
Hospital; School of Public Health,
University of Sydney, Australia

Helen Boardman,
Lecturer in Pharmacy Practice,
Division of Social Research in
Medicines and Health,
School of Pharmacy,
University of Nottingham, UK

Adriana Paola Botello,
Research Fellow, Aberdeen Pain
Research Collaboration (Health
Services Research Unit),
University of Aberdeen,
Aberdeen, UK

Frances Boyle,
Director, Patricia Ritchie Centre for
Cancer Care and Research, Mater
Hospital, North Sydney; University
of Sydney, Australia

Julie Bruce,
Senior Research Fellow, Aberdeen Pain
Research Collaboration (Epidemiology
Group), University of Aberdeen,
Aberdeen, UK

Dag Bruusgaard,
Professor in Social Medicine,
Department of Health and Society,
University of Oslo, Norway

Rachelle Buchbinder,
Director, Monash Department of Clinical
Epidemiology at Cabrini Hospital;
Professor, Department of Epidemiology
and Preventive Medicine, School of Public
Health and Preventive Medicine,
Monash University;
Melbourne, Victoria, Australia

Peter Croft,
Professor of Primary Care Epidemiology,
Arthritis Research UK Primary Care Centre,
Keele University, UK

Clermont E. Dionne,
Director, Population Health Research Unit
(URESP), Research Centre
of the Laval University Affiliated Hospital,
Québec City, Canada

Michael Doherty,
Professor of Rheumatology,
Academic Rheumatology,
University of Nottingham, UK

Kate Dunn,
Senior Lecturer in Epidemiology,
Wellcome Trust Research Career
Development Fellow, Arthritis Research UK
Primary Care Centre,
Keele University, UK

Gene Feder,
Professor of Primary Health Care,
University of Bristol, UK

Harry Hemingway,
Professor of Clinical Epidemiology,
Department of Epidemiology and Public
Health, University College London, UK

Camilla Ihlebæk,
Professor of Public Health,
Research Group for Nature,
Health and Quality of Life,
University of Life Sciences,
Ås, Norway, and Unit for Stress,
Health and Rehabilitation,
Uni Health, Bergen, Norway

Anthony K.P. Jones,
Professor of Neuro-Rheumatology,
Human Pain Research Group
Clinical Sciences Building,
Hope Hospital, Salford, UK

Gareth T. Jones,
Senior Lecturer in Epidemiology,
Aberdeen Pain Research Collaboration
(Epidemiology Group),
University of Aberdeen,
Aberdeen, UK

Yusman Kamaleri,
Research Scientist, SINTEF Technology
and Society, Department of Global Health
and Welfare, Oslo, Norway

Gary J. Macfarlane,
Professor of Epidemiology, Aberdeen Pain
Research Collaboration (Epidemiology
Group) University of Aberdeen,
Aberdeen, UK

Alex MacGregor,
Professor of Genetic Epidemiology
Consultant Rheumatologist,
University of East Anglia, Norwich, UK

Chris J. Main
Professor of Clinical Psychology
(Pain Management),
Arthritis Research UK Primary Care Centre,
Keele University, UK

John McBeth,
Reader in Epidemiology, Arthritis Research
UK Primary Care Centre,
Keele University, UK

Bård Natvig,
Senior Research Fellow,
Department of Health and Society,
University of Oslo, Norway, and National
Resource Centre for Rehabilitation in
Rheumatology, Diakonhjemmet Hospital,
Oslo, Norway

H. Susan J. Picavet,
Senior Public Health Researcher,
Centre for Prevention and Health Services
Research, National Institute of Public Health
and the Environment, Bilthoven,
The Netherlands

Andrea Power,
Clinical Scientist,
Human Pain Research Group,
Clinical Sciences Building,
Hope Hospital, Salford, UK

Heiner Raspe,
Professor of Social Medicine,
Director of Institute of Social Medicine,
University at Lübeck, Germany

Blair H. Smith,
Professor of Primary Care Medicine,
Aberdeen Pain Research Collaboration
(Centre of Academic Primary Care),
University of Aberdeen,
Aberdeen, UK

Elaine Thomas,
Reader in Biostatistics,
Arthritis Research UK Primary Care Centre,
Keele University, UK

Nicola Torrance,
Research Fellow, Aberdeen Pain Research
Collaboration (Centre of Academic Primary
Care), University of Aberdeen,
Aberdeen, UK

Danielle van der Windt,
Professor of Primary Care Epidemiology,
Arthritis Research UK Primary Care Centre,
Keele University, UK

Gwenllian Wynne-Jones,
National Institute for Health Research
(NIHR) Fellow, Arthritis Research UK
Primary Care Centre,
Keele University, UK

M. Justin S. Zaman,
Clinical Lecturer in Cardiology, Division
of Medicine, University College,
London, UK

Weiya Zhang,
Associate Professor in Musculoskeletal
Epidemiology, Academic Rheumatology,
University of Nottingham, UK

Section 1

Basic ideas

Chapter 1

Chronic pain as a topic for epidemiology and public health

Peter Croft, Fiona M. Blyth, and Danielle van der Windt

Epidemiology is the study of the distribution and determinants of illness and disease in populations. It informs clinical practice, but its main application is in public health to guide policy and practice in the prevention of disease and its consequences in populations.

To be considered a public health problem, a disease or health state or event has to be viewed from a population perspective. This implies that there is a measurable and important impact on the population of interest – be it a community or a whole country. For this to be so, the health condition has to be common (affecting large numbers of people, across multiple sections of the community), but it also has to matter – because it limits life, diminishes the enjoyment of it, or has a heavy cost – in direct (e.g. cost of care) or indirect terms (e.g. reduced productivity at work or at home).

The epidemiology of chronic pain can be briefly summarized. Chronic pain is common and universal; it occurs at all ages and in all populations and has been reported throughout recorded history.

From a public health perspective, chronic pain has a major impact on the physical and mental capacity to function in everyday life, the quality of that daily life, and the economic balance-sheet of populations.

So, first we consider why chronic pain is not more widely recognized as an important public health problem, and whether chronic pain can be framed as a suitable topic for population epidemiology and a public health approach.

Pain is a condition in its own right

In medical textbooks, pain has a dual nature. It is both a classic manifestation of, and signpost to, diagnosis in many different diseases and, at the same time, a symptom in its own right needing relief and attention.

Its most important role in the medical tradition has been as a 'symptom of something'. Pain provides a pointer to a diagnosis, to an underlying pathology, which can be investigated, treated, or cured. 'Sudden tight crushing chest pain' is taught to medical students and translated into public health education programmes as a signal of a possible heart attack. Relief of this acute pain is regarded as a satisfying event for both patient and doctor, but even more important is the diagnosis of the underlying medical problem (disease of the coronary arteries resulting in myocardial infarction – 'acute damage to the muscle of the heart' – the classic heart attack) and the action needed to reduce the immediate threat it poses to life.

However, should pain only be regarded as an issue secondary to the important work of diagnosis and attempts at cure of the underlying disease? Siddall and Cousins have argued that the range of unique pathological processes, initiated by stimulation of the sensory nerves ('nociceptive' pain) or damage to nerve fibres ('neuropathic' pain), qualifies chronic pain to be regarded as a disease entity in its own right (Siddall and Cousins, 2004). Aronowitz has pointed out how social and cultural factors have often influenced whether a symptom came to be regarded historically as a disease or not (Aronowitz, 2001). The argument in this book is that, regardless of where pain is placed conceptually on the pathology-symptom spectrum, it can properly and helpfully be viewed as a 'condition in itself'. Epidemiology and public health should be concerned to make the phenomenon of pain – and more specifically chronic or persistent pain – a proper object of concern, study, and policy.

The concept of acute pain as a public health problem

Pain is by definition a subjectively felt experience, and as such raises a challenge to epidemiological science seeking objectively to measure the occurrence of events in populations. When pain is a direct result of an acute diagnosable disease, as in the myocardial infarction example above, objective changes on an electrocardiogram or in levels of cardiac enzymes in the blood can be used to define the event for epidemiological investigation and for public health interventions and policy-making about prevention and best care. To the extent that effective prevention and care of the underlying disease can be put into practice, the level of suffering in a population associated with pain, e.g. the acute pain of myocardial infarction, will be reduced.

In general, this is true of the many situations in which pain arises from an immediate pathological condition, such as trauma, infection, infarction, or inflammation. Relief of the pain is seen as an immediate priority by the sufferer and by the professionals caring for them, and this will be achieved both by pain-reducing procedures (such as medications, embrocations, or distraction techniques) and by tackling the underlying problem. However, for epidemiological and public health purposes, such events are traditionally counted by a defined measure or proxy of the causal disease (e.g. electrocardiographic changes in myocardial infarction) and the pain itself is arguably lost from view. The epidemiology linked with pain and suffering becomes the epidemiology of car accidents, meningitis, heart attacks, or gout.

Despite this, there is no reason why a subjective experience, such as the pain experienced when a bone is fractured, should not be the primary topic of epidemiological investigation. Studying pain complaints in populations through the use of carefully constructed questionnaires, which standardize aspects of the reports of this subjective experience, makes for objective science. In Chapter 5, Dionne discusses this issue in depth and explores methodological approaches to applying such a construct in population studies of pain.

However, this book is concerned with a much broader issue than describing and measuring the experience of pain as a response to acute events in the body. If it were only concerned with the latter problem, then such an aim or objective would remain secondary and subservient to the main business of describing and measuring the occurrence of the underlying event. The public health philosophy would still be summed up as: 'if we can prevent accidents and heart attacks and gout, then the problem of the pain they cause would also be prevented'. Although this book considers (in Section 5) examples of the extent to which this approach is indeed relevant to pain as a population problem, its central thesis is that chronic pain poses a very different and additional challenge for population epidemiology.

The concept of chronic pain as a public health problem

The basic definition of chronic pain – pain which persists beyond the immediate event which precipitated it – does not, on the surface, disturb the standard medical textbook concern with 'pain as a symptom of something'. The pain which persists after a fracture would not be there if the fracture had not happened in the first place.

However, the measurement of the symptom of chronic pain inevitably becomes more concerned with a state – persistence of pain over time – than with the original acute precipitating event. This persistence is traditionally measured in population studies by the estimated duration of a pain complaint. The complexities involved in doing this are considered in the chapters of Section 2, but all approaches start from the position that persistence over time is an essential dimension in defining chronicity of pain.

The epidemiological perspective might still remain firmly focussed on the underlying disease – rheumatoid arthritis as the cause of chronic joint pain for example. Public health strategies might still be concerned with prevention or treatment of this underlying problem as the way to prevent the persisting pain – e.g. prevent or effectively treat rheumatoid arthritis as a means to prevent both chronic joint pain and the restricted activity associated with it. Yet it is clear that not all persons who suffer pain from a particular pathological condition will develop persistent symptoms (e.g. some people get more continuing pain from a healing fracture than others) and not all chronic pain can easily be attributed to underlying pathological causes (back pain being one common example, and more surprisingly angina is another, as Hemingway and colleagues illustrate in Chapter 20).

This is the great puzzle of chronic pain – how it so often appears to be a 'condition in itself' distinct from any obvious immediate cause. Written about elegantly in texts such as those by the late Patrick Wall (Wall, 1999), this puzzle has been the object of spectacular and innovative scientific advances in the field of neurobiology for many decades now, and in Chapter 9 Jones and colleagues consider the example of chronic widespread pain from the perspective of these advances.

This puzzle provides one explanation of why chronic pain has been neglected in the public health agenda and yet needs to be placed clearly on it. The assumption has been that, as a symptom, it will be studied and sorted under the diseases which are presumed to cause it. Surveys of those diseases, which include clinical examinations and investigations, are preferred to surveys based on symptom report alone as the basis for global estimates of the disease burden of chronic pain (Mathers et al., 2006) and this approach has almost certainly underestimated the global burden of chronic pain. Pain conditions are poorly captured in internationally used disease-coding classifications such as the International Classification of Diseases (ICD) (Buchbinder et al., 1996), and yet the extent to which chronic pain has a life of its own makes it a distinct, independent, and important cause of distress and disability in daily life. Concepts and methods are needed in order to study it from the population perspective as a condition in its own right.

Expanding the concept of chronic pain for public health

The story outlined above takes pain, acute or chronic, as a symptom of something or a condition in itself, to a point where it is still 'pain' – a single symptom dependent on subjective report. Persons with chronic pain, however, have a syndrome that usually involves more than self-reported pain in a particular location. In Heiner Raspe's phrase 'back pain is more than pain in the back' (Raspe et al., 2003).

The character of the pain itself (e.g. its severity, or how widespread it is) and the extent of its impact on activities of daily life provide two obvious ways in which the distinctiveness of the symptom as a 'condition in its own right' can be defined and measured in populations.

Although such characteristics can be used to develop simple core definitions of chronic pain for purposes of descriptive epidemiology, Raspe in Chapter 6 describes the evidence that chronic pain, as a measurable phenomenon in populations, consists of a constellation of problems, of varying number, type, and severity, which together represent the 'amplification' of pain into a much broader syndrome than pain alone.

The idea of amplification lines up with evidence and ideas about the evolution and maintenance of chronic pain in sufferers, which draws on disciplines from biology through psychology to sociology. From an epidemiological perspective, this means that the event being counted and studied is a cluster of problems focussed on chronic pain, the whole thing being a distinctive 'condition in itself'. This 'chronic pain syndrome' has its own causes and consequences, which may be independent of, or additional to, the causes and consequences of the identifiable and possibly preventable diseases which precipitated the pain in the first place. This idea is summarized in Figure 1.1.

Individuals, however, will vary in the extent to which their pain is amplified into a broader syndrome and in the way in which the experience, severity, and impact of pain may change over time. For this, the population and public health approach needs a perspective couched in terms of risk and probability.

The concept of risk applied to chronic pain

The likelihood that a person will develop chronic pain can be considered partly independent of the disease that precipitates the pain. Clearly, diseases such as an expanding tumour or recurrent episodes of inflammation in arthritis provide continuing peripheral sensory input into the nervous system over time. However, regardless of whether the active underlying disease is still present or not, a certain propensity or level of risk for developing chronic pain exists in persons prior to their experience of a pain-triggering disease or event, and independent of whether the trigger continues or not. The probability that a person will develop chronic pain, after the onset of acute pain, is then a product of this prior propensity and the nature of the acute or recurrent pain experience.

This picture provides the basis for a way of describing the occurrence of chronic pain in populations which is more dynamic than simple cross-sectional prevalence of the chronic pain syndrome, although closely related to it. One such 'prognostic definition' has been characterized by Von Korff and colleagues and is discussed in the introduction to Section 2. It concerns people who have pain at a point in time, and uses the estimated probability that such people will have pain in the future as the basis for defining current pain status as chronic.

A certain propensity or level of risk for developing chronic pain also applies to people who do not have pain at a particular point in time. Most people experience pain in the course of any single year, and they will carry a certain risk of developing the 'chronic pain syndrome' if they are exposed to a triggering event. This risk will be influenced by the nature, severity, and circumstances of any pain they experience, and by their underlying propensity to develop chronic pain. So, a second way of fitting pain into a traditional epidemiological and public health model is to view it, similarly to blood pressure or cholesterol, as something which everyone experiences to a certain extent and as one risk factor for the development of the chronic pain syndrome. An example of a candidate factor for use as a continuously distributed marker of risk for 'chronic pain syndrome' in populations – namely the number of self-reported sites of pain in the body – is discussed by Natvig et al. in Chapter 7.

Comparator public health problems

Diseases with high public health profile because of their mortality risk, such as cancer, acquired immune deficiency syndrome (AIDS), and cardiovascular disease, can cause pain which is clearly of huge importance to the individual, and deserves and demands treatment by the best means possible, especially if the disease itself cannot be cured. However, the high mortality rates, and the comparatively low prevalence, of these diseases compared with common chronic pain syndromes such as musculoskeletal pain, headache, or widespread pain, mean that the time spent in chronic pain which is directly attributable to such continuing disease only contributes a small part of the burden of chronic pain in populations. The traditional epidemiological view would be to deduce that the fraction of chronic pain in the general population which is attributable to the effects of diseases such as cancer is small.

However, this view is becoming less true as the survival rate from these conditions improves. Blyth and colleagues investigate this view in Chapter 21. Reduction in the fatality rate of many diseases, and improved treatments, mean that people are living for longer with diagnosed conditions such as AIDS, cardiovascular disease, and cancer – resulting in more people living for longer periods with pain which is potentially less 'terminal' as death is delayed. Their experience therefore becomes closer to the experience of pain as a chronic morbidity.

The argument could still be made that this is chronic pain caused by AIDS or road traffic accidents or cancer, and that these conditions are themselves the real public health problem. However the reality, as fatality rates for such diseases fall, is that there is a distinctive and separate epidemiological and public health question about who gets long-term pain amongst the survivors and why. A number of authors in this book consider the evidence that chronic pain might be initiated, and maintained, by tissue damage (e.g. neuropathic pain following surgery). However, even with the most clear-cut examples of regional pathological causes of pain prior predisposition to developing chronic pain may be the important determining factor in its persistence. This principle is summarized in Figure 1.1.

Sick individuals, sick populations

The population perspective can be seen as a view of aggregated individual experience – for example, counting the individuals with chronic pain in order to estimate population frequency and burden. A crucial rationale for providing such population occurrence figures for chronic pain, regardless of cause, is to identify the need for health care and treatments, the impact on health care systems, and the potential to reduce long-term persistence of pain through effective care. Pain is such a common problem in primary care that effective treatments in that setting

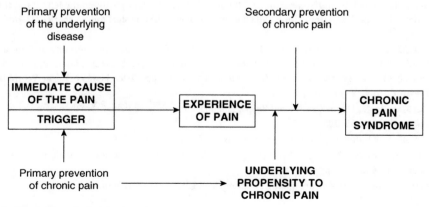

Fig. 1.1 Development of chronic pain

are in essence public health interventions, since so many of the population seek and receive treatment there.

However, the lack of long-term effective treatments and the sheer scale of the problem highlight that the primary prevention goal of public health remains crucial. Here too, the population perspective can focus on the aggregation of individual characteristics in order to define a distribution of risk in the population, and from there determine cause and identify targets for primary prevention of chronic pain.

There is a second population perspective on risk, however, that focusses on what Geoffrey Rose has called sick populations rather than sick individuals (Rose, 1985). Rose was referring to the capacity to make differences by improving a whole population's or community's distribution of levels of risk of disease. An example is cholesterol – shifting the population distribution of this factor would have large effects which would be difficult to replicate if only symptomatic individuals were treated or if people were screened for early disease and treated. The challenge and excitement of a public health view of pain relates to the extent to which populations might be characterized by their risk for chronic pain, and to the potential for those risks to be reduced by population-level interventions on factors such as cultural beliefs about pain, social circumstances, weight, or physical activity. Such interventions might shift the population curve towards lower risk of chronic pain without taking away the need for optimal and available care. Reducing injury rates or population average body mass index are two examples.

Chronic pain as a public health problem

The traditional uses of epidemiology are to provide a description of the occurrence of a disease and to determine causes of its distribution in populations. The aims are to characterize the importance of the disease as a public health problem, provide the basis for policies of prevention, and estimate the need for and effectiveness of health care. This book as a whole is designed to present some examples and illustrations of the extent to which chronic pain is an important public health problem. What we have argued in this introduction is that the important conceptual step is the definition of chronic pain as a 'problem in itself' and the possibility of setting it in traditional epidemiological frameworks of individual and population risk.

References

Aronowitz, R.A. 2001: When do symptoms become a disease? *Ann Intern Med* **134**, 803–8.

Buchbinder, R.A., Goel, V. and Bombardier, C. 1996: Lack of concordance between the ICD-9 soft tissue disorders of the neck and upper limb and chart review diagnosis: one steel mill's experience. *Am J Ind Med* **29**, 171–82.

Mathers, C.D., Lopez, A.D. and Murray, C.L.J. 2006: The Burden of Disease and Mortality by Condition: Data, Methods, and Results for 2001. In: Lopez, A.D., Mathers, C.D., Ezzati, M., Jamison, D.T. and Murray, C.J.L. (eds): *Global Burden of Disease and Risk Factors*, pp 45–93. New York: The World Bank and Oxford University Press.

Raspe, A., Matthis, C., Heon-Klin, V. and Raspe, H. 2003: Chronic back pain: more than pain in the back. *Rehabilitation* **42**, 195–203.

Rose, G. 1985: Sick individuals and sick populations. *Int J Epidemiol* **14**, 32–8.

Siddall, P.J. and Cousins, M.J. 2004: Persistent pain as a disease entity: implications for clinical management. *Anaesth Analg* **99**, 510–20.

Wall, P. 1999: *Pain: The Science of Suffering*. London: Weidenfeld and Nicolson.

Chapter 2

The global occurrence of chronic pain: an introduction

Peter Croft, Fiona M. Blyth, and Danielle van der Windt

The Black Report on Inequalities in Health in 1980 highlighted the paucity and unreliability of morbidity data for describing the burden of disease and ill-health in populations and estimating the variation in disease and illness occurrence between populations (Townsend and Davidson, 1982). The authors contrasted this with the availability and ease of interpretation of mortality data. Feachem and colleagues later re-emphasized the same point from an international perspective (Feachem et al., 1992). They pointed out that, whilst the mortality rate remains an important indicator of general health status of a population, the health priorities of a country, particularly in adults, may not be reflected in the causes of death. Important causes of morbidity may be different to the causes of mortality.

This is particularly true of chronic pain. While commonly occurring conditions such as back pain are important contributors to population morbidity burden, they do not contribute much to the major drivers of population mortality rates or years of life lost to death. Conversely, the enduring goal of reducing the risk of premature mortality in a population will have little impact on the density of severe chronic pain.

Writing in 1992, Feachem and his co-authors concluded that valid and reliable measurement of morbidity in developing and industrialized countries was an ideal not achievable at that time to a standard that could make for meaningful comparisons of morbidity over time or across communities. Chronic pain and many important conditions linked with pain, such as musculoskeletal disease, provide particular challenges for population measurement, compared with other established public health conditions such as cancer or cardiovascular disease, because case definition is more problematic (Dionne et al., 2008; Griffith et al., 2007), and there are often no population disease registries to provide supplementary evidence of disease burden (Silman, 2008). Targets for surveys or surveillance considered by Feachem et al. to represent options for measuring population morbidity included self-reported health status, clinical measurements and observer-generated diagnoses.

Self-reported health in particular reflects both underlying pathology or disease and individual or community perceptions and behaviour related to health and illness. Chronic pain, derived from a mixture of underlying precipitating pathology, propensity and social and psychological influences, represents an important and clear example of a morbidity most appropriately measured, monitored and compared at a population level by self-report.

Types of study

Studies that explore chronic pain as a public health problem (i.e. that estimate population burden) take different forms. Broadly speaking, we can distinguish between studies that focus exclusively or primarily on pain, and general health surveys which include pain as one of several health conditions of interest. *Pain-focussed studies* typically provide insights on the risk factors, natural history and pain burden within specified populations (e.g. geographical areas, primary care-seekers, age subgroups such as children or the elderly or occupational subgroups). *General health surveys* provide crucial information on the frequency of chronic pain compared with other conditions and on the overall impact of chronic pain in society. Put simply, pain-focussed studies give chronic pain a 'shape' in the public health arena, while general health surveys give chronic pain a 'place'. Both are needed to give pain a 'voice'.

The growth and usefulness of general health surveys to measure population burden of disease and ill-health have been encouraged by the development of general health-status measures based on self-report. Many, such as the Short-Form 36 (Ware et al., 1992) and Short-Form 12 (Ware et al., 1996), incorporate some measure of pain and the extent to which it interferes with daily life.

Helpful estimates of the occurrence of chronic pain can be derived also from *routinely collected health-care data*. Such data is a mixture of one component of self-perceived health (perceived need and demand for health care) and measures of disease and treatment recorded by health-care practitioners. The selective nature of health-care use by the general population means that it is a flawed measure of actual morbidity for comparative purposes, especially between countries which have differing ways to access health care, and contrasting cultures of how such care is used. However, primary care data in particular can provide useful indicators of chronic pain occurrence or proxy markers for severe pain such as rates of prescribed analgesic therapy.

Cross-national or international health surveys are worth special consideration because of three important characteristics. Firstly, for developing countries with poor health infrastructure and few (if any) internal capacities to measure chronic disease burden, such studies may provide the only avenue for obtaining prevalence estimates of chronic pain. Secondly, such studies provide the opportunity to look for consistencies in the relationships between pain and demographic characteristics or other health-related factors. If such associations endure across cultures and countries, this is indirect evidence of robust underlying mechanisms of association. Thirdly, difference in occurrence between cultures and countries, although more difficult to interpret, are also informative, particularly about potential causes of disease.

Most international studies of this type are based on general surveys that include questions on pain. A good example is provided by the World Health Organization (WHO) World Mental Health Surveys, which have applied standard instruments across a variety of countries in a co-ordinated series of population surveys incorporating questions on pain (Kessler and Ustun, 2008). Recent publications from these surveys have shed light on consistent associations between pain and a variety of mental health disorders (Demyttenaere et al., 2007).

Another example is the Community Oriented Program for Control of Rheumatic Diseases (COPCORD) series of studies in more than 17 developing and developed countries. These studies have provided unique insights into the morbidity burden of painful musculoskeletal conditions (including back and knee pain) in both developing and developed countries (Brooks, 2006).

Prevalence of self-reported chronic pain

Estimates below are mostly based on questionnaires among samples drawn from the general population. Cross-national comparisons rely on standardization of the question, common understanding or interpretation of the question and what it represents, similar sampling frames and comparable response validity. Few studies guarantee all this, but attempts to provide an overall picture can be made.

The prevalence of chronic pain, defined by duration, in the WHO World Mental Health Surveys was 37% in developed countries (Tsang et al., 2008). This is higher than some other estimates from Denmark (20%), Norway (24%) and one US study (33%) (Sjøgren et al., 2009; Rustøen et al., 2004; Portenoy et al., 2004, respectively), similar to the estimate from the Netherlands as reported in Chapter 12 (36%) and lower than some other estimates from the USA (43%), Israel (46%), Scotland (50%) and Sweden (55%) (Arnow et al., 2006; Neville et al., 2008; Elliott et al., 1999; Andersson, 1994). These differences are likely to reflect differences in the populations chosen for sampling and the precise definitions used for chronic pain.

The WHO Mental Health Surveys provide an estimate of chronic pain for developing countries of 41% (Tsang et al, 2008). Many other individual studies in developing countries draw their samples from population subgroups, but evidence suggests emerging consistency of the chronic pain experience – Brazil (41%), Nepal (47%) and South African women (45%) (Blay et al., 2007; Bhattarai et al., 2007; Naidoo et al., 2009).

If the focus is narrowed to more disabling pain, prevalence estimates are naturally lower, but appear more consistent. König et al. reported on a comparison of the EuroQol or EQ-5D in six European countries. This instrument contains a brief question enquiring about pain or discomfort, rated as none, moderate or severe. The study estimated the prevalence of persons with current moderate-or-severe pain across those general population samples to be 25% of adults (König et al., 2009). Similar estimates are found in Scotland (prevalence of chronic disabling pain 26%), the Netherlands (24%) and USA (24%) (Elliott et al., 1999; van der Windt in Chapter 12; Covinsky et al., 2009).

Narrowing the focus further to severe disabling chronic pain provides estimates of 6% (Scotland), 9% (the Netherlands), 10% (USA), 12% (Australia), 13% (Sweden) and 14% (Nepal) (Elliott et al., 1999; van der Windt in Chapter 12; Blyth et al., 2001; Andersson, 1994; Bhattarai et al., 2007). These figures are similar to those for the more specific problem of chronic widespread pain, consistently ~12% of adult populations (e.g. Bergman et al., 2001; also see Chapters 9 and 15). Variation in these figures is again likely to reflect difference in definitions and sampling frames or source populations.

Age and gender variations in chronic pain prevalence are remarkably consistent across countries and populations (i.e. women consistently report higher prevalence of chronic pain than men, and pain that interferes with life increases with age). This is reviewed in detail in Chapters 10, 12 and 16.

There are two other clear and consistent messages from population surveys of chronic pain in developed and developing countries:

1 *Musculoskeletal pain, notably back and joint pain, is the dominant single type of chronic pain* (see, e.g. the WHO World Mental Health Surveys (Demyttenaere et al., 2007) and Elliott et al., 1999).

2 *Most people with chronic pain have multiple sites of pain* (see, e.g. Chapter 12).

These two facts explain why population surveys of chronic pain in individual sites, especially musculoskeletal sites such as the back, but also headache and other common pain syndromes, often provide prevalence figures close to those for 'all chronic pain', as in the examples shown above.

The presence of multiple pains is also closely associated with pain severity, disability in daily living and associated features of the 'chronic pain syndrome' (see Chapter 6), which explains why population prevalence figures for severe chronic pain are similar to those for severe chronic back pain or chronic widespread pain. For example, most back pain that is chronic and disabling will be accompanied by pain at other body sites and would qualify also as chronic widespread pain. Although we consider different pain syndromes in this book, it is our view that there is substantial overlap between most chronic pain syndromes, and also between chronic pain and many other conditions of chronic ill-health, notably mental illness (see, e.g. Demyttenaere et al., 2007, and van der Windt's Chapter 12).

The summary above hides much variation between individual studies, although the tighter the definition (e.g. of chronic disabling pain or chronic widespread pain), the more consistent the figures tend to become. Although prevalence estimates do differ between countries in surveys such as the WHO studies, they are difficult to explore as classic population differences because potential methodological explanations of the differences (e.g. response, sampling methods or interpretation of questions) pose a barrier to realistic comparison. Currently, trans-national comparisons are more useful to stress the general consistency between countries in their overall frequency of self-reported chronic pain (Figure 2.1).

Dionne, in Chapter 5, highlights the opportunities to perform classic epidemiological analyses of differences between population groups if standard questions can be developed for use in different settings and languages.

One recent example of consistency was a survey of chronic widespread pain in men in eight European countries conducted as part of the European Male Ageing Study (Macfarlane et al., 2009). There was substantial variation in survey completion rates and in prevalence estimates. However, the associations between chronic widespread pain and other characteristics (e.g. age, psychological distress) were similar across countries. Adjusting for the varying distribution of these other factors between the countries explained most, although not all, of the trans-national differences in chronic widespread pain prevalence (notably the higher rates in eastern Europe), and so deals with issues of 'aggregation bias'.

Prevalence of chronic pain based on health care data

Large computerized databases of recorded morbidity seen in primary care consultations have provided estimates of the workload related to painful conditions. A major challenge to this endeavour is that codes and diagnoses in primary care are not organized with respect to chronic pain.

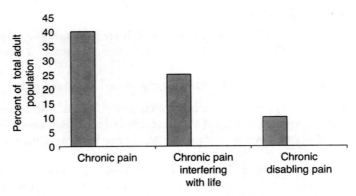

Fig. 2.1 Crude summary figures for chronic pain prevalence (adults).

Hasselstrom et al. met this challenge by classifying all consultations in a year made by a population sample of 14 000 persons in Sweden, according to whether pain was a reason for attending or not (Hasselstrom et al., 2002). They identified that 30% of patients were consulting about pain; half of these contacts were concerned with chronic or recurrent pain, and two-thirds were about musculoskeletal conditions. Koleva et al. recruited 89 general practitioners in Italy to identify contacts concerning pain during two working weeks – one-third of all reported contacts were about pain, i.e. similar to the Hasselstrom estimate; the main complaints were musculoskeletal and abdominal, and, again similarly to the Swedish study, half were about chronic pain. In both studies, two-thirds of the pain consultations resulted in a prescription for some sort of analgesic medication (Koleva et al., 2005). Caudill-Slosberg et al. analysed office visits for musculoskeletal pain in a US Health Maintenance Organization, and found that 28% of adult visits in 2000 were related to musculoskeletal pain (Caudill-Slosberg et al., 2004).

Evidence from population surveys which have included self-report questions about use of health care indicates that not all people with a specific chronic disabling pain in the community will consult primary care health professionals about it in any one year (e.g. Jinks et al., 2004). So primary care consultation data has to be interpreted carefully as a measure of population period prevalence. Moreover, they are only available as population-based measures in a limited number of countries. However, if we assume that consulting populations represent the patterns of pain in the general population, the finding that 30–33% of patients consulting in one year in primary care in Europe will be seeking help for chronic pain does align reasonably with the population estimates of chronic pain from self-report surveys discussed in the previous section. Both estimates of course may suffer from the same 'bias': people without any health problem will not seek health care, but may also be less inclined to respond to a health survey.

Global burden of chronic pain

The impact of chronic pain can be measured simply for epidemiological purposes by questions which focus on troublesome or interfering pain. Worldwide this approach aligns with the perspective taken to calculate population Disability-Adjusted Life Years (DALYs) related to individual diseases. The DALY combines years of life lost (YLL) with years lived with disability (YLD), where disability is estimated by measures such as SF36 or EQ5D (Murray and Lopez, 1996). This means that conditions such as headache and osteoarthritis, which are not linked to premature mortality at the population level, can contribute substantially Chapter 17 to population DALY scores because of the sum of years they contribute to living with chronic pain-related disability. However, DALYS are designed to relate to the population impact of individual diseases, and so will also reflect the mortality of diseases underlying chronic pain (e.g. cancer or ischaemic heart disease) as much as the long-term cumulative public health impact of chronic pain on YLD exemplified by conditions such as arthritis, back pain and headache.

By 2006, the four leading contributors to the Global Burden of Disability, according to DALYs, were human immunodeficiency virus (HIV)-acquired immune deficiency syndrome (AIDS), unipolar depression, coronary heart disease and road traffic accidents – all linked with chronic pain. Injury is a major contributor to the global burden of disease, and occurs predominantly in younger age groups and commonly in developing countries (Mathers et al., 2006). Chronic pain often arises from traumatic injury, and yet is rarely documented in trauma registries as an important sequel of injury (see Chapter 17).

Although the DALYs of the four conditions mentioned above will have substantial components from YLD, there is obviously continuing significant premature mortality related to all four also, and so their impact is the combination of YLD and mortality. There is a case for arguing that DALYs have underestimated the overall health impact of painful conditions, even though pain is one of the domains included in calculating the disability weights. YLD might be the best single measure of chronic pain impact *per se* on population health.

Empirical support for the importance of YLD comes from papers such as those of Melzer, Mottram and Covinsky (Melzer et al., 2005; Mottram et al., 2008; Covinsky et al., 2009). These population-based studies all identified the strong association in adults in their middle years between pain and locomotor disability (Figure 2.2 shows data from Mottram's study). Covinsky identified that people in the age range of 50–59 years with significant pain have a similar prevalence of functional limitation as people from the same population in the age range of 80–89 years who report no pain – a clear indication of the potential impact of chronic pain on YLD.

A second reason why the most recent estimations of the global burden of disease have underestimated the contribution of chronic pain conditions is because of the disease-based model underlying the calculations. A restricted subset of conditions was used as the basis for the calculations, which excluded many of the common regional musculoskeletal pain syndromes

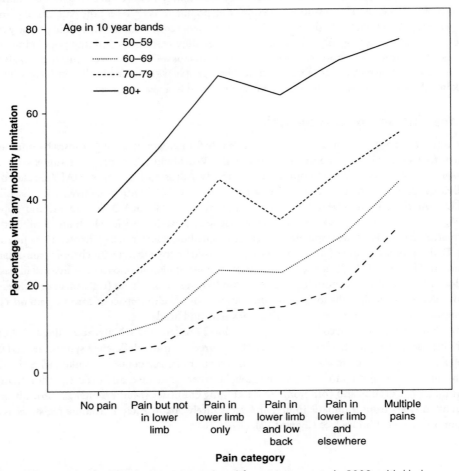

Fig. 2.2 Pain, limited mobility and age. Reproduced from Mottram et al., 2008, with kind permission from Springer Science+Business Media.

that dominate global pain prevalence (Mathers et al., 2006). Osteoarthritis still emerged as one of the 20 leading contributors to the global burden of disease.

In a comparison of chronic conditions among eight developed countries, arthritis consistently had the biggest effect on the SF-36 pain score (Alonso et al., 2004). Chronic lung disease, ischaemic heart disease and congestive cardiac failure all had similar effects to arthritis on physical functioning (i.e. they were the four conditions associated with the worst physical function scores), but the impact of arthritis on physical functioning was the most consistent finding across the different countries.

More recent modelling of health survey data in Europe to produce disability projections for the next 30 years has adopted the measure of disability-free life expectancy. This has identified musculoskeletal conditions as the major and most rapidly accelerating potential cause of future restrictions in total years spent in healthy living (Jagger et al, 2006).

Time trends of pain in populations

The study of historical changes in pain also has to deal with issues of uncertain validity of comparisons – methodological variation in the content and style of questions between surveys undertaken at different points in time makes the study of secular change difficult; nevertheless, attempts have been made.

Results from two cross-sectional population surveys conducted 40 years apart in the North of England (between 1956 and 1995) were compared (Harkness et al., 2005). The authors highlighted the increase in prevalence of low back pain, shoulder and widespread pain and the switch in the gender association in the latter two conditions (from male to female predominance). Earlier investigation of two UK-wide population surveys noted a rise in the prevalence of low back pain between 1986 and 1996, although the prevalence of more severe disabling back pain had not changed (Palmer et al., 2000). By contrast, US researchers have more recently noted a rise in the prevalence of chronic severe impairing back pain in North Carolina in USA from 4% to 10%, between two population surveys conducted in 1992 and 2006 respectively. The increases were similar in whites and blacks, and linked with a rise in health-care use during a period when general health-care use had not increased (Freburger et al., 2009). Low back pain prevalence in random samples of the adult Stockholm county population was measured every 4 years between 1990 and 2006. Investigators using this data noted an increase in pain-related problems generally, and in women in particular (Burström et al., 2007).

The conclusions of the authors of these papers all include an acceptance that sampling bias might be contributing to their findings, but they infer that some of the observed change is real. However, the changes are not necessarily attributable to an increase in underlying disease – rather the authors highlight possible explanations related to rising expectations and increasing availability of investigations and treatments, heightened symptom awareness and changes in sickness-benefit systems.

Benefit or invalidity payments for work loss due to chronic illness provide another way to monitor secular changes in pain over time, although, as with the use of primary care data to monitor pain occurrence, the selectivity of the samples needs to be taken into account. Steenstra et al. investigated trends in occupational disability due to back pain in the Netherlands between 1980 and 2000 (Steenstra et al., 2006). The authors noted that occupational disability attributed to non-specific back and neck pain had increased, whilst attribution of more specific diagnoses declined; they considered this reflected changes in attitudes towards management, and away from clinicians diagnosing 'disease' to an acceptance of the pain as the problem.

Between 1996 and 2003 in Norway, Ihlebaek found poor concordance between sickness-absence rates, which had increased during this time, and self-reported prevalence of symptoms in

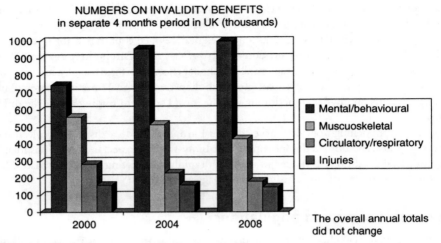

Fig. 2.3 Time trends in sickness benefits for chronic disease

Norwegian population surveys, which had been stable during the same period (Ihlebaek et al., 2006). This is evidence for what Waddell highlighted in his classic book on back pain: population rates of sickness absence and benefit payments for chronic back pain are a separate phenomenon to the occurrence of the symptom itself (Waddell, 1998). Waddell described the historical rise in rates of low back sickness-absence and invalidity rates from the 1950s through to 1990s in the USA, UK and Sweden. Although it now seems likely that this was accompanied by some increase in self-reported prevalence of low back pain in the community, the changes in sickness-certification and invalidity benefit-payment rates far exceeded estimates of the likely changes in general reporting of the symptom.

In another analysis of the Stockholm population survey data 1990–2006, referred to above, a particular increase in the prevalence of combined low back pain and psychological distress in both men and women was identified (Leijon and Mulder, 2009). Although this subgroup represents only a minority of low back pain sufferers, the authors suggested that changes in pain prevalence in recent years reflect alterations in the distress component of chronic pain. This accords with more recent findings from UK invalidity benefit data, shown in Figure 2.3, which shows a decline in musculoskeletal conditions (and other chronic diseases) and a steady rise in mental ill-health as the attributed reasons for not working throughout the period 2000–08 (calculated from open access data on the UK Department of Work and Pensions website).

Conclusion

Population surveys suggest that self-reported chronic pain occurs to a similar extent in many parts of the world. Chronic pain is emerging as an important component of the global burden of disability. Musculoskeletal pain and headaches dominate in terms of frequency and overall impact, but the more severe end of the spectrum is mostly about multiple pains. There is evidence that the reporting of chronic pain has increased in recent decades.

References

Alonso, J., Ferrer, M., Gandek, B., Ware Jr, J.E., Aaronson, N.K., Mosconi, P., et al. and the IQOLA Project Group. 2004: Health-related quality of life associated with chronic conditions in eight countries: Results from the International Quality of Life Assessment (IQOLA) Project. *Qual Life Res* **13**, 283–98.

Andersson, H.I. 1994: The epidemiology of chronic pain in a Swedish rural area. *Qual Life Res* **3**, S19–26.

Arnow, B.A., Hunkeler, E.M., Blasey, C.M., Lee, J., Constantino, M.J., Fireman, B., et al. 2006: Comorbid depression, chronic pain, and disability in primary care. *Psychosom Med* **68**, 262–268.

Bergman, S., Herrström, P., Högström, K., Petersson, I.F., Svensson, B. and Jacobsson, L.T. 2001: Chronic musculoskeletal pain, prevalence rates, and sociodemographic associations in a Swedish population study. *J Rheumatol* **28**, 1369–1377.

Bhattarai, B., Pokhrei, P.K., Tripathi, M., Rahman, T.R., Baral, D.D., Pande, R. et al. 2007: Chronic pain and cost: an epidemiological study in the communities of Sunsari district of Nepal. *Nepal Med Coll J* **9**, 6–11.

Blay, S.L., Andreoli, S.B., Dewey, M.E. and Gastal, F.L. 2007: Co-occurrence of chronic physical pain and psychiatric morbidity in a community sample of older people. *Int J Geriatr Psychiatry* **22**, 902–908.

Blyth, F.M., March, L.M., Brnabic, A.J., Jorm, L.R., Williamson, M. and Cousins, M.J. 2001: Chronic pain in Australia: a prevalence study. *Pain* **89**, 127–134.

Brooks, P.M. 2006: The burden of musculoskeletal disease – a global perspective. *Clin Rheumatol* **25**, 778–781.

Burström, K., Johannesson, M. and Rehnberg, C. 2007: Deteriorating health status in Stockholm 1998-2002: results from repeated population surveys using the EQ-5D. *Qual Life Res* **16**, 1547–53.

Caudill-Slosberg, M.A., Schwartz, L.M. and Woloshin, S. 2004: Office visits and analgesic prescriptions for musculoskeletal pain in US: 1980 vs 2000. *Pain* **109**, 514–519.

Covinsky, K.E., Lindquist, K., Dunlop, D.D. and Yelin, E. 2009: Pain, functional limitations, and aging. *J Am Geriatr Soc* **57**, 1556–61.

Demyttenaere, K., Bruffaerts, R., Lee, S.,et al. 2007: Mental disorders among persons with chronic back or neck pain: Results from the world mental health surveys. *Pain* **129**, 332–342.

Dionne, C.E., Dunn, K.M., Croft, P.R. et al. 2008: A consensus approach toward the standardization of back pain definitions for use in prevalence studies. *Spine* **33**, 95–103.

Elliott, A.M., Smith, B.H., Penny, K.I., Smith, W.C. and Chambers, W.A. 1999: The epidemiology of chronic pain in the community. *Lancet* **354**, 1248–1252.

Feachem, R.G.A., Kjellstrom, T., Murray, C.J. L., Over, M. and Phillips, M.A. 1992: *The health of adults in the developing world*. New York: Oxford University Press.

Freburger, J.K., Holmes, G.M., Agans, R.P., Jackman, A.M., Darter, J.D., Wallace, A.S., et al. 2009: The rising prevalence of chronic low back pain. *Arch Intern Med* **169**, 251–258.

Griffith, L.E., Hogg-Johnson, S., Cole, D.C., Krause, N., Hayden, J., Burdorf, A., et al. and Meta-Analysis of Pain in the Lower Back and Work Exposures (MAPLE) Collaborative Group. 2007: Low-back pain definitions were categorized for a meta-analysis using Delphi consensus methods. *J Clin Epidemiol* **60**, 625–633.

Harkness, E.F., Macfarlane, G.J., Silman, A.J. and McBeth, J. 2005: Is musculoskeletal pain more common now than 40 years ago?: two population-based cross-sectional studies. *Rheumatology* **44**, 890–895.

Hasselstrom, J., Liu-Palmgren, J. and Rasjo-Wraak, G. 2002: Prevalence of pain in general practice. *Eur J Pain* **6**, 375–385.

Ihlebaek, C., Hansson, T.H., Laerum, E., Brage, S., Eriksen, H.R., Holm, S.R., et al. 2006: Prevalence of low back pain and sickness absence: a "borderline" study in Norway and Sweden. *Scand J Public Health* **34**, 555–558.

Jagger, C., Matthews, R., Spiers, N., Brayne, C., Comas-Herrera, A., Robinson, T., et al. 2006: *Compression or expansion of disability? Forecasting future disability levels under changing patterns of diseases*. Wanless Social Care Review Research Report, Leicester Nuffield Research Unit, University of Leicester.

Jinks, C., Jordan, K., Ong, B.N. and Croft, P. A brief screening tool for knee pain in primary care (KNEST). 2: Results from a survey in the general population aged 50 and over. *Rheumatology* **43**, 55–61

Kessler, R.C. and Ustun, T.B. (eds). 2008: *The WHO World Mental Health Surveys*. Cambridge: Cambridge University Press.

Koleva, D., Krulichova, I., Bertolini, G., Caimi, V. and Garattini, L. 2005: Pain in primary care: an Italian survey. *Eur J Public Health* **15**, 475–479.

König, H.H., Bernert, S., Angermeyer, M.C., Matschinger, H., Martinez, M., Vilagut, G., et al. and ESEMeD/MHEDEA 2000 Investigators. 2009: Comparison of population health status in six European countries: results of a representative survey using the EQ-5D questionnaire. *Med Care* **47**, 255–261.

Leijon, O. and Mulder, M. 2009: Prevalence of low back pain and psychological distress over a 16 year period. *Occup Environ Med* **66**, 137–139.

Macfarlane, G.J., Pye, S.R., Finn, J.D., Wu, F.C., Silman, A.J., Bartfai, G., et al. and European Male Ageing Study Group. 2009: Investigating the determinants of international differences in the prevalence of chronic widespread pain: evidence from the European Male Ageing Study. *Ann Rheum Dis* **68**, 690–695.

Mathers, C.D., Lopez, A.D. and Murray, C.L.J. 2006: The Burden of Disease and Mortality by Condition: Data, Methods, and Results for 2001. In: Lopez, A.D., Mathers, C.D., Ezzati, M., Jamison, D.T. and Murray, C.J.L. (eds): *Global Burden of Disease and Risk Factors* pp 45–93. New York: The World Bank and Oxford University Press.

Melzer, D., Gardener, E. and Guralnik, J.M. 2005: Mobility disability in the middle-aged: cross-sectional associations in the English Longitudinal Study of Ageing. *Age Ageing* **34**, 594–602.

Mottram, S., Peat, G., Thomas, E., Wilkie, R. and Croft, P. 2008: Patterns of pain and mobility limitation in older people: cross-sectional findings from a population survey of 18,497 adults aged 50 years and over. *Qual Life Res* **17**, 529–539.

Murray, C.J. and Lopez, A.D. (eds). 1996: *The Global Burden of Disease*. Cambridge MA: Harvard University Press.

Naidoo, S., Kromhout, H., London, L., Naidoo, R.N. and Burdorf, A. 2009: Musculoskeletal pain in women working in small-scale agriculture in South Africa. *Am J Ind Med* **52**, 202–209.

Neville, A., Peleg, R., Singer, Y., Sherf, M. and Shvartzman, P. 2008: Chronic pain: a population-based study. *Isr Med Assoc J* **10**, 676–680.

Palmer, K.T., Walsh, K., Bendall, H., Cooper, C. and Coggon, D. Back pain in Britain: comparison of two prevalence surveys at an interval of 10 years. *BMJ* **320**, 1577–1578.

Portenoy, R.K., Ugarte, C., Fuller, I. and Haas G. 2004: Population-based survey of pain in the United States: differences among white, African American, and Hispanic subjects. *J Pain* **5**, 317–328.

Rustøen, T., Wahl, A.K., Hanestad, B.R., Lerdal, A., Paul, S. and Miaskowski, C. 2004: Prevalence and characteristics of chronic pain in the general Norwegian population. *Eur J Pain* **8**, 555–565.

Silman, A.J. 2008: Forty six million Americans have arthritis. True or false? *Arth Rheum* **58**, 1220–1225.

Sjøgren, P., Ekholm, O., Peuckmann, V. and Grønbaek, M. 2009: Epidemiology of chronic pain in Denmark: an update. *Eur J Pain* **13**, 287–292.

Steenstra, I.A., Verbeek, J.H., Prinsze, F.J. and Knol, D.L. 2006: Changes in the incidence of occupational disability as a result of back and neck pain in the Netherlands. *BMC Public Health* **6**, 190.

Townsend, P. and Davidson, N. 1982: *Inequalities in health: the Black Report*. London: Penguin Books.

Tsang, A., Von Korff, M., Lee, S., Alonso, J., Karam, E., Angermeyer, M.C., et al. 2008: Common chronic pain conditions in developed and developing countries: gender and age differences and comorbidity with depression-anxiety disorders. *J Pain* **9**, 883–891.

Waddell, G. 1998: *The back pain revolution*. Edinburgh: Churchill Livingstone.

Ware, J.E. Jr. and Sherbourne, C.D. 1992: The MOS 36-item short-form health survey (SF-36). I. Conceptual framework and item selection. *Med Care* **30**, 473–483.

Ware, J. Jr., Kosinski, M. and Keller, S.D. 1996: A 12-Item Short-Form Health Survey: construction of scales and preliminary tests of reliability and validity. *Med Care* **34**, 220–233.

Chapter 3

The demography of chronic pain: an overview

Fiona M. Blyth

Cardiovascular disease, cancer, and injury dominate the public health agenda of many developed countries and increasingly in developing countries as well. It is the thesis of this book that chronic pain should be afforded at least some of the status of these public health giants. As part of drawing this picture, the core demography needs to address how frequent chronic pain is in populations (see Chapter 2), identify the groups in whom it is most often found, and explore why some population subgroups experience higher rates of pain than others. In this way the burden can be estimated, the health care needs identified, cause investigated, and prevention planned.

Disease occurrence in populations is generally described in terms of distribution by age and sex, two fundamental characteristics by which humans vary. Age and sex, separately and combined, provide us with a method for mapping chronic pain across the complex terrain of biology and life experience. Differences in occurrence of chronic pain across the lifespan and between sexes can provide important insights into aetiology, as well as defining which population groups bear the greatest risk and burden of chronic pain.

Along with age and gender, socioeconomic circumstances are powerful harbingers of human health. Historically, the field of public health emerged in response to diseases that were socially patterned – i.e. they were unequally distributed according to social circumstances, with the greatest load being carried by the most socially disadvantaged. Major public health problems tend to be unequally distributed within populations, and we need to know if chronic pain is similar to that too.

Age distribution

There are two useful frameworks for thinking about pain in relation to age. The first, which is more commonly used, is a static framework that examines the occurrence of pain in defined age-groups within a population at a given point or period in time. This provides a snapshot of pain burden that can be compared with other characteristics of that population (demographic and health/disease profile). The second framework is a dynamic one that tracks the development and progress of pain burdens across time.

Prospective studies of pain are still relatively uncommon and rarely continue for more than 3 years, although exceptions are now appearing as long-established cohorts, birth and adult, are being analysed for pain-relevant data. A particular type of prospective study is the life-course study, which uses the human lifespan as its timeframe and is used to evaluate the effects of biological and psychosocial exposures on the onset of chronic conditions in adult life, with a central emphasis on the timing of these exposures in relation to critical developmental periods and the possible effects of accumulation of exposures over time (Ben-Shlomo and Kuh, 2002).

To date, most of the literature on pain burden and age has described changes in pain with age in cross-sectional studies. These studies have often included insufficient numbers of the very young or very old to provide reliable estimates of pain burden at the extremes of age. There are compounding problems thrown up by the difficulties in accurately assessing this burden in young children and older people with cognitive impairment.

Helme and Gibson (1999) have examined the potential explanations for the commonly observed phenomenon of chronic pain peaking or plateauing in middle age. Some factors would lead to an increase in prevalence with increasing age (e.g. increasing morbidity in older age), while others would lead to a decline (e.g. a tendency of older people to discount the importance of pain, age-related decline in nociception, or general reduction in activity with age). More recently, the view that pain decreases in old age has been challenged in a systematic review of back-pain prevalence studies (Dionne et al., 2007). This showed that the prevalence of lower severity back pain tapers off in late middle age, while the prevalence of more severe forms of back pain continues to rise into old age. A similar phenomenon was observed in a large prospective population study of osteoarthritis, which found that the onset of disabling pain continued to rise into the oldest age groups in the study (and was more common in women), while the onset of pain *per se* had no clear relationship with age (Thomas et al., 2007).

The epidemiology of pain in young and older age-groups, and the life-course approach to chronic pain studies, are considered in more detail in later chapters.

Gender distribution

The evidence for sex (biological) and gender (role) differences in pain experience comes from a wide range of sources – animal studies, experimental and clinical studies in humans, and population studies. In addition to many individual studies, there are several reviews of this topic (Unruh, 1996; LeResche, 1999; Fillingim, 2001; Craft et al., 2004; Craft, 2007; Greenspan et al., 2007). Consistent themes have emerged – women tend to report more persistent pain, pain of greater intensity and more pain-related disability than men. Women also tend to report more pain at multiple sites, and respond differently to some classes of analgesia, compared with men. In addition, there are specific pain conditions that occur more often in women (e.g. migraine, temporomandibular joint disease, fibromyalgia) or in men (e.g. gout or cluster headache). There are sex-specific pain conditions – e.g. dysmenorrhoea in women and prostatitis in men. However, for back pain, which contributes so much to the overall population burden of chronic pain, there is little consistent evidence of strong gender-related prevalence differences.

However, many important questions remain unanswered. Why do women report more chronic pain – is it due to greater incidence, duration, or both? Do women seek treatment for pain more than men do because their pain is worse or because women more generally seek help for health problems than men do? To what extent are these phenomena due to biological factors, socio-cultural factors or some interplay of both? What is the influence of time, notably critical developmental periods such as puberty, the menstrual cycle, pregnancy, menopause, and andropause? Why do these differences in pain burden between men and women tend to diminish with age?

Dworkin et al. (1992) delineated three ways in which epidemiological studies could help unpick this puzzle – by providing a population approach that does not rely on treatment-seeking as a criterion for study entry, by providing a developmental perspective that can help disentangle aspects that vary with age (e.g. critical developmental periods); and finally by providing an ecological perspective that examines environmental exposures that are particularly relevant to gender-role considerations (e.g. social roles, educational and work trajectories).

The first major review article of gender, sex, and pain was published in 1996 (Unruh, 1996). This review described (i) the prevalence of common recurrent pains (headache and migraine, orofacial pain, musculoskeletal pains, back pain, and abdominal pain) by gender; (ii) gender variations in pain from common health care procedures (e.g. venepuncture, post-surgical pain); (iii) disease-related pain (e.g. osteoarthritis and cancer) by gender and gender-specific pain syndromes (e.g. pain arising from female reproductive tract functions such as menstruation and childbirth; and for men pain from infantile circumcision or pain arising in the male genital organs); (iv) gender aspects of the relationship of stress and depression with pain; disability due to pain; coping with pain; medication use; and health care utilization. While the likely importance of the interplay between biological and psychosocial factors was highlighted in the interpretation of gender variations, the evidence base for explanatory biological mechanisms and psychosocial mechanisms was small.

Unruh (1996) identified five key areas for advancing research in this area. These were (i) explicit exploration of the extent to which gender is associated with fundamental aspects of pain experience, such as pain frequency, duration, and severity; (ii) understanding the relationship between gender, age, and pain experience; (iii) understanding how men and women differentially interpret and evaluate pain experiences; (iv) examining how gender relates to presentation for treatment and treatment pathways; (v) quantifying gender differences in responses to treatment interventions; and (vi) improving knowledge of sex-based differences in the biological mechanisms of pain experience.

In the ensuing decade, growing interest in this field led to an increased research focus on the biological basis for apparent sex differences in pain experiences (Craft et al., 2004; Craft, 2007). As population studies of pain will increasingly offer the opportunity to incorporate biological data collection within the framework of representative study populations (Smith et al., 2007), such studies of the biological mechanisms of pain will become more directly relevant to aetiological and clinical studies.

In 2007 the Special Interest Group on Sex, Gender and Pain within the International Association for the Study of Pain (IASP) produced a consensus report on studying sex and gender differences in pain and analgesia (Greenspan et al., 2007). While the research agenda articulated in this report relates in greatest detail to animal and experimental human research models, there are several aspects that are immediately relevant to the population study of chronic pain. These include specific consideration of the potential that age-related changes in prevalence of some pain conditions relate to the hormonal changes of puberty and/or menopause; the relationship between co-morbid pain burden, specific 'non-pain' co-morbidities (e.g. anxiety and/or depression) and both pain occurrence and pain-related disability; and explicit exploration of how, when, and why the over-representation of women (and/or the under-representation of men) in seeking treatment for pain occurs (even allowing for the greater prevalence of chronic pain in women in the community). Perhaps the most important area outlined in future directions is the one also highlighted by the earlier review (Unruh, 1996): – that the greatest differences are seen in chronic pain syndromes, and hence risk factors for chronicity itself may form an important area of inquiry for those interested in understanding sex differences in pain experience.

The broader context for thinking about sex and gender differences in pain is that of gender, sex, and health. As Krieger (2003) has pointed out, the concept of gender has appeared relatively recently in the health literature, and for much of that time there has been widespread confusion between the constructs of sex-linked biology and gender relations. Others have emphasized that asking how sex and gender matter and when they do or do not matter in health and clinical practice are increasingly important questions (Gesenway, 2001). In population studies, results are sometimes reported by sex, or sex is used as an adjustment variable in modelling (either on its own or as part of an interaction term). While disaggregation by sex can be a useful starting point, none of these techniques is sufficient to explore complex sex/gender relationships (Rolfs et al., 2007; Ruiz-Cantero et al., 2007).

An important aspect of the growing interest in sex, gender, and health has been the attention drawn to the under-representation of women in clinical trials, particularly in early-phase trials of new drugs where dosage and toxicity data were collected (Bartlett et al., 2005; Gesenway, 2001; Ruiz-Cantero et al., 2007). In addition, identifying studies that focus on gender differences in health is hampered by poor indexing within major bibliographic databases (Ruiz-Cantero et al., 2007). In the first major review of the literature on pain and gender referred to above, Unruh (1996) also identified the problem of studies that were not designed with large-enough sample sizes or adequate numbers of men and women to detect gender differences in pain experiences, or reported incidental instances of gender variations in pain experiences.

In Chapter 10 of this book, Picavet explores in detail epidemiological evidence for the mechanisms that might underlie the excess of chronic musculoskeletal pain in women.

Socioeconomic status distribution

It is not, perhaps, surprising that chronic pain occurrence shows distinct social patterning and an inverse relationship with material wealth; in this it joins many other causes of morbidity and mortality, whether this is conceptualized as general health or disability, or as specific diseases (Eachus et al., 1999). While primary interest in the relationship between pain and socioeconomic status is relatively recent (Blyth, 2008; Poleshuck et al., 2008;), the relationship between socioeconomic status and health has long engaged health researchers.

There are continuing lively debates, e.g. about the relative role of material circumstances (and the structural causes of this) versus perceived inequality or social status in causing health inequalities in developed societies (Lynch et al., 2000; Krieger and Davey Smith 2004; Wilkinson and Pickett, 2008; Marmot and Siegrist, 2004), and the relationship between socioeconomic status and race. Gender differences in pain are recognized to interconnect with socioeconomic status, as are racial and cultural factors (Cañizares et al., 2008; Fuentes et al., 2007; Green et al., 2003), and early life exposures exert influence into adult life (Lynch et al., 2000).

Paralleling these is an equally energetic debate about whether these patterns represent the sum of individual poor circumstances (where the level of inquiry is how to intervene to help individuals) or if these patterns reflect factors operating at the population or group level (where population interventions may help more vulnerable individuals) or both.

However, in many parts of the world, absolute poverty underpins poor population health, often acting adversely in conjunction with gender differences. The previous chapter discussed that, even in parts of the world with developing economies or economies in transition, there is evidence that pain is common and problematic, and that chronic non-communicable diseases in general are increasingly important, as evidenced by a recent review article highlighting that back pain is common and increasing in prevalence in Africa (Louw et al., 2007).

Population-based studies of chronic pain have consistently shown that chronic pain occurrence is inversely related to socioeconomic status, and almost equally consistently have not explored the nature of this relationship. Many markers of individual socioeconomic status, such as level of education, occupation, employment status, income, housing status, access to a car, and health insurance status, have been used (Brekke et al., 2002; Eachus et al., 1999; Poleshuck et al., 2008; Blyth, 2008; Croft and Rigby, 1994), often as a single variable. Rarely has socioeconomic status been conceptually centre stage. Yet, each of these markers maps to different components of socioeconomic status, and reflects different influences on it. For example, poor adult-onset health (a correlate of chronic pain) may adversely and rapidly affect employment status and income (Lindholm et al., 2002), while having relatively little effect on educational attainment. A simple marker of educational attainment on the other hand, such as years spent in school and higher education, is more stable and established earlier in life, and hence more likely to reflect long-term socioeconomic status in adulthood (Eachus et al.,1999; Latza et al., 2000).

The most appropriate measure of socioeconomic status in older people is undecided. Recent work from the English Longitudinal Study of Ageing suggests that subjective social status measured on an ordinal scale correlates with a wide range of subjective and clinical health indicators in older people, but relates differently to more conventional socioeconomic indicators (Demakakos et al., 2008).

The relationship between chronic pain and socioeconomic status importantly includes pain severity. Persons living in adverse socioeconomic circumstances not only experience more pain, they also experience more severe pain (Brekke et al., 2002; Eachus et al., 1999). This phenomenon is seen for other health conditions, producing what has been termed the 'double suffering' (Blank et al., 1996) of not only higher levels of occurrence but also higher levels of severity. Added to this is the greater burden of disease co-morbidity, which itself is linked with socioeconomic status (Latour-Perez, 1999; Eachus et al., 1999). This suggests that the relationship between pain severity and socioeconomic status is not an exclusive one, and the search for explanations must have a correspondingly broad focus (Latour-Perez, 1999). In addition, evidence from birth-cohort studies suggests that chronic pain conditions 'run in families', so that children of parents with chronic pain conditions are more likely to develop pain conditions themselves (Waldie and Poulton, 2002; Grøholt et al., 2003). This is discussed in detail in Chapters 14 and 15.

Studies examining how pain and socioeconomic status relate to one another fall into two categories: those that test this at the individual level and those that test it at the group or population level. In the pain literature, most commonly, the individual level is used in analysis, and such studies have tended to show that individual-level risk factors for pain only partially explain the inverse relationship between pain and socioeconomic status (Croft and Rigby, 1994; Latza et al., 2000). More generally, socially patterned differences in health are more than the sum of individuals (Pearce, 1996). That is to say, poor risk-factor profiles in individuals do not, in general, account for socioeconomic status differences in health.

A few studies have included measures of the relative affluence or deprivation of the area where subjects live, based on their residence. These area-based indices are composite measures that include several indicators of socioeconomic status, including car ownership, level of unemployment, levels of crime, and access to health care (Urwin et al., 1998; Jordan et al., 2008). Exploration of population-level relationships between pain and socioeconomic status has been undertaken using such area-level measures. What distinguishes these studies are multi-level modelling analytic techniques that simultaneously but explicitly explore individual-level and area-level socioeconomic influences on pain, as well as joint effects of both.

Cañizares et al. (2008) have shown that low-income Canadians living in areas with higher proportions of low-income families were more likely to report having arthritis than low-income Canadians living in areas with better income profiles. In other words, area income levels moderated the effects of individual-level income. Similarly, Fuentes et al. (2007) found that higher neighbourhood socioeconomic status was associated with better chronic pain outcomes in American adults aged 50 or older and presenting for tertiary-level pain management. In the UK, Jordan et al. (2008) demonstrated that an older adult's risk of developing disabling pain varies with the deprivation characteristics of their area of residence. Such area-level variation is only partially explained by the individual risk factor profiles of those individuals who develop disabling chronic pain, although the group of studies of area-level influences on the occurrence of chronic widespread pain by the Manchester group suggest that individual variations in the prevalence of psychological factors explain much apparent area-level contrasts in pain prevalence (Davies et al., 2009).

Such studies throw up questions of analytic complexity, and importantly they require *a priori* specification of what matters, and at what level (Blyth et al., 2007).

Implications for prevention and management

Public health interventions are concerned with prevention and control at a population level (Rose, 1985). This implies a broader scope than the typical clinical approach of dealing with individuals who are at high risk of an adverse outcome, or who have already experienced an adverse outcome. Interventions at a population level generally aim to lower the overall risk of that population (and consequently reduce the pool of high-risk individuals requiring clinical care). These two approaches are not mutually exclusive propositions. The concept and assessment of population-level and individual-level risk depend on variations in those risks, i.e. higher and lower levels of risk exposure between populations or individuals, which are related to pain occurrence.

Age and gender patterns of chronic pain prevalence (and other measures of population pain burden) are informative in several ways. Separately and together they identify which groups within a given population carry the greatest burden of pain, and provide clues to the aetiology of particular pain conditions. When consistent patterns span markedly different populations, this points to a likely biological underpinning. The last chapter noted an impressive consistency of sex- and age-linked patterns across populations.

Age and sex are also common metrics for comparing the burden of chronic pain to other commonly occurring health conditions within populations, and for helping to connect chronic pain to other big public health problems such as injury (particularly in developing countries). Age and sex frameworks also help to map out which health outcomes are important – e.g. recent prospective studies are providing evidence that pain importantly compromises independent physical functioning in older people (Leveille et al., 2002; Soldato et al., 2007; Mottram et al., 2008), a key outcome in this age group.

Socioeconomic gradients in pain are a critical indicator that population-level factors are involved in the occurrence and consequences of chronic pain. They fit with evidence from population-level intervention studies that community beliefs about pain and other measures of pain disability (e.g. workers' compensation claims for back pain) are at least in part influenced by group-level factors (Buchbinder et al., 2004), even though many questions remain about the mechanism of such effects (Buchbinder et al., 2008). A public health approach by definition requires the development of population or societal-level interventions.

The size of the community burden of chronic pain, the dynamic natural history of persistent pain, and evidence that population-level influences matter, together suggest that a high-risk approach of identifying those individuals most at risk of developing chronic pain, or of those most at risk of poor pain outcomes, will be insufficient to lower the overall population burden. Most health problems occur along a continuum of risk-factor/disease-exposure patterns, so that a high-risk group is not a separate entity but part of this continuum – so the potential for high-risk group membership is always there, unless the whole population's risk is reduced. The most easily identified individual risk factors (those with the highest measures of association with pain) are not necessarily those that contribute most to the population burden of pain – unless they are also commonly found within populations (Rose, 1985). Even then, ignoring population-level risk factors, and how both individual and societal level risk factors interact, will inevitably lead to interventions that, at best, may help some but not many.

Population-level factors, such as socioeconomic inequality, are often described as 'upstream' or 'distal', giving the impression of less aetiological force. However, this may be a false impression. Such factors can have augmenting effects by influencing a whole range of more 'downstream' or 'proximal' causes (Krieger, 2008; Pearce, 1999). The perception of these as weaker aetiologically is reinforced by common methods of analysis, which simplify complex interconnections among factors, ignore levels of exposure, and treat proximal and distal variables as the same (Sheppard, 2003; Weitkunat and Wildner, 2002). High-risk and population approaches are not either/or propositions, although much remains unknown about how best to combine the two, and debate is active about how best to develop complex, multi-factorial interventions for complex health problems (Allore et al., 2005; Hawe et al., 2004). Chronic pain, similar to other chronic conditions, arises from interacting causal factors that span different periods of time and act at different levels, and may also be modified by protective factors. Future efforts to reduce the population burden of chronic pain will need to engage with these issues to deliver the best outcomes for the public's health.

References

Allore, H.G., Tinetti, M.E., Gill, T.M. and Peduzzi, P.N. 2005: Experimental designs for multicomponent interventions among persons with multifactorial geriatric syndromes. *Clin Trials* **2**, 13–21.

Bartlett, C., Doyal, L., Ebrahim, S., et al. 2005: The causes and effects of socio-demographic exclusions for clinical trials. *Health Technol Assess* **9**, (38).

Ben-Shlomo, Y. and Kuh, D. 2002: A life course approach to chronic disease epidemiology: conceptual models, empirical challenges and interdisciplinary perspectives. *Int J Epidemiol* **31**, 285–293.

Blank, N. and Diderechsen, F. 1996: Social inequalities in the experience of illness in Sweden: A "double suffering". *Scand J Soc Med* **24**, 81–89.

Blyth, F.M. 2008: Chronic pain – is it a public health problem? *Pain* **137**, 465–466.

Blyth, F.M., Macfarlane, G.J. and Nicholas, M.K. 2007: The contribution of psychosocial factors in the development of chronic pain: the key to better outcomes for patients? *Pain* **127**,8–11.

Brekke, M., Hjortdahl, P. and Kvien, T.K. 2002: Severity of musculoskeletal pain: relationship to socioeconomic inequality. *Soc Sci Med* **54**, 221–228.

Buchbinder, R. and Jolley, D. 2004: Population-based intervention to change back pain beliefs: three year follow up population survey. *BMJ* **328**, 321.

Buchbinder, R., Gross, D.P., Werner, E.L. and Hayden, J.A. 2008: Understanding the characteristics of effective mass media campaigns for back pain and methodological challenges in evaluating their effects. *Spine* **33**, 74–80.

Ca izares, M., Power, J.D., Perruccio, A.V. and Badley, E.M. 2008: Association of regional racial/cultural context and socioeconomic status with arthritis in the population: a multi-level analysis. *Arth Rheum* **59**, 399–407.

Craft, R.M., Mogil, J.S. and Aloisi, A.M. 2004: Sex differences in pain and analgesia, the role of gonadal hormones. *Eur J Pain* **8**,397–411.

Craft, R.M. 2007: Modulation of pain by estrogens. *Pain* **132**, S3–S12.

Croft, P.R. and Rigby, A.S. 1994: Socioeconomic influences on back pain in the community in Britain. *J Epidemiol Community Health* **48**, 166–-170.

Davies, K.A., Silman, A.J., Macfarlane, G.J., Nicholl, B.I., Dickins, C., Morriss, R., Ray, D. and McBeth, J. 2009: The association between neighbourhood socio-economic status and the onset of chronic widespread pain: results from the EPIFUND study. *Eur J Pain* **13**, 635–40.

Demakakos, P., Nazroo, J., Breeze, E. and Marmot, M. 2008: Socioeconomic status and health: The role of subjective social status. *Soc Sci Med* **67**, 330–40.

Dionne,C.E., Dunn, K.M. and Croft, P.R. 2007: Does back pain prevalence really decrease with increasing age? A systematic review. *Age Ageing* **35**, 229–234.

Dworkin, S., Von Korff, M., and LeResche, L. 1992: Epidemiologic studies of chronic pain: A dynamic-ecologic perspective. *Ann Behav Med* **14**, 11–13.

Eachus, J., Chan, P., Pearson, N., Propper, C. and Davey-Smith, G. 1999: An additional dimension to health inequality: disease severity and socioeconomic position. *J Epidemiol Community Health* **53**, 603–611.

Fillingim, R.B. 2001: *Sex, gender, and pain*. Seattle, IASP Press.

Fuentes, M., Hart-Johnson, T. and Green, C.R. 2007: The association among neighborhood socioeconomic status, race and chronic pain in Black and White older adults. *J Nat Med Assoc* **99**, 1160–1169.

Gesenway, D. 2001: Reasons for sex-specific and gender-specific study of health topics. *Ann Int Med* **135**,935–938.

Green, C.R., Anderson, K.O., Baker, T.A., et al. 2003: The unequal burden of pain: confronting racial and ethnic disparities in pain. *Pain Med* **4**, 277–294.

Greenspan, J.D., Craft, R.M., LeResche, L., et al. 2007: Studying sex and gender differences in pain and analgesia. A consensus report. *Pain* **132**,S26–S45.

Grøholt, K.E., Stigum, H., Nordhagen, R. and Köhler, L. 2003: Recurrent pain in children, socio-economic factors and accumulation in families. *Eur J Epidemiol* **18**, 965–975.

Hawe, P., Shiell, A. and Riley, T. 2004: Complex interventions – how "out of control" can a randomised controlled trial be? *BMJ* **328**,1561–1563.

Helme, R. and Gibson, S. 1999: Pain in older people. In Crombie, I.K., Croft, P., Linton, S., LeResche, L. and Von Korff, M. (eds.). *Epidemiology of Pain*. Seattle, IASP Press.

Jordan, K.P., Thomas, E., Peat, G., Wilkie, R. and Croft, P. 2008: Social risks for disabling pain in older people: A prospective study of individual and area characteristics. *Pain* **137**, 652–661.

Krieger N 2003. Gender, sexes, and health, what are the connections – and why does it matter? *Int J Epidemiol* **32**, 652–657.

Krieger, N. and Davey Smith, G. 2004: "Bodies count" and body counts: social epidemiology and embodying inequality. *Epidemiol Rev* **26**, 92–103.

Krieger, N. 2008: Proximal, distal, and the politics of causation: what's level got to do with it? *Am J Public Health* **98**, 221–230.

Latour-Perez, J. 1999: Social inequalities in severity of illness. *J Epidemiol Community Health* **53**, 599–600.

Latza, U., Kohlmann, T., Deck,R. and Raspe, H. 2000: Influence of occupational factors on the relation between socioeconomic status and self-reported back pain in a population-based sample of German adults with back pain. *Spine* **25**, 1390–7.

LeResche, L. 1999: Gender considerations in the epidemiology of chronic pain. In Crombie, I.K., Croft, P., Linton, S., LeResche, L. and Von Korff, M. (eds.). *Epidemiology of Pain*. Seattle, IASP Press.

Leveille, S.G., Bean, J., Bandeen-Roche, K., Jones, R., Hochberg, M. and Guralnik, J.M. 2002: Musculoskeletal pain and risk for falls in older disabled women living in the community. *J Am Geriatr Soc* **50**, 671–678.

Lindholm, C., Burström, B. and Diderechsen, F. 2002: Class differences in the social consequences of illness? *J Epidemiol Community Health* **56**, 188–192.

Louw, Q.A., Morris, L.D. and Grimmer-Somers, K. 2007: The prevalence of back pain in Africa: a systematic review. *BMC Musculoskeletal Disorders* **8**, 105.

Lynch, J.W., Davey Smith. G., Kaplan, G.A. and House, J.S. 2000: Income inequality and mortality: importance to health of individual income, psychosocial environment, or material conditions. *BMJ* **321**, 1200–1204.

Mottram, S., Peat, G., Thomas, E., Wilkie, R. and Croft, P. 2008: Patterns of pain and mobility limitation in older people: cross-sectional findings from a population survey of 18,497 adults aged 50 years and over. *Qual Life Res* **17**, 529–539.

Pearce, N. 1996: Traditional epidemiology, modern epidemiology and public health. *Am J Pub Health* **86**, 678–683.

Pearce, N. 1999: Epidemiology as a population science. *Int J Epidemiol* **28**, S1015–S1018.

Poleshuck, E.L. and Green, C.L. 2008: Socioeconomic disadvantage and pain. *Pain* **136**, 235–238.

Rolfs, I., Borrell, C., Artazcoz, L. and Escribà-Ag ir. 2007: The incorporation of gender perspective into Spanish health surveys. *J Epidemiol Community Health* **61**(suppl II), ii46–ii53.

Rose, G. 1985: Sick individuals and sick populations. *Int J Epidemiol* **14**, 32–35.

Ruiz-Cantero, M.T., Vives-Cases, C., Artazcoz, L., et al. 2007: A framework to analyse gender bias in epidemiological research. *J Epidemiol Community Health* **61**(suppl II), ii20–ii25.

Sheppard, L. 2003: Insights on bias and information in group-level studies. *Biostatistics* **4**, 265–278.

Siegrist, J. and Marmot, M. 2004: Health inequalities and the psychosocial environment – two scientific challenges. *Soc Sci Med* **58**, 1463–1473.

Smith, B., Macfarlane, G.J. and Torrance, N. 2007: Epidemiology of chronic pain, from the laboratory to the bus stop, time to add understanding of biological mechanisms to the study of risk factors in population-based research? *Pain* **127**,5–10.

Soldato, M., Liperoti, R., Landi, F., et al. 2007: Non malignant daily pain and risk of disability among older adults in home care in Europe. *Pain* **129**, 304–310.

Thomas, E., Mottram,S., Peat, G., Wilkie, R. and Croft, P. 2007: The effect of age on the onset of pain interference in a general population of older adults: Prospective findings from the North Staffordshire Osteoarthritis Project (NorStOP). *Pain* **129**, 21–27.

Unruh, A. 1996: Gender variations in clinical pain experience. *Pain* **65**, 123–167.

Urwin, M., Symmons, D., Allison, T., et al. 1998: Estimating the burden of musculoskeletal disorders in the community : the comparative prevalence of symptoms at different anatomical sites, and the relation to social deprivation. *Ann Rheum Dis* **57**, 649–655.

Waldie, K.E. and Poulton, R. 2002: Physical and psychological correlates of primary headache in young adulthood: A 26 year longitudinal study. *J Neurol Neurosurg Psychiatry* **72**, 86–92.

Weitkunat, R. and Wildner, M. 2002: Exploratory causal modelling in epidemiology: are all factors created equal? *J Clin Epidemiol* **55**, 436–444.

Wilkinson, R.G. and Pickett, K.E. 2008: Income Inequality and Socioeconomic Gradients in Mortality. *Am J Pub Health* **98**: 699–704.

Basic epidemiological concepts applied to pain

For readers who are not epidemiologists, this appendix is intended to serve as an introduction or reminder of some common epidemiological terms and definitions. For readers already familiar with epidemiology, this appendix contains some reflections on the problems and challenges of applying epidemiological concepts and methods to the measurement and study of pain.

Basic measures of occurrence

The first aim of epidemiology is to measure patterns of illness and disease in populations and provide the basic public health descriptions of a phenomenon such as chronic pain.

The core epidemiological concept is the frequency or occurrence of an event or status (a symptom, an illness or disease). The standard measure involved is a ratio of the number of such events (numerator) to the total number of people (the population denominator) who might have or develop them.

Prevalence

Prevalence is the simplest measure of occurrence and represents the proportion of all the people in a particular population who have the problem. The prevalence of chronic pain could be described as "The proportion of UK adults who report pain that has lasted for at least 3 months is 33%".

Even this example is not so simple when the fluctuating nature of pain is considered.

Prevalence could start with one point in time ("point prevalence" e.g. have you got the pain today?) and then identify the sub-group of people who have had it for 3 months in order to estimate the point prevalence of chronic pain.

More helpful and usual is to ask people to recall pain experience over a period of time to allow for the fluctuations which might mean that they do not have it on the particular day they are being surveyed but they have had it, for example, for a period of at least 3 months during the past year ("period prevalence" e.g. "The proportion of people who experience pain during the course of one year which lasts for at least 3 months").

Von Korff introduced a helpful refinement of this measure to account for the fluctuating and uneven course of pain experience over time. The recall for period prevalence of chronic pain is based on the number of days in pain recalled over a specified period such as 3 or 6 months (Von Korff et al., 1992).

Point prevalence will tend to be lower than period prevalence, especially if the period is extended to one year or longer, because the snapshot at one point in time leaves out people who have experienced it in that same year but who do not have it on that day.

Incidence

Incidence measures the frequency of onset of a symptom or illness or disease, and is an estimate of what occurs over a specific period of time. "The incidence of post-herpetic neuralgia in persons who have shingles is about 25 per 100 shingles sufferers per year".

Incidence is important to pain studies because it can capture episodic short-lived pain and recurrence of episodes, as well as the development of chronicity. The denominator population is free of the problem and *cumulative incidence* over a period of time is the proportion of that pain-free population who, for example, develop pain (or chronic pain) during the next 12 months. Because the onset of pain (or chronic pain) is difficult to capture from surveys, this figure is usually calculated in terms of transitions in state (for example from "no pain in the past 3 months" to "pain in the past 3 months") between two fixed survey points, and will tend to underestimate total incidence if the period of recall at the second time point does not cover the whole period between the surveys.

Life-time incidence, or the cumulative prevalence of chronic pain across all ages, is usually calculated in terms of recall ("have you ever..."). Because chronic pain not only tends to be stable for periods of time but also a status from which there is always potential to improve or recover for periods, this figure gives a picture of the likelihood that a person will experience chronic pain at some time in their lives.

A more dynamic expression of the rate of development of pain over time is the *incidence rate or density*. Unlike the rate of events accessible to measurement at the time they occur (myocardial infarction or death for example), true incidence rates are rarely calculated for pain. They would apply for example to the event rate of documented primary care consultations for new acute episodes of back pain over time, in which individuals are regarded as susceptible to a new episode each time they recover from a previous one, and incidence rate is calculated by the number of episodes per person-time.

Incidence generally (cumulative incidence or incidence rate) is more difficult to calculate for pain because:-

a first-ever onset of many common conditions triggering chronic pain (e.g. osteoarthritis) is difficult to ascertain, as also is the first-ever onset of chronic pain syndromes

b the onset of, and recovery from, new episodes of recurrently painful problems (e.g. migraine) is difficult to ascertain, and either recorded events such as health care consultations are used as a proxy for occurrence or, more usually, episodes are summarised over time as a period prevalence.

Cumulative incidence can only be used where the denominator is closed to new members, as in a cohort study, whereas the incidence rate can apply where the denominator has a dynamic fluctuating membership, such as the registered population of a general practice. In practice these two measures are often conflated, without attention to their distinctiveness.

Chronicity

An alternative way to measure cumulative incidence of pain, and in particular chronic pain, is to express its frequency relative, not to the general population, but to the precipitating cause.

In it simplest form, this is the proportion of acute episodes of pain which become chronic – the chronic pain equivalent of a "case-fatality" rate or a conversion or transition rate. This is useful but limited since, unless the underlying rate of acute pain in the general population is known, it does not provide a direct estimate of population occurrence of chronic pain.

More restricted but useful are estimates of the occurrence of pain, and in particular chronic pain, related to specific diseases which trigger their onset, for example the proportion of HIV-AIDS patients who develop chronic pain in the course of a year. This figure (the "pain-linkage rate" of a particular disease) has to be used with caution because its generalisability depends on the selectivity of the patients being studied. However if generalisability can be established, and if the incidence or prevalence of the triggering disease in the general population can be reliably estimated, then the population incidence or prevalence of chronic pain related to this condition can be calculated.

Risk and odds

Risk is another term for incidence – it expresses the average likelihood of developing an illness or disease for a member of a specified population or group. Since incidence is expressed as the ratio of the number of events to the total population number who might develop the event during a specified time, the denominator of risk includes the numerator – "out of every 100 adults in the UK who are free of chronic pain at the start of a year, there will be 11 who develop an episode of pain lasting for 3 months or longer during that year". The risk is 11 per 100 per year, or 0.11.

Odds are slightly different. These are a ratio of the number of people who have an event to the number of people who do not. In the example in the previous paragraph, the odds of developing chronic pain in the year will be 11 divided by 89, or 0.12. This figure illustrates the general point that, if the incidence is not high, then risk and odds will be similar. Conversely the higher the occurrence figure, odds estimates become higher than the risk calculation. For example, if the period prevalence of chronic pain in the population is 33 per 100 persons (a "risk" of having chronic pain of 0.33), the odds of chronic pain are 33:67, or 0.49.

Estimates of effect

The second aim of epidemiology is to study causes and prognosis of illness and disease to inform public health interventions and monitor their outcome.

To do this, epidemiologists can either draw on estimates of occurrence, and, by comparing different people in different places across different times, make inferences about aetiology and prevention; or they can set up studies specifically designed to determine links between illness and disease and potential causal factors, or to study characteristics related to poor outcome. The observed relation between risk factor and illness or disease is known as the effect estimate.

Risk ratio

The basic effect estimate used by the epidemiological scientist is the *risk ratio* (or relative risk). Risk is the estimated incidence of illness or disease in a particular group. The risk ratio is the risk in the group exposed to a risk factor (for example female gender) divided by the risk in a comparator group not exposed to the risk factor (i.e. men), to give the intuitively sensible estimate of the number of times more or less likely the exposed group is to develop the illness or disease in question, compared with the unexposed group. In the example above, if the incidence of chronic pain in one year in UK adult women is 14 per cent, and in men it is 10 per cent, then the risk ratio is 1.4 – women are 1.4 times more likely than men to develop chronic pain over a year (assuming ages are comparable). The ratios of odds in the two groups will give odds ratios, but if the outcome is common then these will be overestimates of the risk ratios. This is important because many statistical approaches to modelling risks draw on the odds ratio rather than the risk ratio. The absolute value of the odds ratio however can cause problems in pain epidemiology because of the frequency of events – the assumption that the odds ratio can simply be interpreted as an estimate of a person's risk of developing a particular outcome is often flawed. Although the presence of an association between risk factor and outcome can still be assumed, the interpretation of its strength cannot.

Absolute risk

More useful for clinical practice is the absolute risk. This is the extra occurrence of the illness or disease in the group "exposed" to a particular risk factor, over and above the occurrence observed in the unexposed group.

The absolute annual risk of developing chronic pain in UK adult women would, from the figures in the previous section, be 14% minus 10%, i.e. an extra 4% of annual risk over and above the annual risk in adult men. Here the thinking is that the unexposed group (i.e. men 'unexposed' to characteristics related to being female) provides an estimate of the underlying risk of the problem due to factors than sex and gender. These causes are assumed to be common to both groups. So subtracting this underlying risk from the total incidence in the exposed group provides the additional, excess or attributable risk. This excess risk can be expressed as a proportion of the total risk in the population exposed (in this case, women): 4% relative to 14%, i.e. 0.28 of the total annual risk of developing chronic pain in women is attributable to some aspect of being female.

Interpretation must be fluid and critical. In this example, it might be some protective aspect of maleness that is the factor, and it is likely that more of the risk in both men and women might be attributable to things that differ between the sexes.

Population attributable risk

Finally, for the public health view, the crucial step is to introduce an estimate of the population frequency (or prevalence) of exposure. The absolute risk of chronic pain is high in an individual exposed to multiple myeloma, and this is an important cause of pain for individual sufferers. However multiple myeloma remains a relatively rare problem compared to many other causes of pain and, from a public health perspective, is not a target in the sense that if multiple myeloma were cured or prevented, this would not have a major impact on population rates of chronic pain. (That is not to say that multiple myeloma is not an important target for prevention for other reasons, but, from a societal rather than an individual perspective, targeting it is not a strategy to achieve substantial reductions in chronic pain in the population).

The *population attributable risk, or the more usually calculated population attributable proportion,* are more appropriate effect measures to grasp this "population effect from a societal perspective". The proportion takes the number of extra cases of the problem which can be attributed to the exposure, and expresses this as a proportion of the numbers with the problem in the whole population. So it can indicate the proportion of all cases in the population that would be prevented if the exposure was removed. For example, Jinks has calculated that a modest reduction in body mass index in all persons who are overweight or obese might prevent the development of one-fifth of all new cases of chronic knee pain in older persons (Jinks et al., 2006).

The population attributable risk or proportion summarise the focus and orientation of this book. We are interested in chronic pain as a public health experience and we assume that, from some aspects, the disabling chronic pain experienced by back pain sufferers is as important a target for public health prevention as the chronic pain experienced by road traffic accident victims for example. It may be that preventing road traffic accidents is more important for other reasons (mortality or disability unrelated to pain for example), or that preventing back pain is more important for other reasons (the costs to the economy for example), but in terms of the chronic pain experience per se, the public health concern is equivalent. So the issue of how common the underlying problem is and what can be done to prevent it is paramount. And the potential for general exposures to be tackled (for example obesity as a factor promoting chronicity in all later-onset pain) may be the most important thing from a public health perspective, because of their high frequency, compared to the effects on population levels of chronic pain achieved through tackling individual diseases which trigger pain.

Internal and external validity

Bias in epidemiology is any systematic distortion of the truth or validity of a particular estimate of occurrence or association. It can be *internal* to a study – i.e. the figure produced is incorrect. An example of this might be that an individual, in response to a survey question, no longer remembers a pain in childhood for which they were hospitalised.

Extensive sections of this book on public health aspects of pain are concerned with estimates of population occurrence of the symptom. Discussion of bias in pain studies is often dominated by issues of internal validity relating to the subjectivity of the symptom and potential problems of recall and classification. We take the view in this book that a subjective symptom such as pain - variable, uncertain, subject to the vagaries of influences such as mood and culture – can be studied as a phenomenon epidemiologically. In all its variability, pain is no different to blood pressure – an objectively measured phenomenon equally influenced by such vagaries as the colour of the coat the observer is wearing and how quickly the person has walked to the measurement setting.

However, even if each of a series of population estimates of pain occurrence is in itself free of internal bias (i.e. there is a standard questionnaire, good response, clear sample), studies which compare pain prevalence between populations often have problems. For comparisons of occurrence (prevalence or incidence) between population groups (countries or sociodemographic classes for example) and drawing on different studies, variation arises from differences in study methods such as the definitions of pain used, settings and samples used, and methods of measurement.

The figure produced by a study may be correct for the study population, and therefore free of internal bias, but its extrapolation or interpretation outside the study population may be incorrect, i.e. it lacks *external validity*. An example would be an accurate estimate of pain prevalence in a group of patients in a hospital outpatient setting, which is mistakenly taken to be a true estimate of the population prevalence of pain. Such patients may be a highly selective group sociodemographically, especially with respect to the likelihood of having conditions predisposing to pain, and so prevalence in this group is unlikely to be a true representation of pain experience in the wider community.

In estimating measures of association and effect within one study, however, *internal validity* remains the concern. For example, if two socially diverse groups are compared, follow-up rates in the two groups need to be reasonably similar or, if they are different, there needs to be evidence that the differences are not systematic – for example people in one social group who improve may be less likely to attend for follow-up than people in the other social group when they improve. Concluding that improvement relates to social group may be a biased step because of the differential loss to follow-up.

Confounding is a special case of bias when differences in outcome between the exposed and unexposed groups are related to factors other than the main group differences under study. For example, differences in pain outcomes are observed between manual and clerical workers, but these partly disappear when the higher levels of stress and depression in the manual workers are taken into account. Stress and depression ("confounders") in this situation partly explain the observed relation between type of work and pain outcomes.

But caution needs to be used in assuming that confounding is necessarily a bias. If, in the work example, the poor outcomes were attributed directly and entirely to doing manual work, then stress or depression are confounding factors. However, if something about manual work leads workers to become more depressed, which then subsequently results in more pain, this becomes explanation rather than confounding – the target for prevention may be the psychosocial environment of manual work as the cause of pain rather than the physical side of the labour involved, for example.

Finally *effect modification* is not about bias but about the possibility that two or more different variable or protective or risk factors interact when they co-occur, and influence disease or illness in different ways to when they are acting alone. In chapter 10, for example, Picavet examines the possibility that occupational risks may have different effects in women compared with men.

References

Jinks, C., Jordan, K. and Croft, P. 2006: Disabling knee pain- another consequence of obesity: results from a prospective cohort study. *BMC Public Health* **6**, 258.

Von Korff, M., Ormel, J., Keefe, F.J. and Dworkin, S.F. 1992: Grading the severity of chronic pain. *Pain* **50**, 133–49.

Definition and measurement of chronic pain for population studies

Chapter 4

Introduction

Peter Croft, Kate Dunn, Fiona M. Blyth, and Danielle van der Windt

In Section 1, we referred to the difficulties of defining pain for population studies. In Chapter 5, Dionne presents a response to this, reviews concepts and available instruments, and describes an approach to developing standard core definitions of pain for measurement in epidemiological studies which can be used for comparative epidemiology and estimates of occurrence and burden.

The other two chapters in this section consider the issues involved in developing broader concepts of chronic pain (Raspe) and potential methods to measure the population risk of chronic pain for population studies (Natvig et al.).

In this introduction, we draw on all three chapters to highlight general points about defining chronic pain as a public health issue.

A core definition of chronic pain for public health

The meaning of the word 'chronic' encompasses notions of time, especially long duration, and some of the distinctiveness of chronic pain can be simply captured from an epidemiological perspective by adding a measure of duration to standardized self-report questions about pain.

There is no universal consensus about how long a definitive duration should be, but the International Association for the Study of Pain (IASP) has characterized chronic pain as 'pain which has persisted beyond normal tissue healing time', which, 'in the absence of other criteria, is taken to be 3 months' (IASP, 1986). This reflects the most widely accepted time period. The use of the 3-month duration to define chronic pain in epidemiological studies has been challenged on empirical (Dunn and Croft, 2006) and conceptual (Von Korff and Dunn, 2008) grounds – see also the other chapters in this section. Despite this, it provides a practical and simple cut-off for basic descriptions of occurrence in populations.

Duration alone is a marker, albeit crude, of the extended or 'amplified' chronic pain syndrome in general population studies. However, simple expansions of the basic definition that include, for example, a measure of the significance or impact of the pain, can get closer to the extended concept of a chronic pain syndrome. An early example of this, applicable to population studies, was the Chronic Pain Grade, based on combining a measure of pain severity with a measure of impact in one scale (Von Korff et al., 1992).

Another approach is offered by the single question from the Short Form-36 (SF-36) questionnaire ['During the past 4 weeks, how much did pain interfere with normal work (including work both outside the house and housework)?'] (Ware and Kosinski, 2001). In Chapter 16, Thomas takes the example of pain in older people to explore how this simple definition works in practice. Such a question is no less subjective than the reporting of pain itself, and is a marker of 'perceived' interference, as compared with an objectively measured reduction in activity, for example.

In population studies it correlates with components of Raspe's amplified model (Chapter 6). So at the level of populations, it can be regarded as a simple proxy measure of the 'chronic pain syndrome'.

Other chapters in this book provide detailed accounts of different epidemiological definitions for different purposes in relation to different examples of chronic pain conditions. We propose, however, that a simple core definition of chronic pain for epidemiological purposes can be represented as 'pain which has persisted for 3 months or more and which interferes with activities of daily life'. How this is best measured is the topic of Chapter 5.

Expanding the concept of time

This core definition is sufficient to provide a static cross-sectional estimate of the point prevalence of chronic pain based on recalled duration and reported impact. It has a single unitary concept of time, provided as a framework for a respondent's recall and summary of their experience.

However, pain is rarely a stable continuous state over time, and although longitudinal studies of pain have only relatively recently begun to appear in any number, available evidence suggests that dynamic cycles of recurrence of symptoms, and flare-ups in the severity of pain, often occur. This has led to proposals to think of continuous and episodic pain together under the umbrella term of 'persistent pain'. In this book we use the term 'chronic' to mean 'recurrent episodes' as well as 'continuous' pain.

The implication of this instability for estimating the burden of chronic pain is that the composition of a chronic pain cohort in a population will be affected by the length of time used to define chronicity, by the choice of which patterns of recurrence are considered to belong to the same episode of 'chronic pain', and by the actual time period over which this is ascertained.

The few studies which document first onset and continuing patterns of chronic pain suggest it incorporates a fluctuating course with acute exacerbations (or flare-ups) and periods of relatively few symptoms, as well as persistence (Von Korff, 1994; Carey et al., 1999). A typical chronic pain prevalence study (which asks about chronic pain at one point in time) may only include a proportion of all persons with chronic pain depending on the timing of data collection in relation to this ongoing cycle (Smith et al., 2004). It is also apparent that there are different trajectories and patterns of progression to chronicity, so that another approach to capturing the dynamic nature of chronic pain is to identify these and consider them separately (Von Korff and Saunders, 1996; Croft et al., 2006; Dunn et al., 2006). Dunn et al (2006) used latent class analysis of monthly pain reports to classify back pain patients into groups defined by their pain trajectories over a 6-month period. Chronic pain experience over this time period was summarized in one of four possible pathways: recovery, continuing low severity, continuing high severity, and fluctuating severity. The average course of almost all individuals could be represented by membership of one of the four pathways (see Figure 4.1), even though, within each pathway, individuals varied as to their exact course over the series of monthly pain assessments (six in total).

Almost two decades ago now, Von Korff pointed to a simple expansion of the prevalent recall question, which enquired about the number of days on which pain is experienced over a specified period of time. Although the measure relies on recall (retrospective self-assessment), it allows for the short-term episodic or fluctuating nature of pain to be incorporated. This approach introduces a requirement that the recall period used is simultaneously long enough to capture the characteristic patterns of chronic pain in its different forms, while being short enough to minimize the risk of inaccurate recall.

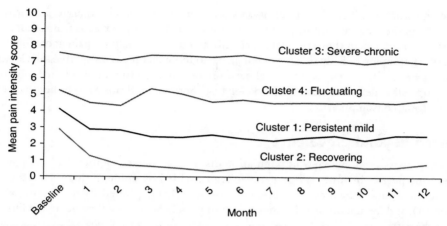

Fig. 4.1 Pain Pathways: based on monthly pain reports following a primary care consultation for back pain. Adapted from Dunn et al., 2006, with permission from Oxford Journals.

Expanding the concept of pain

The conceptualization of the burden of chronic pain can be expanded further in population studies by adding severity components. For acute pain, severity is often characterized as level of pain intensity, a feature which varies between different acute episodes and is one measure of the likelihood that an acute episode will develop into chronic pain (e.g. Eisenach et al; 2008). From a public health perspective, our interest is rather more with how chronic pain intrudes on and detracts from quality of life and ability to function in daily-life tasks, as well as the impact of chronic pain on societal structures, such as the health care system, workers compensation system, and disability support services (e.g. van Leeuwen et al., 2006). More severe chronic pain is seen as pain that has a measurable consequence in one or more of these domains; pain intensity alone is not a sufficiently strong marker of this aspect of chronic pain. The challenge is to provide a sufficiently convincing definition of the problem we wish to study without confusing or mixing it up with the impact and consequences we wish to measure.

One solution is to include some components of this extended or 'amplified' chronic pain syndrome in the core definition – at its simplest this would be the measure of pain interference in daily life suggested above. Ways to measure this are reviewed by Dionne in Chapter 5; Raspe, in Chapter 6, explores the amplification of pain in full and provides constructs and concepts for putting extended definitions into practice.

The epidemiological challenge is to identify the simplest markers of this amplified chronic pain syndrome for use in population studies. One candidate for this is the extent of distribution of pain complaints in the body. In Chapter 7, Natvig and his colleagues summarize their population-based work based on analysis of the number of reported pain areas. The average number of areas per person affected in 1 year by pain, as recalled by participants in their adult Norwegian population sample, was three. The distribution of this frequency was associated with the frequency of other components of the amplified chronic pain syndrome, such that the authors proposed that chronic pain limited to one site appeared to be a different syndrome to pain at that site when accompanied by other pains.

Natvig's work highlights how population studies of chronic pain vary, either implicitly or explicitly, in the types of chronic pain that are captured. The range extends from studies that include all chronic pain (however that is defined), to those that focus on pain at one body site (or a select grouping of body sites, e.g. joint pain), to those that focus on specific aetiologies of chronic pain (e.g. trauma or occupational overuse), or that consider pain in selected subgroups of the population defined by disease association (e.g. those with arthritis pain) or health care use (e.g. analgesic consumption).

Moving beyond prevalence

The static cross-sectional view of population disease and illness, captured at one point or across one period in time, is one perspective provided by epidemiology. However, we need to incorporate the idea of a developing or underlying 'propensity to chronicity' (see Chapter 1), and the notion that the impact of chronic pain at any one time lies in the future as well as the past.

The potential for measuring chronic pain in terms of current prognosis for future continuing chronic pain has been explored in a series of publications by Von Korff and colleagues (see, e.g. Von Korff and Miglioretti, 2005; Von Korff and Dunn, 2008). The conceptual leap proposed by the authors is that chronic pain can be defined in terms of the likelihood of what will happen in the future and that this is more helpful than defining it only in terms of what has happened previously. Current status becomes focussed on the probability that 'clinically significant pain will be present at a future time'. This fits with the ideas of propensity and risk discussed in the introduction to this book.

In a series of empirical investigations, these authors tested a risk score which integrates pain intensity, pain interference with daily activity, and days unable to carry out usual activities (all from the Graded Chronic Pain scale), days in pain in the past 6 months, number of pain conditions at sites other than the index (out of five specified), and depressive symptom score. In studies of a range of pain conditions (e.g. back pain, orofacial pain, headache, knee pain), in different clinical settings in the USA and UK, they assessed the capacity of the risk score to predict 'clinically significant pain', defined primarily by grades II–IV on the Chronic Pain Grade at a time in the future ranging from 6 months to 5 years. Other outcomes, such as the SF-36 Physical Function score, ratings of worry about pain, medication use, and employment, were also investigated. The score had superior prognostic value and consistency in predicting these outcomes than a measure of baseline pain duration alone (days in pain in the previous 6 months), which persisted after adjusting for baseline days in pain.

The authors highlighted important features about this approach to defining chronic pain:

- It is multidimensional, incorporating components of the 'amplified' chronic pain syndrome, such as impact on daily activity and psychological aspects of pain, as discussed above and in Chapter 6.
- It is a dynamic definition of current status – it implies probability and risk and therefore the potential for change, rather than the static view of chronic pain defined by past duration with its implication of 'unlikely to change'.

Thus far, this model has been mostly applied to persons who present with pain to primary health care. This means that it is as yet untested as a means to define chronic pain in populations, although that work is currently in progress (Dunn, personal communication). It relates closely to the approach to extended definitions of pain discussed in Chapters 5 and 6, but also to ideas of population risk or propensity for chronic pain.

Moving towards measuring risk and defining chronic pain propensity in the whole population

The previous section underlined the dynamic nature of chronic pain and the proposal that at any one time the chronic status of the individual in pain may best be measured by the probability that the amplified chronic pain syndrome will continue in the future. This is important for public health in defining prevalence and population impact, identifying opportunities for secondary and tertiary prevention, and characterizing the potential demand and need for health care. Such 'prognosis', however, also applies to people who are not in pain or who do not yet have the amplified chronic pain syndrome. Traditional epidemiology is concerned with cause and the potential for prevention in public health. From a public health perspective, it is helpful to investigate the onset of a condition as a target for primary prevention. Here the target of interest is propensity to chronic pain in the general population.

In formal epidemiological terms, the onset of chronic pain can be regarded as the point at which pain has persisted for longer than a certain specified time (3 months in most classifications as discussed above). Under the expanded definition, it would represent the point of transition to the amplified 'chronic pain syndrome', or, using our core definition, transition to a state of 'persistent pain which interferes with daily life'. It is just one of the many challenges in bringing chronic pain into an epidemiological framework that this incidence point of chronic pain is difficult to ascertain directly because of the fluctuating subjective nature of the problem.

Unless individuals are monitored closely for long periods of time, proxy markers of onset will be needed. These might include the transition in status between two time points without knowing precisely the in-between point when onset actually occurred. Another alternative is to use a measure of health care, such as primary health care consultations, recorded as events at the time they occur, as an expression, albeit selective, of incidence. Raspe, in Chapter 6, likens this process of transition to the staging of a disease such as cancer, and refers to 'stages' in the amplification of chronic pain. Similarly, with reference to Figure 4.1, it is possible that individuals progress from one trajectory to another, rather than the trajectories representing only differences between individuals. However, there are no prospective empirical studies of this as yet.

For population incidence studies and the overall public health picture, it is the onset of the chronic pain syndrome which is the crucial instantaneous event when 'underlying propensity'-plus-'trigger event' results in onset of chronic pain syndrome. This is an arbitrary point in time but allows the syndrome to be placed in an epidemiological framework. In Susser's (1973) and Rothman and Greenland's (1998) analyses of causality in epidemiology, this distinction equates to usually necessary, but insufficient, causes (propensity) and contributing, and occasionally sufficient, causes (disease or triggers of acute pain).

The proposal put forward by Natvig and colleagues in Chapter 7 is to use one component of the amplified chronic pain syndrome (number of pain sites) as a simple measure of future risk of continuing chronic pain syndrome in the whole general population.

Moving beyond pain

This book is about chronic pain. The chronic pain syndrome is not unique in its collection of characteristics and symptoms – some of the arguments apply to fatigue and other functional symptoms, although with less clear-cut underlying biological mechanisms of causality and chronicity.

One perspective is that chronic pain syndrome is on a spectrum of more-or-less linkage with other symptoms or syndromes. The more severe the pain (as measured, e.g. by its widespreadness or bothersomeness), the more likely other symptoms are to be concurrently reported. At one end of this spectrum is chronic widespread pain (or its more clinically specific subgroup of fibromyalgia) and syndromes such as irritable bowel and chronic fatigue which co-occur in the population (Kanaan et al., 2007; Schur et al., 2007). In the middle of the spectrum, as van der Windt illustrates in Chapter 12, is the simple co-occurrence of multiple symptoms in the same individuals in the general population and the primary care clinic.

All three sets of authors in this section argue that this pattern of concurrence may be distinctive enough in population terms to be added to the definition of the amplified chronic pain syndrome. This inclusivity underlines the importance and distinctiveness of Raspe's model as a basis for epidemiology and public health. Macgregor and Jones and colleagues (Chapters 8 and 9) point to genetic and stress-related mechanisms to explain why such overlap of symptoms and syndromes might happen. It seems logical for the current risk and prognosis models of Von Korff and Natvig to be extended to include 'number of non-pain symptoms', as a means to refine and add predictive utility to 'number of pain sites' or prognostic summary scores in predicting risk of chronic pain-related disability and participation restriction in the general population.

The conclusion is that in population terms we have to regard the chronic pain syndrome as a multi-morbid or co-morbid phenomenon, and that it is only by this means that we can make sense of epidemiological studies of individual pain syndromes. The challenge in public health is less about preventing individual syndromes of pain than in preventing the development of multiple problems in the same person – or in Raspe's terms preventing the onset and progression of the amplified chronic pain syndrome.

References

Carey, T.S., Garrett, J.M., Jackman, A.M. and Hadler, N.M. 1999: Recurrence and care seeking after acute back pain: results of a long-term follow-up study. North Carolina Back Pain Project. *Med Care* **37**, 157–164.

Croft, P.R., Dunn, K.M. and Raspe, H. 2006: Course and prognosis of back pain in primary care: the epidemiological perspective. *Pain* **122**, 1–3.

Dunn, K.M. and Croft, P.R. 2006: The importance of symptom duration in determining prognosis. *Pain* **121**, 126–132.

Dunn, K.M., Jordan, K. and Croft, P.R. 2006: Characterising the course of low back pain: a latent class analysis. *Am J Epidemiol* **163**, 754–761.

Eisenach, J.C., Pan, P.H., Smiley R., Lavand'homme P., Landau, R. and Houle, T.T. 2008: Severity of acute pain after childbirth, but not type of delivery, predicts persistent pain and postpartum depression. *Pain* **140**, 87–94.

International Association for the Study of Pain Subcommittee on Taxonomy. 1986: Classification of chronic pain. Descriptions of chronic pain syndromes and definitions of pain terms. *Pain* Suppl **3**, S1–S226.

Kanaan, R.A., Lepine, J.P. and Wessely, S.C. 2007: The association or otherwise of the functional somatic syndromes. *Psychosom Med* **69**, 855–859.

Rothman, K., and Greenland, S. 1998: *Modern Epidemiology*. 2nd edn. Philadelphia: Lippincott-Raven.

Schur, E.A., Afari, N., Furberg, H., Olarte, M., Goldberg, J., Sullivan, P.F. and Buchwald, D. 2007: Feeling bad in more ways than one: comorbidity patterns of medically unexplained and psychiatric conditions. *J Gen Intern Med* **22**:818–821.

Smith, B.H., Elliott, A.M., Hannaford, P.C., Chambers, W.A. and Smith, W.C. 2004: Factors related to the onset and persistence of chronic back pain in the community: results from a general population follow-up study. *Spine* **29**,1032–1040.

Susser, M. 1973: *Causal Thinking in the Health Sciences. Concepts and Strategies in Epidemiology*. New York: Oxford Univerity Press.

Van Leeuwen, M.T., Blyth F.M., March, L.M., Nicholas, M.K. and Cousins, M.J. 2006: Chronic pain and reduced work effectiveness: the hidden cost to Australian employers. *Eur J Pain* **10**, 161–166.

Von Korff, M. 1994: Studying the natural history of back pain. *Spine* **19**, 2041S–2046S.

Von Korff, M. and Dunn, K.M. 2008: Chronic pain reconsidered. *Pain* **138**, 267–276.

Von Korff, M. and Miglioretti, D.L. 2005: A prognostic approach to defining chronic pain. *Pain* **117**, 304–313.

Von Korff, M., Ormel, J., Keefe, F.J. and Dworkin, S.F. 1992: Grading the severity of chronic pain. *Pain* **50**, 133–149.

Von Korff, M. and Saunders, K. 1996: The course of back pain in primary care. *Spine* **21**, 2833–2837.

Ware Jr., J.E. and Kosinski, M. 2001: *SF-36 Physical and Mental Health Summary Scales: A Manual for Users of Version 1*. 2nd edn. Lincoln Rhode Island, QualityMetric Inc.

Chapter 5

Measuring chronic pain in populations

Clermont E. Dionne

This chapter reviews ways in which chronic pain has been measured in epidemiological studies, and will summarize a simple approach which emphasizes the need for core standard definitions to describe pain presence and persistence, i.e. a discussion of the principles underlying our work on a core definition of back pain and how they might be rolled out to epidemiological definitions of chronic pain generally.

Introduction

Pain is frequent and accompanies the human experience. While the eradication of all pain is commendable, it is not yet a reasonably achievable goal. However, it is pain that is severe and persistent that stands out as the source of the largest part of the burden.

In this chapter, I adopt the general approach to chronic pain outlined in the most recent (1994) International Association for the Study of Pain (IASP) definition: 'a persistent pain that is not amenable, as a rule, to treatments based upon specific remedies, or to the routine methods of pain control such as non-narcotic analgesics' (Merskey and Bogduk, 1994). The crucial feature here that differentiates acute and chronic pain is not the duration of the pain, but the inability of the body to restore its original functions (Loeser and Melzack, 1999). It must be remembered, however, that chronic pain takes several guises that may be of variable interest to the clinician, the health policy decision-maker, the researcher, or the public health specialist, and epidemiologist.

This chapter starts with a reflection on the purposes of measuring chronic pain in populations. I then expose the complex character of pain as the core of the main challenge to measuring pain from the population health perspective, and follow with a summary of evidence-based, current knowledge on chronic pain measurement. Then, I suggest a simple approach to address the complexity of measuring chronic pain in populations.

Purposes of chronic pain measurement in populations

In the clinical context, the focus is on one individual. Specific measures aim at diagnosing, treating, and assessing the evolution of pain within this single individual. Such measures are often part of a physical examination and, most of the time, are not applicable to studies with large numbers of subjects and repeated measures that characterize many epidemiological investigations. The population health perspective thus adopts a very different approach to health conditions compared to the clinical perspective. While measuring a health condition in populations, the public health eye will focus on summary and variability measures of the typical person, time and place characteristics, in an effort to capture the nature, source, extent, evolution, and consequences of the condition in this population.

Measuring chronic pain in populations allows:

1 Surveillance: estimation of the frequency of chronic pain in specific populations and its evolution,

2 Aetiological investigations: identification of specific factors that influence onset, persistence, recurrence, and consequences of chronic pain,

3 Evaluation of treatment: identification of the most effective and efficient interventions for chronic pain,

4 Characterization of health policies: better allocation of resources to address chronic pain.

Measuring chronic pain in populations implies comparisons between groups that must have demonstrable validity.

The nature of the beast: addressing the complexity of pain

Defining and measuring health conditions always constitute a challenge for clinicians and researchers. For pain syndromes though, the challenge is bolder than for most other health conditions for three main reasons:

1 pain is complex, essentially subjective, and multidimensional,

2 pain syndromes are extremely variable in their manifestations, and

3 pain varies considerably with time.

This high level of complexity implies important limits for the valid measurement and comparison of figures for chronic pain frequency within and between populations. The problem takes on greater importance when one considers the limits pain measurement imposes in the context of questionnaires that often only allow a small space or of interviews in a finite time, e.g. as in national health surveys. One solution to this important problem is to standardize our definitions of pain and the instruments used to measure its frequency, with the goal of minimizing the 'noise' variability and capturing only the variability that matters, i.e. true differences between groups, places, and time periods. The study of such differences is part of the traditional epidemiological contribution to insight into the phenomenon itself (in this case, pain), better allocation of resources, more effective interventions, and diminution of the collective burden of pain. Although clearly desirable, this standardization is not easy to achieve. Important efforts in that direction are, however, essential if we want public health to contribute significantly to diminish the enormous burden of chronic pain in populations.

Summary of the scientific evidence in chronic pain measurement

In most epidemiological studies, chronic pain is measured with interviews and questionnaires that rely on self-report. This is not a problem, since pain is a subjective, internal, and personal experience that cannot be directly observed by others (Buenaver and Edwards, 2007); pain is thus what the patient or individual who suffers from pain says it is (McCaffrey and Beebe, 1989). These interviews and questionnaires must, however, meet the basic requirements of reliability, validity and, if they are to be used in longitudinal studies, responsiveness (Guyatt et al., 1989). To meet these requirements, the instruments and their application first need to be standardized.

A first essential step in measuring any construct is to define it clearly and to identify its components. The adequacy of this process will result in high face and content validity. As an individual phenomenon, pain could be characterized by several elements: its 'symptoms' (e.g. irradiation, paraesthesia), its 'intensity' (importance of the perception), its 'site' (region of the body that is affected), the 'time frame' of reference (when it happens), its 'consequences' (e.g. work disability, interference with daily activities, financial costs), its 'frequency' (how often it happens), its 'duration' (how long it lasts), and its 'source' (e.g. pain from cancer). Furthermore, 'severity' is another key element of pain that can be defined by some levels of the other elements (e.g. intensity) or different combinations of them (e.g. pain intensity and interference with daily activities). There are also other dimensions of pain that include its affective and evaluative qualities (Melzack, 1975). The multidimensional character of pain constitutes a major challenge for its valid measurement, especially at the population level.

Since the early works of Melzack and Wall in 1983, several instruments have been designed to measure some dimensions of pain, the psychometric qualities of which have often been studied and compared. This body of work provides us with the scientific evidence to underpin the challenge of measuring pain in populations.

Symptoms of pain

The literature shows considerable variability as to pain symptoms that are measured in epidemiological studies. For instance, ache, complaint, deformity, discomfort, insufficiency, pain, joint swelling, stiffness, and tiredness have all been used, alone as well as in combination (e.g. ache, pain or discomfort; pain or swelling). There is no clear evidence as to the choice of wordings for symptoms of pain; this choice varies with the objectives of the study. However, here, as in other circumstances, considerations of validity are paramount.

Pain intensity

Pain intensity (or magnitude) is typically measured with pain-rating scales, of which at least 22 different versions exist (Strong et al., 1991). Horizontally oriented (Ogon et al., 1996) Visual Analogue Scales (VAS) and Verbal Rating Scales (VRS) have been shown to constitute reliable, valid, and responsive instruments to measure pain intensity. Numerical Rating Scales (NRS) are however more easily understood, more reliable and responsive than VAS and VRS (Bolton and Wilkinson, 1998; Grotle et al., 2003), and thus have been recommended as the scales of choice to measure pain intensity in patients with pain (Strong et al., 1991). Jensen et al. (1994) have also shown that an NRS using 11 points is as sensitive as an NRS with more points on the scale (Jensen et al., 1994). NRS can be administered in written or verbal form and, unlike the VAS, difficulty with the scale does not appear to be associated with age (Jensen et al., 1986). A composite pain-intensity score calculated as the mean of 12 ratings taken on 4 days is more reliable and valid than a single measure of average pain (Jensen and McFarland, 1993). Among elders with cognitive impairments, pain-behaviour observation has been shown to be a valid assessment method (Weiner et al., 1996).

Pain site

When pain is measured over the phone (without supporting documents), one must rely solely on a description of the affected site, that should be as specific and univocal as possible. An example for low back pain was adapted from Anderson (1986):

> Any report of pain that occurs between the gluteal folds inferiorly and the line of the 12th rib superiorly, plus sciatica and cruralgia even if there are no concurrent symptoms in the back.
>
> (Dionne, 1999)

One can appreciate that such a definition, although it can be easily understood by clinicians, needs to be worded in lay terms in most applications, which may be difficult.

Non-specific terms such as 'back', 'low back', 'lower back', and 'lower part of the back' may have variable interpretations. For instance, 'back pain' may include neck pain for some individuals, while it is restricted to the lumbar area for others.

When the measurement is taken with a self-report questionnaire or during a face-to-face interview, body diagrams and schemas could be used to further standardize the pain-site description. Such a diagram is included in the Nordic Questionnaire (Kuorinka et al., 1987). When possible, such tools may be mailed in advance to participants to a telephone survey or be made available on the Internet. A recent study has shown slightly higher prevalences with a diagram compared to detailed written questions, but globally there was a high agreement between both (sensitivity of the diagram: 62–81%) as to the prevalence of musculoskeletal pain at nine anatomical sites. The agreement was, however, lower for the low-educated and oldest age groups (van den Hoven et al., 2010).

Time frame of reference

The time frame of the pain measure is one of the most variable elements of pain definitions in the literature. It goes from 'today' (point prevalence) to 'ever' (lifetime period prevalence), with 1-week, 2-week, 1-month, 3-month, 6-month, 1-year, 5-year and 10-year prevalence figures as the most often reported. Annual incidence (in person-years) and cumulative incidence are more rarely found. Because researchers often need to document pain retrospectively, recall bias can affect the validity of chronic pain measures (Haythornwaite and Fauerbach, 2001; Gendreau et al., 2003). However, there is scientific evidence that supports the validity of retrospective reports of pain intensity, duration, and associated disability for at least a 3-month recall period (Salovey et al., 1992; Von Korff, 2001).

Pain consequences

There are few available specific measures of work disability besides the usual measures of absence from/presence at work and the number of days of work absence. Some new, more developed measures are, however, promising (Beaton and Kennedy, 2005; Dionne et al., 2005).

Several instruments exist to measure interference of pain with daily activities (e.g. Roland–Morris Disability Questionnaire (RMDQ; Roland and Morris, 1983), Oswestry Disability Index-(ODI; Fairbank et al., 1980), Short Form-36 (SF-36; Ware, 1993)). Results from daily diary studies and prior research on the internal consistency and convergent validity of pain-disability measures also suggest that retrospective reports of interference with daily activities provides useful information (Von Korff, 2001).

There are no published standardized measures of the individual financial consequences of pain.

Pain frequency

Frequency refers to the number of repetitions of a periodic process per unit of time (e.g. number of episodes last year (e.g. 0, 1–2, 3–6, >6); just once/a few spells/frequent spells/never got better). This is a characteristic of pain that seems not to have been scrutinized.

Pain duration

There is some evidence that measures of duration can be useful to characterize chronic pain: the following categories of patient-reported symptom duration have been found to be associated with differences in pain severity, disability, and psychological status: 0–6 months, 7 months to 2 years, and 3 years and more (Dunn and Croft, 2006).

Alternative definitions exist, which can also be applied to duration of health care episode for pain (Demmelmaier et al., 2008; Hinkley and Jaremko, 1994). However, the meaning of recalled duration of symptoms is a continuing topic of discussion, and this has implications for the interpretation of duration in population epidemiology (see Chapter 4).

In many publications, pain is defined as 'acute' (<3 months) and 'chronic' (>3 months) according to the duration of symptoms. Although it has some pragmatic advantages in summarizing currently available population data, this definition is becoming obsolete as more flexible definitions develop (Loeser and Melzack, 1999; Von Korff and Dunn, 2008).

Source of pain

Source of pain is, most of the time, self-reported in epidemiological studies. The most frequent approach used in such circumstances is to identify some specific sources of pain the investigators want to exclude (e.g. pain from feverish illness, menstruation, paralysis or exertion, pain linked with a previous medical diagnosis of fibromyalgia or systemic rheumatic disease). When participants are recruited in medical settings, however, it may be possible to exclude other specific causes of pain (e.g. for back pain, those with 'red flags' suggesting non-mechanical spinal conditions: fractures, infections, malignancies, inflammatory arthritis, cauda equina syndrome, or visceral disease; Nachemson et al., 2000).

Pain severity

Pain severity is probably the element most often found in pain definitions after symptoms, site of pain, and time frame of the measure. It has been defined in different ways: duration >3 months (Merskey and Bogduk, 1994), pain that is severe enough to seek treatment, disabling pain [e.g. ODI (Fairbank et al., 1980) >25], pain that is 'bad enough to limit your usual activities or change your daily routine for more than one day', pain that is significantly bothersome, (Dunn and Croft, 2005), and 'pain that troubled you'. The Graded Chronic Pain Scale combines pain intensity and activity limitation (Von Korff et al., 1992; Von Korff et al., 1990; Penny et al., 1999), with pain self-reported on a continuum – background pain/mild/moderate/severe/hyper-severe pain (Borkan et al., 1995). In post-operative pain patients, Bodian et al. (2001) and Jensen et al. (2003) have identified the cut-off to define severe pain on an 11-point VAS around 7/10.

Generic pain-measurement instruments

Generic pain-measurement instruments can be used to measure pain in different and/or multiple anatomical sites. Such instruments include the 15-item Profile of Chronic Pain: Screen (PCP: S; Ruehlman et al., 2005), the Chronic Pain Experience Instrument (CPEI; Davis, 1989), the Glasgow Pain Questionnaire (Thomas et al., 1996), the Level of Expressed Need (LEN; Smith et al., 2001), the McGill Pain Questionnaire (MPQ; Melzack and Wall, 1983) and, its short version, the Short-form McGill Pain Questionnaire (Melzack, 1987), the Nordic Questionnaire (Kuorinka et al., 1987), the Pain Module of the Standard Evaluation Questionnaire (SEQ Pain; Muller et al., 2008), the SF-36 Bodily Pain scale (Von Korff, 2001; Ware, 1993; Brazier et al., 1992), and the Troublesomeness Grid (Parsons et al., 2006). These instruments are especially useful to provide a complete picture of pain syndromes, as pain in one site is often accompanied by pain symptoms in other sites (Croft et al., 2007; Croft 1996). They have, however, the disadvantage of being long and are sometimes complicated to administer properly. These instruments do not necessarily measure all the dimensions of pain mentioned previously.

Specific pain-measurement instruments

Specific pain-measurement instruments are intended to be applied to individuals with a specific pain syndrome or pain that is limited to a single anatomical site. These instruments include, for arthritis: the Arthritis Impact Measurement Scales (Meenan et al., 1980; Meenan et al., 1982); for hip pain: the Harris Hip Score, (Harris, 1969) and the Merle D'Aubigne Score (D'Aubigne and Postel, 1954); for knee pain: the American Knee Society Score (Liow et al., 2000); for migraine: the Migraine Disability Assessment Scale (MIDAS; Stewart and Lipton, 2002); for musculoskeletal pain: the Pain Disability Questionnaire (PDQ; Anagnostis et al., 2004); for neck pain: the Copenhagen Neck Functional Disability Scale (Jordan et al., 1998); for neuropathic pain: the Neuropathic Pain Scale (NPS; Galer and Bensen, 1997); for pain from osteoarthritis of the knee or hip: the Western Ontario and McMaster Universities Index (WOMAC; Bellamy et al., 1988); for shoulder pain: the Constant Score (Constant and Murley, 1987), the Disability of the Shoulder and Hand (DASH) Score (Hudak et al., 1996), the Shoulder Pain Disability Index (SPADI; Roach et al., 1991), and the University of California at Los Angeles Rating System (UCLA) Score (Kay and Amstutz, 1988); for low back pain: the Graded Chronic Pain Scale (GCPS; Von Korff, 2001; Von Korff et al., 1992; Penny et al., 1999; Underwood et al., 1999), the Japan Low Back Pain Evaluation Questionnaire (JLEQ; Shirado et al., 2007), the Oswestry Low Back Pain Disability Index (ODI; Fairbank et al., 1980), the Roland–Morris Disability Questionnaire (RMDQ; Roland and Morris, 1983; Jensen et al., 1992), and the Quebec Pain Scale (Kopec et al., 1996; Kopec et al., 1995). Again, these instruments do not necessarily measure all the elements or dimensions of pain mentioned previously.

Summary

There is no shortage of pain-measurement instruments, but rather there is a plethora of these for use in population research. Most of them have been shown to possess proper psychometric qualities. This variety of instruments constitutes a richness and is the fruit of the labour of numerous pain investigators and methodologists. For internal validity purposes, i.e. measuring pain with one instrument within a single population, these instruments cover a wide spectrum of research needs. However, when external validity is at stake, i.e. when one wants to study different populations (e.g. compare or summarize the prevalence of pain measured with different instruments in two or more countries), this variety has a high cost: since almost every instrument is based on its own definition of pain, assesses only some of its dimensions, and hence provides a different measure, the resulting figures cannot be validly compared or summarized.

The chronic pain literature shows extreme variation in the definitions and measures of pain used. For instance, while examining 51 papers that addressed the prevalence of low back pain among older adults as part of a systematic review on the relationship between age and the prevalence of back pain (Dionne et al., 2006), we found such a wide range of definitions of back-pain prevalence that it was almost impossible to pool the results. Other authors have reported similar difficulties (Loney and Stratford, 1999; Leboeuf-Yde and Lauritsen, 1995; Bressler et al., 1999). This problem is even more important when one considers other sources of heterogeneity across pain studies, most of them methodological (e.g. differences in study design, sampling frame, analysis). If regional and international comparisons of population studies are to be used to investigate the causes and consequences of pain and to determine the influence of different health care systems on the occurrence of pain syndromes, there needs to be highly standardized information to compare.

Consensual definitions as an answer to external validity problems

Although each investigator, given the context and objectives of a study, has a unique insight into the best measurement instrument to use for measuring chronic pain, a broader picture requires the adoption, by the pain-research community, of a core standard definition and corresponding measurement instrument. To address the specifics of population studies, these must have some basic characteristics: 1) they need to be simple enough for individuals of average education to understand the questions and answer validly, 2) the measurement should be short, so that it can be used in large surveys, and 3) the instrument must be adaptable to different study contexts and objectives. While each investigator can continue to choose a definition and an instrument to address these characteristics, the challenge lies in achieving consensus on one or a few definitions and instruments that could be widely used thereafter, opening new possibilities of worldwide comparisons and research synergies. It must be stressed, however, that achieving minimal consensus on core definitions and instruments does not exclude or discourage each investigator from adding other measurement instruments to address their specific internal research questions and requirements.

This challenge has recently been attempted for low back pain (Dionne et al., 2008). I take this as an example, and summarize below the methods that were used and the outcomes of this process, so as to demonstrate the perspective of measuring chronic pain more widely and comparatively in population studies.

In order to identify standard definitions of low back pain for use in epidemiological prevalence studies, an international panel of experts in back pain was invited to participate in a Delphi procedure to agree on at least two definitions of low back pain:

1 A 'minimal' definition, for use in large population-based general surveys, where there are many constraints and space for only one or two questions, and

2 An 'optimal' definition for use in focussed studies where the investigators have space or time for multiple questions.

In a first step, the definitions found in 51 papers reporting the results of back pain population-based studies (Dionne et al., 2006) were examined to identify the different definitions of the elements presented above. Using the definitions of low back pain found in the 51 articles, 77 different definitions of these elements were identified (time frame: 12, site: 8, symptoms: 26, duration: 13, frequency: 7, severity: 8, and source: 3). These items were listed, grouped by element, in a questionnaire that asked Delphi participants to rate each of them on an 11-point rating scale where 0 meant 'Not at all suitable for a standard definition of low back pain' and 10 meant 'Would definitely use for a standard definition of low back pain'. The rating had to be done twice: once for an 'optimal' definition of low back pain and once for a 'minimal' definition. The questionnaire offered the opportunity to write general as well as specific comments and to add new definitions for each of the elements. The questionnaire for Round 1 of the Delphi was sent by email, with two reminders.

Distributions of individual scores of panel members in Round 1 were established, and items that did not reach an *a priori* determined consensual median score of at least 6/10 were excluded. New items suggested by the participants in Round 1 were added to the list. The same instructions as for Round 1 were used for Round 2 of the Delphi. Median and individual scores of Round 1 were provided to each participant.

Distributions of individual scores of panel members in Round 2 were established and items that did not reach the consensual median score of at least 6/10 were excluded from further consideration. In a third round, participants were asked to choose only one item in each element, for each definition.

A workshop was organized at the 2006 International Forum VIII for Primary Care Research on Low Back Pain held in Amsterdam to present the results of Rounds 1–3 and discuss them with the participants. Before the workshop, two definitions (minimal and optimal) were built, using the items remaining following Rounds 1–3. Participants in the workshop were provided with these definitions and the list of all items considered in Rounds 1–3, along with the median scores obtained and specific comments. Results of the workshop were integrated with those of the first three rounds and compared with the scientific evidence. When a definition was not coherent with the scientific evidence after the workshop, a change was suggested to the panel members with an explanation. During a fourth round, participants were asked to vote for or against one minimal definition and one optimal definition. They were encouraged to provide specific comments, especially when they voted against a proposal.

It was finally agreed that a minimal definition must be truly minimal and that a diagram (body manikin with shaded area for low back pain) should be used when possible to identify site of pain. A severity criterion ('bad enough to limit your usual activities or change your daily routine for more than one day') was thought to be essential for a minimal definition; otherwise the minimal definition would result in extremely high prevalence of back pain that would not be meaningful. Finally, the time frame was judged the third essential feature of a minimal definition. 'Past month' was considered ambiguous (for instance, on 15 February, 'past month' may be interpreted as the period between January 15 and February 14 or the period between January 1 and 31). It was suggested to use 'past 4 weeks' instead.

It was also agreed that an optimal definition would be built from the minimal definition by adding other elements.

The final results of this Delphi process are presented in Tables 5.1 and 5.2. Table 5.3 presents examples of use of the optimal definition.

Table 5.1 Final minimal definition of low back pain that resulted from the Delphi study. The diagram should be used in face-to-face interviews and questionnaires (a), and the wording alone used in telephone surveys (b). Reprinted with permission from Dionne et al., 2008.

a) For face-to-face interviews and paper or online questionnaires:

In the past 4 weeks, have you had pain in your low back (in the area shown on the diagram)?
Yes ☐ No ☐

If yes, was this pain bad enough to limit your usual activities or change your daily routine for more than one day?
Yes ☐ No ☐

LOW BACK

b) For telephone surveys:

In the past 4 weeks, have you had pain in your low back?
Yes ☐ No ☐

If yes, was this pain bad enough to limit your usual activities or change your daily routine for more than one day?
Yes ☐ No ☐

Table 5.2 Final optimal definition of low back pain that resulted from the Delphi study. Elements can be combined as investigators see fit to provide different specific definitions (see examples in **Table 5.3**). Reprinted with permission from Dionne et al., 2008.

Time frame: In the past 4 weeks,

Site and symptoms:[1] have you had pain in your low back (in the area shown on the diagram)?

Yes ☐   No ☐

LOW BACK

If yes, was this pain bad enough to limit your usual activities or change your daily routine for more than one day?

Yes ☐   No ☐

Sciatica: have you had pain that goes down the leg?

Yes ☐   No ☐

If yes, has this pain spread below the knee?

Yes ☐   No ☐

Exclusions: Please do not report pain from feverish illness or menstruation.

Frequency:[2] If you had pain in your low back in the past 4 weeks, how often did you have the pain?

On some days ☐   On most days ☐   Every day ☐

Duration:[2] If you had low back pain in the past 4 weeks, how long was it since you had a whole month without any low back pain? (Please tick only one box).

Less than 3 months ☐
3 months or more but less than 7 months ☐
7 months or more but less than 3 years ☐
3 years and more ☐

Severity:[2,3] If you had low back pain in the past 4 weeks, please indicate what was the usual intensity of your pain on a scale of 0 to 10, where 0 means "no pain" and 10 means "the worst pain imaginable" (Please circle your answer).

| 0 | 1 | 2 | 3 | 4 | 5 | 6 | 7 | 8 | 9 | 10 |
No pain   Worst pain

[1] The diagram should be used in face-to-face interviews and paper or online questionnaires and omitted in telephone surveys, as detailed in the minimal definition (Table 5.1).

[2] Questions on frequency, duration, and severity can be used for sciatica by replacing 'low back pain' by 'pain that goes down the leg'.

[3] For reporting, categories are: *"Mild= <7/10"* and *"Severe ≥7/10)"*.

It is very important to stress that the key feature of the approach used in this study was the consensus of experts in the field of back pain prevalence research and primary care of back pain; hence, the intent was not to find 'the best' low back pain definitions nor to present the final definitions as 'the only' low back pain definitions. The goal was simply to bring leading back-pain experts together to agree as much as possible on definitions that could be published and suggested for free use in future epidemiological studies. The crucial issue for the purposes of this book is that there was acceptance and general agreement that the definitions were being moulded for epidemiological purposes and so could afford to be simple in their content and language.

Table 5.3 Examples of optimal definitions of low back pain built from the items presented in **Table 5.2**. Reprinted with permission from Dionne et al., 2008.

Example 1. If the investigator is interested in the prevalence of severe long-standing low back pain and conducts a survey using postal questionnaires, the following questions should be asked:

Q1-In the past 4 weeks, have you had pain in your low back (in the area shown on the diagram)? Please do not report pain from feverish illness or menstruation.

Yes ☐   No ☐

LOW BACK

Q2-If yes, was this pain bad enough to limit your usual activities or change your daily routine for more than one day?

Yes ☐   No ☐

Q3-If you had low back pain in the past 4 weeks, how long was it since you had a whole month without any low back pain? (Please tick only one box).

Less than 3 months   ☐
3 months or more but less than 7 months   ☐
7 months or more but less than 3 years   ☐
3 years and more   ☐

Q4-If you had low back pain in the past 4 weeks, please indicate what was the usual intensity of your pain on a scale of 0 to 10, where 0 means "no pain" and 10 means "the worst pain imaginable" (Please circle your answer).

          0   1   2   3   4   5   6   7   8   9   10
No pain   Worst pain

Example 2. If the investigator is interested in the prevalence of sciatica and conducts a telephone interview, the following questions should be asked:

Q1-In the past 4 weeks, have you had pain that goes down the leg?

Yes ☐ No ☐

Q2-If yes, was this pain bad enough to limit your usual activities or change your daily routine for more than one day?

Yes ☐ No ☐

Q3-If you had pain that goes down the leg in the past 4 weeks, has this pain spread below the knee?

Yes ☐ No ☐

Q4-If you had pain that goes down the leg in the past 4 weeks, how often did you have the pain?

On some days ☐   On most days ☐   Every day ☐

Clinicians on the consensus panels accepted that this meant ignoring the complexities and variation which individual sufferers experience from their back pain and which might be crucial characteristics in the clinical assessment of such individuals. It is the purpose to which definitions are to be put that determines the rules for their development – and pain is no different in this to other more 'disease-focussed' examples. For epidemiological or population-study purposes, the definitions of conditions such as hypertension, asthma, or prostatism, or of influences on health such as exercise or diet, are often extreme simplifications of how a clinician or a physiologist might characterize and define them for other purposes.

As a whole, the work on low back pain should be considered as a step towards better standardization of definitions for epidemiological, population, and public health purposes, and as a template for consensus development of comparable epidemiological definitions of other chronic pain syndromes. The use of these definitions will allow the comparison of low back pain prevalence figures from different countries, age groups, settings, and occupational groups, among others, and will facilitate meta-analysis of results of epidemiological studies of back pain, which is currently difficult or impossible. They are suitable for regular inclusion in national surveys. Validation work and continuing use will allow researchers to test these definitions and improve them, as evidence for the validity of specific elements emerges (updated definitions and cultural adaptations are posted on a website: *www.uresp.ulaval.ca/backpaindefs*). Maintaining the wording and presentation of the definitions will allow maximum benefit to be gained from the research conducted.

One important strength of the study is that it included several international back-pain investigators, many of whom are multilingual. This maximizes the possibilities for cross-cultural adaptations.

This approach to reaching a consensus definition of back-pain prevalence could certainly be applied to other chronic pain syndromes.

Public health implications

Measuring chronic pain in large population studies requires substantial resources, time, and energy. Such an investment should provide benefits that go beyond the immediate objectives of the study. It is unfortunate that many large studies in the pain field cannot be used at a 'meta' level in conjunction with the results of other national and international studies to allow comparisons and summaries. Relatively simple to realize, comparisons and summaries present a huge potential for advancing our understanding of chronic pain, e.g. developing a public health perspective of the sort that transformed approaches to prevention of cancer and coronary heart disease, and taking steps towards prevention and better management of this common and disabling condition. The consensus approach I have presented in the previous section is a proposal that holds serious promise to improve this situation, but needs to be applied widely to other pain syndromes and to be used as a core set of questions across surveys in different populations. Although they cannot answer the needs of all situations, consensual definitions can be easily used in conjunction with more specific definitions without losing their usefulness. The opportunity to rigorously study global variations in chronic pain as a means to identify causes and targets for prevention and intervention beckons pain scientists willing to adopt this consensual epidemiological approach to measuring pain symptoms in different populations and different social and cultural settings.

Conclusions

The field of pain research is moving forward rapidly in many disciplines, and there are likely to be many innovations in measurement, explanatory models, prevention, and treatment in the coming years. However, whatever advances there are in the measurement techniques of pain, the true benefits of their application to population studies will always be subsidiary to our capacity to use the results for the efficient surveillance of pain in populations, better allocation of resources, and more effective interventions. This will be better accomplished if investigators use comparable core pain measurements. I believe this methodological issue, closely linked to the multidimensional nature of pain, is crucial for the field. Of course, efforts must continue to be made to gain a better understanding of pain and improve the construct validity of measurement techniques. In the meantime though, I am convinced that for investigators to agree on standard definitions and measures of pain, even imperfect and limited ones, is the most profitable option for the epidemiological and public health investigation of chronic pain in populations.

References

Anagnostis, C., Gatchel, R.J. and Mayer, T.G. 2004: The pain disability questionnaire: A new psychometrically sound measure for chronic musculoskeletal disorders. *Spine* **29**, 2290–2303.

Anderson, J.A. 1986: Epidemiological aspects of back pain. *J Soc Occup Med* **36**, 90–94.

Beaton, D.E. and Kennedy, C.A. 2005: Beyond return to work: Testing a measure of at-work disability in workers with musculoskeletal pain. *Qual Life Res* **14**, 1869–1879.

Bellamy, N., Buchanan, W.W., Goldsmith, C.H., Campbell, J. and Stitt, L.W. 1988: Validation study of WOMAC: A health status instrument for measuring clinically important patient relevant outcomes to antirheumatic drug therapy in patients with osteoarthritis of the hip or knee. *J Rheumatol* **15**, 1833–1840.

Bodian, C.A., Freedman, G., Hossain, S., Eisenkraft, J.B. and Beilin, Y. 2001: The visual analog scale for pain: Clinical significance in postoperative patients. *Anesthesiology* **95**, 1356–1361.

Bolton, J.E. and Wilkinson, R.C. 1998: Responsiveness of pain scales: A comparison of three pain intensity measures in chiropractic patients. *J Manipulative Physiol Ther* **21**, 1–7.

Borkan, J., Reis, S., Hermoni, D. and Biderman, A. 1995: Talking about the pain: A patient-centered study of low back pain in primary care. *Soc Sci Med* **40**, 977–988.

Brazier, J.E., Harper, R., Jones, N.M., O'Cathain, A., Thomas, K.J., Usherwood, T. et al. 1992: Validating the SF-36 health survey questionnaire: New outcome measure for primary care. *BMJ* **305**, 160–164.

Bressler, H.B., Keyes, W.J., Rochon, P.A. and Badley, E. 1999: The prevalence of low back pain in the elderly. A systematic review of the literature. *Spine* **24**, 1813–1819.

Buenaver, L. and Edwards, R. 2007: Measurement of pain, in Ernst E, Pittler MH, Wider B (eds) *Complementary therapies for pain management: An evidence-based approach*, pp.37–46. Mosby Elsevier, Toronto.

Carey, T.S., Garrett, J., Jackman, A., Sanders, L. and Kalsbeek, W. 1995: Reporting of acute low back pain in a telephone interview. Identification of potential biases. *Spine* **20**, 787–790.

Constant, C.R. and Murley, A.H. 1987: A clinical method of functional assessment of the shoulder. *Clin Orthop Relat Res* **214**, 160–164.

Croft, P. 1996: The epidemiology of pain - the more you have, the more you get. *Annals Rheum Dis* **55**, 859–860.

Croft, P., Dunn, K.M. and Von Korff, M. 2007: Chronic pain syndromes: You can't have one without another. *Pain* **131**, 237–238.

Croft, P. and Raspe, H. 1995: Back pain. *Baillieres Clin Rheumatol* **9**, 565–583.

D'Aubigne, R.M. and Postel, M. 1954: Functional results of hip arthroplasty with acrylic prosthesis. *J Bone Joint Surg Am* **36**, 451–475.

Davis, G.C. 1989: Measurement of the chronic pain experience: Development of an instrument. *Res Nurs Health* **12**, 221–227.

Demmelmaier, I., Lindberg, P., Asenlof, P. and Denison, E. 2008: The associations between pain intensity, psychosocial variables, and pain duration/recurrence in a large sample of persons with nonspecific spinal pain. *Clin J Pain* **24**, 611–619.

Dionne, C.E. 1999: Low back pain, in Crombie IK, Croft PR, Linton SJ, LeResche L, Von Korff M (eds) *Epidemiology of pain*, pp.283–97. IASP Press, Seattle, WA.

Dionne, C.E., Bourbonnais, R., Fremont, P., Rossignol, M., Stock, S.R. and Larocque, I. 2005: A clinical return-to-work rule for patients with back pain. *CMAJ* **172**, 1559–1567.

Dionne, C.E., Dunn, K.M. and Croft, P.R. 2006: Does back pain prevalence really decrease with increasing age? A systematic review. *Age Ageing* **35**, 229–234.

Dionne, C.E., Dunn, K.M., Croft, P.R., Nachemson, A.L., Buchbinder, R., Walker, B.F. *et al*. 2008: A consensus approach toward the standardization of back pain definitions for use in prevalence studies. *Spine* **33**, 95–103.

Dunn, K.M. and Croft, P.R. 2005: Classification of low back pain in primary care: Using 'Bothersomeness' to identify the most severe cases. *Spine* **30**, 1887–1892.

Dunn, K.M. and Croft, P.R. 2006: The importance of symptom duration in determining prognosis. *Pain* **121**, 126–132.

Fairbank, J.C., Couper, J., Davies, J.B. and O'Brien, J.P. 1980: The Oswestry low back pain disability questionnaire. *Physiotherapy* **66**, 271–273.

Ferraz, M.B., Quaresma, M.R., Aquino, L.R., Atra, E., Tugwell, P. and Goldsmith, C.H. 1990: Reliability of pain scales in the assessment of literate and illiterate patients with rheumatoid arthritis. *J Rheumatol* **17**, 1022–1024.

Galer, B.S. and Jensen, M.P. 1997: Development and preliminary validation of a pain measure specific to neuropathic pain: The Neuropathic Pain Scale. *Neurology* **48**, 332–328.

Gendreau, M., Hufford, M.R. and Stone, A.A. 2003: Measuring clinical pain in chronic widespread pain: Selected methodological issues. *Best Pract Res Clin Rheumatol* **17**, 575–592.

Grotle, M., Brox, J.I. and Vollestad, N.K. 2003: Cross-cultural adaptation of the norwegian versions of the Roland-Morris Disability Questionnaire and the Oswestry Disability Index. *J Rehabil Med* **35**, 241–247.

Guyatt, G.H., Deyo, R.A., Charlson, M., Levine, M.N. and Mitchell, A. 1989: Responsiveness and validity in health status measurement: A clarification. J Clin Epidemiol **42**, 403–438.

Harris, W.H. 1969: Traumatic arthritis of the hip after dislocation and acetabular fractures: Treatment by mold arthroplasty. An end-result study using a new method of result evaluation. *J Bone Joint Surg Am* **51**, 737–755.

Haythornwaite, J.A. and Fauerbach, J.A. 2001: Assessment of acute pain, pain relief, and patient satisfaction, in Turk DC, Melzack R (eds) *Handbook of pain assessment*, 2nd edn, pp.417–430. Guilford Press, New York, NY.

Hinkley, B.S. and Jaremko, M.E. 1994: Effects of pain duration on psychosocial adjustment in orthopaedic patients: The importance of early diagnosis and treatment of pain. *J Pain Symptom Manage* **9**, 175–185.

Hudak, P.L., Amadio, P.C. and Bombardier, C. 1996: Development of an upper extremity outcome measure: The DASH (Disabilities of the Arm, Shoulder and Hand). The Upper Extremity Collaborative Group (UECG). *Am J Ind Med* **29**, 602–608.

Jensen, M.P., Chen, C. and Brugger, A.M. 2003: Interpretation of visual analog scale ratings and change scores: A reanalysis of two clinical trials of postoperative pain. *J Pain* **4**, 407–414.

Jensen, M.P., Karoly, P. and Braver, S. 1986: The measurement of clinical pain intensity: A comparison of six methods. *Pain* **27**, 117–126.

Jensen, M.P. and McFarland, C.A. 1993: Increasing the reliability and validity of pain intensity measurement in chronic pain patients. *Pain* **55**, 195–203.

Jensen, M.P., Strom, S.E., Turner, J.A. and Romano, J.M. 1992: Validity of the Sickness Impact Profile Roland scale as a measure of dysfunction in chronic pain patients. *Pain* **50**, 157–162.

Jensen, M.P., Turner, J.A. and Romano, J.M. 1994: What is the maximum number of levels needed in pain intensity measurement? *Pain* **58**, 387–392.

Jordan, A., Manniche, C., Mosdal, C. and Hindsberger, C. 1998: The Copenhagen Neck Functional Disability Scale: A study of reliability and validity. *J Manipulative Physiol Ther* **21**(8), 520–527.

Kay, S.P. and Amstutz, H.C. 1988: Shoulder hemiarthroplasty at UCLA. *Clin Orthop Relat Res* **228**, 42–48.

Kopec, J.A., Esdaile, J.M., Abrahamowicz, M., Abenhaim, L., Wood-Dauphinee, S., Lamping, D.L. et al. 1995: The Quebec Back Pain Disability Scale. Measurement properties. *Spine* **20**, 341–352.

Kopec, J.A., Esdaile, J.M., Abrahamowicz, M., Abenhaim, L., Wood-Dauphinee, S., Lamping, D.L. et al. 1996: The Quebec Back Pain Disability Scale: Conceptualization and development. *J Clin Epidemiol* **49**, 151–161.

Kuorinka, I., Jonsson, B., Kilbom, A., Vinterberg, H., Biering-Sorensen, F., Andersson, G. et al. 1987: Standardised Nordic questionnaires for the analysis of musculoskeletal symptoms. *Appl Ergon* **18**, 233–237.

Leboeuf-Yde, C. and Lauritsen, J.M. 1995: The prevalence of low back pain in the literature: A structured review of 26 Nordic studies from 1954 to 1993. *Spine* **20**, 2112–2118.

Liow, R.Y., Walker, K., Wajid, M.A., Bedi, G. and Lennox, C.M. 2000: The reliability of the American Knee Society score. *Acta Orthop Scand* **71**, 603–608.

Loeser, J.D. and Melzack, R. 1999: Pain: An overview. *Lancet* **353**, 1607–1609.

Loney, P.L. and Stratford, P.W. 1999: The prevalence of low back pain in adults: A methodological review of the literature. *Phys Ther* **79**, 384–396.

McCafferey, M. and Beebe, A. 1989: *Pain: Clinical manual for nursing practice*, The CV Mosby Co, St-Louis, MO.

Meenan, R.F., Gertman, P.M. and Mason, J.H. 1980: Measuring health status in arthritis. The arthritis impact measurement scales. *Arthritis Rheum* **23**, 146–152.

Meenan, R.F., Gertman, P.M., Mason, J.H. and Dunaif, R. 1982: The arthritis impact measurement scales. Further investigations of a health status measure. *Arthritis Rheum* **25**, 1048–1053.

Melzack, R. 1975: The McGill Pain Questionnaire: Major properties and scoring methods. *Pain* **1**, 277–299.

Melzack, R. 1987: The Short-Form McGill Pain Questionnaire. *Pain* **30**, 191–197

Melzack, R. and Wall, P.D. 1983: *The challenge of pain*. Basic Books, New York, NY.

Merskey, H. and Bogduk, N. 1994: *Classification of chronic pain. Definitions of chronic pain syndromes and definition of pain terms*, 2nd edn. International Association for the Study of Pain, Seattle, WA.

Muller, U., Tanzler, K., Burger, A., Staub, L., Tamcan, O., Roeder, C. et al. 2008: A pain assessment scale for population-based studies: Development and validation of the Pain Module of the Standard Evaluation Questionnaire. *Pain* **136**, 62–74.

Nachemson, A.L., Waddell, G. and Norlund, A.I. 2000: Epidemiology of neck and low back pain, in Nachemson AL, Jonsson E (eds). *Neck and back pain: The scientific evidence of causes, diagnosis, and treatment*, pp.165–187. Lippincott Williams & Wilkins, Philadelphia, PA.

Ogon, M., Krismer, M., Sollner, W., Kantner-Rumplmair, W. and Lampe, A. 1996: Chronic low back pain measurement with visual analogue scales in different settings. *Pain* **64**, 425–428.

Parsons, S., Carnes, D., Pincus, T., Foster, N., Breen, A., Vogel, S. et al. 2006: Measuring troublesomeness of chronic pain by location. *BMC Musculoskelet Disord* **7**, 34.

Penny, K.I., Purves, A.M., Smith, B.H., Chambers, W.A. and Smith, W.C. 1999: Relationship between the Chronic Pain Grade and measures of physical, social and psychological well-being. *Pain* **79**, 275–279.

Roach, K.E., Budiman-Mak, E., Songsiridej, N. and Lertratanakul, Y. 1991: Development of a shoulder pain and disability index. *Arthritis Care Res* **4**, 143–149.

Roland, M. and Morris, R. 1983: A study of the natural history of back pain. Part I: Development of a reliable and sensitive measure of disability in low-back pain. *Spine* **8**, 141–144.

Ruehlman, L.S., Karoly, P., Newton, C. and Aiken, L.S. 2005: The development and preliminary validation of a brief measure of chronic pain impact for use in the general population. *Pain* **113**, 82–90.

Salovey, P., Seiber, W., Smith, A., Turk, D., Jobe, J. and Willis, G. 1992: *Reporting chronic pain episodes on health surveys*. National Center for Health Statistics, Hyattsville, MD.

Shirado, O., Doi, T., Akai, M., Fujino, K., Hoshino, Y. and Iwaya, T. 2007: An outcome measure for Japanese people with chronic low back pain: An introduction and validation study of Japan Low Back Pain Evaluation Questionnaire. *Spine* 32, 3052–3059.

Smith, B.H., Penny, K.I., Elliott, A.M., Chambers, W.A. and Smith, W.C. 2001: The Level of Expressed Need--a measure of help-seeking behaviour for chronic pain in the community. *Eur J Pain* 5, 257–266.

Stewart, W. and Lipton, R. 2002: Need for care and perceptions of MIDAS among headache sufferers study. *CNS Drugs* 16 Suppl 1, 5–11.

Strong, J., Ashton, R. and Chant, D. 1991: Pain intensity measurement in chronic low back pain. *Clin J Pain* 7, 209–218.

Thomas, R.J., McEwen, J. and Asbury, A.J. 1996: The Glasgow Pain Questionnaire: A new generic measure of pain; development and testing. *Int J Epidemiol* 25, 1060–1067.

Underwood, M.R., Barnett, A.G. and Vickers, M.R. 1999: Evaluation of two time-specific back pain outcome measures. *Spine* 24, 1104–1112.

van den Hoven, L.H., Gorter, K.J. and Picavet, H.S. 2010: Measuring musculoskeletal pain by questionnaires: The manikin versus written questions. *Eur J Pain* 14, 435–438.

Von Korff, M. 2001: Epidemiologic and survey methods: Chronic pain assessment, in Turk DC, Melzack R (eds) *Handbook of pain assessment*, 2nd edn. pp.603–618. Guilford Press, New York, NY.

Von Korff, M. and Dunn, K.M. 2008: Chronic pain reconsidered. *Pain* 138, 267–276.

Von Korff, M., Dworkin, S.F. and LeResche, L. 1990: Graded chronic pain status: An epidemiologic evaluation. *Pain* 40, 279–291.

Von Korff, M., Ormel, J., Keefe, F.J. and Dworkin, S.F. 1992: Grading the severity of chronic pain. *Pain* 50, 133–149.

Ware, J. 1993: *SF-36 Health Survey: Manual and interpretation guide*. The Health Institute, New England Medical Center, Boston, MA.

Weiner, D., Pieper, C., McConnell, E., Martinez, S. and Keefe, F. 1996: Pain measurement in elders with chronic low back pain: Traditional and alternative approaches. *Pain* 67, 461–467.

Chapter 6

Measuring the impact of chronic pain on populations: a narrative review

Heiner Raspe

Introduction

Any measurement, i.e. any methodical assignment of numbers to empirical phenomena, requires a specification of

- 'what' is to be measured (a certain 'quality'), first in theoretical terms,
- the 'unit of measurement' (to what or to whom does the quality belong – e.g. to a person or a knee joint?) and, which can be different, the 'unit of observation' or 'analysis', i.e. the entity to which results shall ultimately refer,
- the 'aim' of measurement (inter alia, e.g. classification, point estimate of frequency, comparison, change over time, prediction, indication for intervention),
- its 'method' and 'instrument',
- and its 'pragmatic context', its 'why and what for', its usefulness.

Based on these distinctions the following text deals from a social medicine perspective with

- chronic pain and
- a wide range of its implications and consequences ('impact'), using chronic back pain (BP) as a prominent example, and
- a corresponding wide range of dimensions and components referring to its consequences at a population level

The last two aims present particular problems: very few, if any, pain-related measures characterize entire populations as such (i.e. 'all the inhabitants of a given country or area considered together' (Last, 2001)). Virtually all measures refer to single subjects, whose individual measurement results can then be aggregated into sums, various epidemiological rates, means, or other summary statistics. They can be used to distinguish between differently 'sick populations' as a whole (Rose, 2008). However, not every clinically useful variable is relevant within a population and social medicine context.

The finger–floor distance (the measured distance from the tips of fingers to the floor when a person is standing and bending their backs forward as far as they are able), or the straight leg-raising test (the angle to which a person can raise upwards their fully straightened leg when they are lying flat on a plane surface), for instance, are certainly relevant for assessing and monitoring patients with ankylosing spondylitis or sciatica – individually and as a clinical group. Their population average, median, standard deviation, and interquartile range seem, however, to be definitely irrelevant for someone interested in or responsible for the health and welfare of a certain population – in contrast, e.g. to the number and proportion of people in that population who have chronically disabling low back pain, the number of their days off work per 10 000, their loss of quality-adjusted life years (QALYs) or the sum of all back pain-related direct and indirect costs.

To become relevant from a population and social medicine perspective, the chronic disorder and its implications and consequences must become clinically or otherwise visible, interfere with social roles and relations, impact on social institutions, and/or elicit organized responses from the health care, social, and/or welfare system. Such impact indicators are always relevant from a societal and patient perspective, though the average physician may find them of only little interest or relevance to the immediate problem facing them in a clinical setting.

It is this perspective which guides us in presenting and discussing a limited number of variables characterizing the social implications and consequences of chronic pain. Which of the wide range of pain-related dimensions, components, variables, and items will help to monitor, evaluate, and ultimately improve health and welfare of a given 'painful' population?

The dimension of the problem can be simply indicated: in Europe (in 2003) the overall prevalence of moderate or severe chronic pain (incorporating the complex problem of chronic pain) was 19% (Breivik et al., 2006), ranging from 30% in Norway to 11% in Spain. A recent German national health survey found (for 2002–03) a 1-year prevalence of chronic back pain of nearly 19% among adults (Neuhauser et al., 2005). Here, 'chronic pain' was defined as having persisted daily or nearly daily for at least 3 months.

The predicament of chronic pain, using the example of back pain

In order to understand the public health impact of chronic pain, we first have to understand the actual predicament of the condition. Pain can be basically classified with respect to affected regions (e.g. headache, neck pain, pelvic pain). It can be 'graded' according to its actual severity – usually in terms of a combination of pain intensity and interference with daily activities (e.g. Von Korff et al., 1992). In this view, back pain, for instance, is initially not more than pain in a region called 'the back'. CBP then seems to be not more than pain in the back which has been persisting for a predefined period of time, e.g. at least 12 weeks.

However, chronic pain is usually much more than persistent or recurrent pain in a certain region. It is regularly accompanied by, or associated with, a wide range of further pains, unpleasant sensory and emotional experiences, and certain – often dysfunctional – cognitions and behaviours (e.g. Raspe et al., 2003). When regional pain becomes chronic, it more often than not develops into an increasingly complex syndrome with an increasingly poor prognosis.

The syndromic character of back pain was demonstrated early by Hans Valkenburg and co-workers in their famous Epidemiologic Study of Cardiovascular Risk Indicators (EPOZ; Valkenburg and Haanen, 1982): '(combined) pain in the shoulders, neck and low back was present at examination 4 to 6 times as often as could be expected from the frequencies of the separate sites' (p. 19). In other words, back pain was often 'accompanied' by other types of rheumatic pain. Since then, the picture presented in published work has been widening, and the concept of CBP syndrome can now be considered to comprise, besides back and other musculoskeletal pains (Kamaleri et al., 2008),

- a plethora of bodily complaints, probably originating from a centrally heightened proprio- and entero-ceptive awareness (Schmidt et al., 1989; Bacon et al., 1994; Hagen et al., 2006),
- symptoms of cognitive and emotional distress (Flor and Turk., 1988; Meyer et al., 2007),
- dysfunctional pain behaviours (e.g. physical inactivity, bed rest) and, most recently,
- relevant somatic and psychological 'co-morbidities' (see below).

Several studies have found a high prevalence of a wide spectrum of medically certified 'co-morbid' conditions, i.e. conditions which occur concurrently with low back pain (Hestbaek et al., 2003; Hestbaek et al., 2004; Schneider et al., 2007; Hüppe and Raspe, 2009). Some can be understood as underlying conditions (e.g. ankylosing spondylitis) or explained by common and shared risk factors such as smoking, obesity, low physical activity, or unfavourable physical or psychosocial working and living conditions (e.g. chronic obstructive pulmonary disease (COPD), congestive heart disease (CHD), metabolic syndrome). Others may be seen as complications of chronic disabling pain (e.g. depression, impaired cardiovascular fitness) and still others (e.g. asthma, arthritis) can so far only be described as back pain-associated due to some as yet unknown mechanisms. Interestingly, the only chronic disorder consistently not associated with back pain seems to be diabetes mellitus (Hüppe and Raspe, 2009).

While many aspects of these interrelations are still elusive, some elements of the back pain syndrome mentioned above turn out to be associated with a set of risk indicators common to them all, including age, female gender, low social status, and low life and work satisfaction (Aggarwal et al., 2006).

The syndromic character of chronic pain forms the basis of various 'staging' algorithms such as the Mainz Pain Staging and Pain Chronicity Scoring System (MPSS; Gerbershagen, 1996). This system focusses on selected temporal and spatial aspects of the most prominent pain experienced by the person being scored, and additionally assesses the use of, and dependence on, analgesics, as well as the type and amount of previous health care utilization (e.g. physicians, hospitals, operations, rehabilitation). Overall 10 variables are involved. The MPSS has been validated (Wurmthaler et al., 1996), used (Buchner et al., 2007), and criticized (Hueppe et al., 2001).

Our group proposed a different and partly still hypothetical model for assessing the stage of 'amplification' of back pain, to use a term introduced by Barsky in 1979 (Barsky, 1979; Raspe et al., 2003; Hüppe and Raspe, 2009). The model profits from Loeser's multidimensional concept of pain, bears some analogy to the tumour-grading system used in cancer medicine, and exclusively incorporates variables that address 'impairments' according to the International Classification of Functioning, Disability and Health (ICF) of the World Health Organization (2001). The ICF defines impairments as 'problems in body function or structure' including psychological disturbances.

Our conceptual model essentially captures three dimensions of 'amplification' – namely, the extent of pain in time or location on the body, the presence of additional bodily complaints, and the degree of psychological distress. As shown in Table 6.1 the measurement model applies six operationally defined yes/no variables, two to each of the three conceptual dimensions.

A Code 'P_1', 'C_1', and/or 'D_1' is assigned when at least one of the two variables is to be coded 'yes'. Code $P_1C_1D_1$ thus denotes back pain which shows temporal and/or regional spread, reduced vitality and/or somatization, and catastrophizing and/or depressiveness.

The basic idea of the model can be visualized by a drawing (adapted from Loeser (1980) and Waddell (1987)) which may be interpreted as showing a Roman fountain seen from above (cf. C.F. Meyer, who described such a fountain in a 19th century poem (Browning, 1984); cf. Figure 6.1).

The small circle at the bottom of the figure represents the main source at the top of the fountain (pain in the back) which, if not contained, swells over and flows down filling the three basins below, one after the other.

Stage 1 of chronic, i.e. amplified, back pain refers to back pain (ICF b28013) which has spread over time and/or regionally (P-Dimension).

Stage 2 denotes back pain which is additionally accompanied by vital exhaustion and/or multiple bodily complaints (P + C) or follows the pattern P1C0D1, i.e. shows instead symptoms of psychological distress), whereas in Stage 3 all three components are present (see above).

Table 6.1 Impairments as components of chronic, i.e. 'amplified', back pain

Dimension	Component	Operational definition, instrument
Pain	Temporal extension	Back pain in the past 12 months 'ever or nearly daily'
	Regional spread	Distal radiation to above or below the knee
Complaints	Reduced vitality	SF-36, 4-item subscale<20.6 points for males, <15.6 for females
	Somatization	SCL-90-R, 12-item subscale somatization >1.37 males, >1.58 females
Distress	Catastrophizing	Kieler Schmerz Inventar, 5-item subscale *** >3.65 for males and females
	Depressiveness	CES-D 20 items>19.6 males, >23.6 females

Cut-offs represent the 97.5th percentile of the calibration samples *** Hasenbring, 1994;may be substituted by the sub-scale 'Catastrophizing' from Flor and Turk (Flor and Turk, 1988)

SF-36 = Short Form-36 (Ware, 1993); SCL-90-R = Symptom Checklist 90-Revised (Derogatis, 1977); CES-D = Centre for Epidemiologic Studies depression scale (Radloff, 1977).

It can be shown that the three pairs of variables actually meet the requirements of a Gutman scale with a scalability coefficient of >0.90 and fewer than 10% of responses not conforming to the model (in this case, 8.3%). Being in a higher stage is cross-sectionally and prospectively associated with an increasingly impaired subjective health status and an increasing number of medically diagnosed co-morbid conditions (Hüppe and Raspe, 2009).

Staging is one way to overcome the obvious limitations of a mere temporal definition of 'chronicity'. Two others can be mentioned here (see Chapter 4): Von Korff and Miglioretti (2005) proposed 'a prognostic approach to defining chronic pain'; and Dunn et al. (2006) identified 'pain pathways' in the form of four distinct patterns describing the short-term course of low

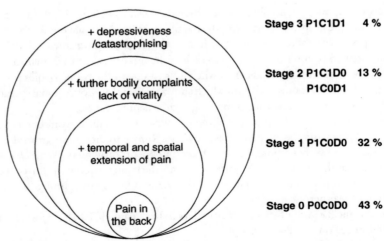

Fig. 6.1 Amplification in non-specific back pain (data from Hüppe and Raspe (2009); n=1,769)

back pain (e.g. 'persistent mild' or 'severe chronic' back pain) which may be extrapolated into the future.

In summary, chronic pain impacts on populations less by its central impairment (i.e. pain *per se*) and more by the aggregate and interactions of all concomitant symptoms, signs, co-morbid disorders, and risky behaviours such as smoking and physical inactivity.

Classifying the impact of chronic pain

To structure the impact of chronic pain on populations, I first refer to the precursor of the ICF, the International Classification of Impairments, Disabilities, and Handicaps (ICIDH), originally proposed by Philip Wood, a UK rheumatic disease epidemiologist (World Health Organisation, 1980). Besides impairments, he distinguished 'disabilities' and 'handicaps' as further 'consequences of disease'. Disabilities were defined as 'restriction or lack of ability to perform an activity in the manner or within the range normal for a human being' and handicaps as limitations in the 'fulfilment of a role that is normal (depending on age, sex, and social and cultural factors) for that individual' (World Health Organization, 1999). It assumed six 'survival roles': orientation, physical independence, mobility, occupation, social integration, and economic self-sufficiency.

The ICF (World Health Organization, 2001) can in part be seen as a refinement of the preceding ICIDH. Various former disabilities and handicaps are now to be classified as activity limitations and/or participation restrictions. In other parts, the ICF follows different principles, concepts, and aims. One important addition, especially in a public health context, pertains to the inclusion of context factors, personal and environmental, as shown in Figure 6.2. It implies a second message: participation restrictions and/or activity limitations can by themselves lead to functional or structural deficits and all interact with context factors bi-directionally.

Against this background, what are, from a population and social medicine perspective, relevant consequences of the highly complex chronic pain syndrome?

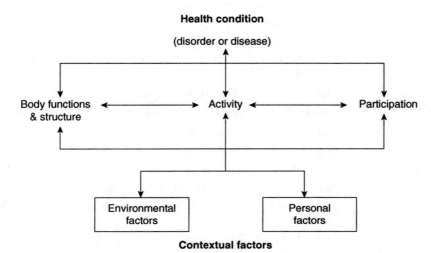

Fig. 6.2 The conceptual structure of the International Classification of Function (ICF). Reproduced from World Health Organization, 2001, with permission.

Consequences of the chronic pain syndrome with population impact, using back pain as the example

As mentioned above, the label 'with population impact and of social medicine relevance' should be attached primarily to variables which refer to consequences of chronic pain which are clinically or otherwise visible, interfere with social roles and relations, impact on social institutions and/or elicit organized social responses, e.g. from the health care sector.

Table 6.2 enumerates dimensions and components which satisfy these criteria and are (with very few exceptions, see below) not by themselves impairments. We do not cover conceptual,

Table 6.2 Consequences of the back pain syndrome on populations

Dimension	Component
Mortality	Specific death rate
	Mortality ratio
	Years of Life Lost
Activity limitation/ participation restriction	Impaired handling of stress and other psychological demands
	Limitations in basic and instrumental activities of daily living
	Impaired leisure-time activities, recreation
	Impaired social (sexual) relations, social isolation
	Disability days, Disability Adjusted Life Years (Murray et al, 2002).
	Loss of household productivity
	Change in work status
	Work disability, absence from work
	Dependence on others/carers
Impaired health-related quality of life	Multidimensional generic or back pain- specific instruments
	Utility measures
	Quality-Adjusted Life Years
Health care utilization	Consultations with primary, secondary, and tertiary care physicians and other clinicians
	Adverse events, side effects of interventions
	Unmet health care needs, under/over-treatment
	Addictive behaviour (e.g. analgesia)
	Dissatisfaction with health care
Financial problems	Loss of family income, individual poverty
Cost	Direct (doctor fee, medication, hospitalization, other clinical services)
	Out-of pocket (Over-the-counter drugs, private physiotherapy, co-payments, individual health services)
	Indirect (productivity loss, absenteeism, disability benefit, disability pension)
Societal	Poverty rate, area deprivation, and poverty
	Dysfunctional back beliefs (e.g. in media)
	Change in legislation
Equity	Increasing social gradients in welfare, health, and health care

technical, and statistical aspects of their measurement (Deyo et al., 1998; Bombardier, 2000; Dworkin et al., 2005; Terwee et al., 2007). Instruments and their metric properties are also outside the scope of this review, as are epidemiological concepts of how to estimate the population impact of certain consequences.

The basis for the qualitative review summarized in Table 6.2 is an observation of, and participation in, back-pain research over the last two decades, here with a main focus on publications of outcome assessment (including disability and health status) as well as those detailing cost of illness, 'correlates of back problems' and 'impact'. Special attention was paid to the ICF (World Health Organization, 2001), its precursor ICIDH (see above), the ICF core sets for low back pain (Cieza et al., 2004), and subsequent studies on their content and construct validity (Sigl et al., 2006; Mullis et al., 2007; Bautz-Holter et al, 2008; Røe et al., 2009).

Mortality (McBeth et al., 2009), activity limitations and participation restrictions, impaired quality of life, health care utilization, financial problems, and different types of costs easily fulfil all four 'impact and relevance' criteria (visibility, interference, impact, and elicitation) and can all be traced back to individual subjects and aggregated into descriptive statistics. Few seem to constitute impairments. Examples of exceptions to this would be certain side effects of medical interventions (e.g. gastric pain) or some sub-dimensions of quality-of-life measures such as loss of 'energy for everyday life' or 'negative feelings such as blue mood, despair, anxiety, depression' [both items from WHO's Quality of Life Questionnaire WHOQOL-Bref (http://www.who.int/substance_abuse/research_tools/whoqolbref/en/)].

Two dimensions, however, refer to supra-individual 'ecological' qualities and characterize entire societies or certain of their segments. As the prevalence and severity of CBP is closely and inversely associated with social class and often implies financial losses, it may add to area deprivation and poverty. This, in turn, contributes to social inequality and inequity, producing even more cases of chronic pain. The incidence of CBP may be further provoked by dysfunctional societal 'back beliefs' (Goubert et al., 2004; Werner et al., 2005; Gross et al., 2006) – often propagated by the media – and the cases may then contribute to an even more 'pathophilic' climate, followed, for instance, by an increase in work disability and disability pensions. Such increases can trigger legislative interventions (e.g. the "epidemics" of repetitive strain injury in Australia and fibromylagia in Norway). This nicely illustrates the potential for interaction between incident back pain, environmental context ('societal attitudes', ICF e460), 'participation restriction in remunerative employment' (d850), and societal reaction ('legal policies', e550).

Such societal beliefs can be the targets for preventive action. For example, Buchbinder and colleagues (2008) have shown that a mass media campaign can be successful in influencing back beliefs and back-pain related behaviours – at least in Victoria, Australia (see Chapter 25).

We have investigated the extent to which the dimensions and components mentioned in Table 6.2 have been used in studies of back pain. To do this, we re-analysed more than a dozen intervention studies mostly concerning CBP, published in 2006 and 2007 (for details see Raspe, 2008). Our specific aim was to determine if these therapeutic studies had addressed the first six dimensions and their components.

The review included 16 studies, covering a wide range of orthodox and heterodox treatments and programmes. Functional capacity was assessed by all 16 studies (mainly by three instruments: Oswestry, Roland–Morris, and Hannover Questionnaire), covering a wide range of basic and instrumental activities of daily living; 12 studies measured quality of life (mostly by the 'generic' SF-36); only nine covered any form of resource use (e.g. taking painkillers, consulting a doctor); and eight screened for psychological distress in the form of depression, anxiety, and/or bothersomeness. Only four included a QALY-estimate and two measured work disability; in contrast, four paid special attention to range of movement measurements, even though the focus of the studies was stated to be non-specific back pain. Six were explicitly aimed at adverse events of their experimental intervention, four systematically assessed patient adherence, and three evaluated treatment satisfaction.

In summary, several of the dimensions enumerated in Table 6.2 are either not covered at all or only partly so in published studies. A clinical orientation prevails in these studies: the concept of participation and participation restriction (or in older terms: handicap) has not yet fully reached the world of therapeutic research in CBP.

'Change we need' – if our studies (and interventions) are to aim at more than the welfare of individual patients. Her or his wellbeing is, and of course must remain, the most prominent concern of any clinician. However, this does, and must, not exclude a broader view which additionally encompasses the impact of chronic pain conditions on populations, through the link between all pain-related impairments and handicaps/participation restrictions via disabilities and activity limitation, moderated by personal and environmental context factors.

References

Aggarwal, V.R., McBeth, J., Zakrzewska, J.M., Lunt, M. and MacFarlane, G. 2006: The epidemiology of chronic syndromes that are frequently unexplained: do they have common associated factors? *Intl J Epidemiol* **35**, 468–476.

Bacon, N.M.K., Bacon, S.F., Atkinson, J.H., Slater, M.A., Patterson, T.L., Grant, I. and Garfin, S.R. 1994: Somatization symptoms in chronic low back pain patients. *Psychosomatic Med* **56**, 118–127.

Barsky, A. 1979: Patients who amplify bodily sensations. *Ann Internal Med* **91**, 63–70.

Bautz-Holter, E., Sveen, U., Cieza, A., Geyh, S. and Røe, C. 2008: Does the International Classification of Functioning, Disability and Health (ICF) Core Set for low back pain cover the patients' problems? A cross-sectional content-validity study with a Norwegian population. *Eur J Physical Rehab Med* **44**, 387–397.

Bombardier, C. 2000: Outcome assessments in the evaluation of treatment of spinal disorders. *Spine* **25**, 3100–3103.

Breivik, H., Collett, B., Ventafridda, V., Cohen, R. and Gallacher, D. 2006: Survey of chronic pain in Europe. *Eur J Pain* **10**, 287–333.

Browning, R.M. 1984: *German Poetry from 1750–1900*. New York, The Continuum Publishing Company.

Buchbinder, R. 2008: Self-management education en masse: effectiveness of the back pain: Don't take it lying down mass media campaign. *MJA* **189**. 29–32.

Buchner, M., Neubauer, E., Zahlten-Hinguranage, A. and Schiltenwolf, M. 2007: The influence of the grade of chronicity on the outcome of multidisciplinary therapy for chronic low back pain. *Spine* **32**, 3060–3066.

Cieza, A., Stucki, G., Weigl, M., Disler, P., Jäckel, W., van der Linden, S. *et al.* 2004: ICF core sets for low back pain. *J Rehabil Med Suppl* **44**, 69–74.

Derogatis, L.R. 1977: *SCL-90-R Manual*. Baltimore, Johns Hopkins School of Medicine.

Deyo, R.A., Battie, M., Beurskens, A.J., Bombardier, C., Croft, P., Koes, B. *et al.* 1998: Outcome measures for low back pain research. A proposal for standardised use. *Spine* **23**, 2003–2013.

Dunn, K.M., Jordan, K. and Croft, P.R. 2006: Characterizing the course of low back pain: A latent class analysis. *Am J Epidemiol* **163**, 756–761.

Dworkin, R.H., Turk, D.C., Farrar, J.T., Haythornthwaite, J.A., Jensen, M.A., Katz, N.P. *et al.* 2005: Core outcome measures for chronic pain clinical trials: IMMPACT recommendations. *Pain* **113**, 9–19.

Flor, H. and Turk, D.C. 1988: Chronic back pain and rheumatoid arthritis: Predicting pain and disability from cognitive variables. *J Behav Med* **11**, 251–265.

Gerbershagen, H.U. 1996: Das Mainzer Stadienkonzept des Schmerzes: Eine Standortbestimmung. In: Klingler D, Morawetz A, Thoden U, Zimmermann M (Hg.): Antidepressiva als Analgetika, pp. 71–95. Aarachne, Wien.

Goubert, L., Crombez, G. and Bourdeaudhuij, I. 2004: Low back pain, disability and back pain myths in a community sample: prevalence and interrelationships. *Eur J Pain* **8**, 385–394.

Gross, D.P., Ferrari, R., Russell, A.S., Bchir, M.B., Battié, M.C. *et al.* 2006: A population-based survey of back pain beliefs in Canada. *Spine* **31**, 2142–2145.

Hagen, E.M., Svensen, E., Eriksen, H.R., Ihelebaek, C.M. and Ursin, H. 2006: Comorbid subjective health complaints in low back pain. *Spine* **31**, 1491–1495.

Hasenbring, M. 1994: Kieler Schmerz Inventar. Bern, Huber.

Hestbaek, L., Leboeuf-Yde, Ch. and Manniche, C. 2003: Is low back pain part of a general health pattern or is it a separate and distinctive entity? A critical literature review of comorbidity wiwth low back pain. *J Manipulative Physiological Therap* **26**, 243–252.

Hestbaek, L., Leboeuf-Yde, C., Ohm Kyvik, K. *et al.* 2004: Comorbidity with low back pain. *Spine* **29**, 1483–1491.

Hueppe, M., Matthießen, V., Lindig, M., Preuss, S., Meier, T., Baumeier, W. *et al.* 2001: Vergleich der Schmerzchronifizierung bei Patienten mit unterschiedlicher Schmerzdiagnose. *Schmerz* **15**, 179–185.

Hüppe, A. and Raspe, H. 2009: Amplifizierte Rückenschmerzen und Komorbidität in der Bevölkerung. *Der Schmerz* **23**, 275–283

Kamaleri, Y., Natvig, B., Ihlebaek, C.M. and Bruusgard, D. 2008: Localized or widespread musculoskeletal pain: Does it matter? *Pain* **138**:41–46.

Last, J.M. (ed) 2001: *A dictionary of epidemiology* 4th edn. New York, Oxford, Toronto: Oxford University Press, 136.

Loeser, J.D. 1980: Perspectives on pain, In: Turner, P. (ed) *Clinical pharmacy and therapeutics*, pp. 313–316. London, Macmillan.

MacFarlane, G. 2009: Musculoskeletal pain is associated with a long-term increased risk of cancer and cadiovascular-related mortality. *Rheumatol* **48**, 74–77.

McBeth, J., Symmons, D.P., Silman, A.J., Allison, T., Webb, R., Brammah, T. and Macfarlane, G. 2009: Musculoskeletal pain is associated with a long-term increased risk of cancer and cardiovascular-related mortality. *Rheumatol* **48**:74–77.

Meyer, T., Cooper, J. and Raspe, H. 2007: Disabling low back pain and depressive symptoms in the community-dwelling elderly: A prospective study. *Spine* **32**, 2380–2386.

Mullis, R., Barber, J., Lewis, M. and Hay, E. 2007: ICF core sets for low back pain: do they include what matters to patients? *J Rehabil Med* **39**, 353–357.

Murray, C.J.L., Salomon, J.A., Mathers, C.D. and Lopez, A.D. (eds) 2002: *Summary measures of population health*. World Health Organization, Geneva.

Neuhauser, H., Ellert, U. and Ziese, T. 2005: Chronische Rückenschmerzen in der Allgemeinbevölkerung in Deutschland 2002/2003: Prävalenz und besonders betroffene Bevölkerungsgruppen. *Gesundheitswesen* **67**, 685–693.

Radliff, L.S. 1977: The CES-D scale: A self-report depression scale for research in the general population. *Applied Psychol Measurement* **1**, 385–401.

Raspe, A., Matthis, C., Héon-Klin, V. and Raspe, H. 2003: Chronische Rückenschmerzen: Mehr als Schmerzen im Rücken. Ergebnisse eines regionalen Surveys unter Versicherten einer Landesversicherungsanstalt. *Rehabilitation* **42**, 195–203.

Raspe, H. 2008: Management of chronic low back pain in 2007–2008. *Curr Opin Rheumatol* **20**, 276–281.

Raspe, H., Hüppe, A. and Matthis, C. 2003: Theorien und Modelle der Chronifizierung: Auf dem Weg zu einer erweiterten Definition chronischer Rückenschmerzen. *Schmerz* **17**, 359–366.

Rose, G. 2008: *Rose's strategy of preventive medicine*. Oxford: Oxford University Press. pp. 90–91

Røe, C., Sveen, U., Geyh, S., Cieza, A. and Bautz-Holter, E. 2009: Construct dimensionality and properties of the categories in the ICF Core set for low back pain. *J Rehabil Med* **41**, 429–437.

Schmidt, A.J.M., Gierlings, R.E.H. and Peters, M.L. 1989: Environmental and interoceptive influences on chronic low back pain behavior. *Pain* **38**, 137–143.

Schneider, S., Mohnen, S.M., Schiltenwolf, M. and Rau, Ch. 2007: Comorbidity of low back oain: Representative outcomes of a national study in the Federal Republic of Germany. *Eur J Pain* **11**, 387–397.

Sigl, T., Cieza, A., Brockow, T., Chatterji, S., Kostanjsek, N. *et al.* 2006: Content comparison of low back pain-specific measures based on the International Classification of Functioning, Disability and Health (ICF). *Clin J Pain* **22**, 147–153.

Terwee, C.B., Bot, S.D.M., de Boer, M.R., van der Windt, D.A.W.M., Knol, D.L. *et al.* 2007: Quality criteria were proposed for measurement properties of health status questionnaires. *J Clin Epidemiol* **60**, 34–42.

Valkenburg, H.A. and Haanen, H.C.M. 1982: The epidemiology of low back pain. In: White AA III, Gordon SL (eds.): Symptoms on idiopathic low back pain. pp. 9–22 Mosby Company, Miami, FL.

Von Korff, M. and Miglioretti, D.L. 2005: A prognostic approach to defining chronic pain. *Pain* **117**, 304–313.

Von Korff, M., Ormel, J., Keefe, F. and Dworkin, S.F. 1992: Grading the severity of chronic pain. *Pain* **50**, 133–149.

Waddell, G. 1987: A new clinical model for the treatment of low back pain. *Spine* **12**, 632–44.

Ware, J. 1993: *SF-36 Health Survey : Manual and interpretation guide*. The Health Institute, New England Medical Center, Boston, MA.

Werner, E.L., Ihlebaek, C., Skouen, J.S. and Laerum, E. 2005: Beliefs about low back pain in the Norwegian general population: Are they related to pain experiences and health professionals? *Spine* **30**, 1770–776.

World Health Organization. 1980: *International Classification of Impairment, Disability and Handicap*. WHO, Geneva.

World Health Organization. 1999: *ICIDH-2: International Classification of Functioning and Disability*. WHO, Geneva.

World Health Organization. 2001: *International Classification of Functioning, Disability, and Health: ICF*. WHO, Geneva.

Wurmthaler, Ch., Gerbershagen, H.U., Dietz, G., Korb, J. *et al.* 1996: Chronifizierung und psychologische Merkmale – Die Beziehung zwischen Chronifizierungssstasdien bei Schmerz und psychophsischem Befinden, Behinderung und familiären Merkmalen. *Z Gesundheitspsychologie Bd.*, **IV**, 2, 113–136.

Chapter 7

Number of pain sites – a simple measure of population risk?

Bård Natvig, Camilla Ihlebæk, Yusman Kamaleri, and Dag Bruusgaard

Introduction

Pain is a usual experience of adult human life. Many apparently distinctive clinical syndromes of pain and dysfunction show considerable overlap in both population and clinical settings (Croft et al., 2003). The majority of studies on chronic musculoskeletal pain have focused on localized pain, resulting in a substantial body of research on low back pain, neck pain, shoulder pain, and knee pain. However, most individuals suffering from musculoskeletal pain report pain at more than just one pain site (Picavet and Schouten, 2003; Croft, 2009). Having pain at one site increases the risk of having pain at other sites, or as formulated by one of the editors of this book: 'Chronic pain syndromes: you can't have one without another' (Croft et al., 2007).

Chronic pain at multiple sites has mostly been studied according to the American College of Rheumatology or Manchester definitions of fibromyalgia and chronic widespread pain (Neumann and Buskila, 2003). These definitions are dichotomous, based on yes/no answers about whether someone meets the criteria or not. There are, however, no natural cut-off points between localized pain and widespread pain. Musculoskeletal pain is better represented by a continuum of 'widespreadness' from a single pain site to multi-site pain (Croft et al., 2006). The question is not 'have you got it?', but 'how much of it have you got?' (Croft, 2009).

In our population-based prospective study in Ullensaker, Norway (The Ullensaker Study), we have used a generic approach to measuring musculoskeletal pain. We have taken 'one step backwards' in order to describe all sorts of musculoskeletal pain, distinguished only by their location, without using diagnostic labels or predefined categories based on assumed aetiology. In particular, we have not used a dichotomous definition of chronic widespread pain, but instead we have described the continuum of 'widespreadness' of pain by a simple count of 'number of pain sites'.

In this chapter we summarize our results from The Ullensaker Study, compare our results to some other studies which have used similar approaches, and consider the application of our findings to a public health view of chronic pain in the general population. We discuss some limitations in our approach and make suggestions for future research.

The Ullensaker study

The Ullensaker study is a cohort study of musculoskeletal pain. Ullensaker is a suburban area northeast of Oslo, Norway (see map – Figure 7.1). There were about 18 000 inhabitants in 1990 and 23 700 in 2004.

In 1990, a self-administered questionnaire was posted to all inhabitants born in 1918–20, 1928–30, 1938–40, 1948–50, 1958–60, and 1968–70 (Ullensaker I). The same sample received the

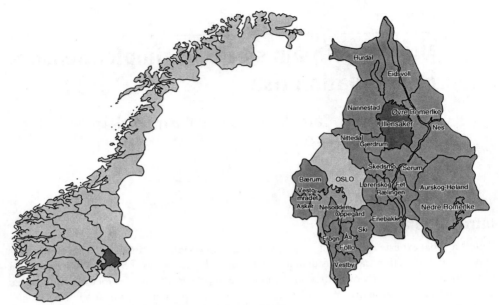

Fig. 7.1 Ullensaker municipality in Akershus County in Norway.

questionnaire again in 1994 (Ullensaker II) and 2004 (Ullensaker III). New inhabitants in 1994 and 2004 belonging to the age cohorts were included in the study sample of the respective years. In 1990, 4050 persons were contacted and 2722 (67.2%) returned the questionnaire. Out of 6108 individuals contacted in 2004, 3325 (54.4%) returned the questionnaire. Among the participants in 1990, 1644 participated again in 2004 (60.4%). A total of 1443 responders participated in all three data collections.

We assessed musculoskeletal pain by a validated self-report questionnaire, the Standard Nordic Questionnaire (SNQ) in 1990, 1994, and 2004 (Kuorinka et al., 1987). The respondents were instructed to report whether they had experienced pain or discomfort in each of 10 different body regions during two time periods: (i) the past 12 months and (ii) the past seven days. The 10 pain sites included: head, neck, shoulder, elbow, hand/wrist, upper back, lower back, hip, knee, and ankle/foot. The checklist was supplemented with a 'pain-region drawing' to illustrate pictorially the 10 body regions referred to in the questionnaire. 'Number of pain sites' (NPS) is the sum of the reported pain sites.

In addition, the questionnaires included demographic and socioeconomic factors, and variables concerning lifestyle, work, function, and psychological status.

Results from the Ullensaker study

Cross-sectional analyses

In our surveys, more than 90% reported some form of musculoskeletal pain or discomfort during the past 12 months, and 70% reported musculoskeletal pain or discomfort during the past 7 days (Kamaleri et al., 2008a; Table 7.1). For each pain site (out of the 10 possible), ≥85% of people who reported pain at that site also reported pain from at least one other pain site (Kamaleri et al., 2008b).

Based on data from Ullensaker I and II, we described univariate cross-sectional associations between number of pain sites and a range of demographic, health, function, and lifestyle variables (Natvig et al., 2000). In the adjusted model there was a strong link between female gender and

Table 7.1 Number of pain sites (NPS) reported for the past 7 days and the past 12 months by gender. Reproduced from Kamaleri et al., 2008a, with permission from Elsevier.

NPS 2004	Past 7 days (%)			Past 12 months (%)		
	Women	Men	Total	Women	Men	Total
0	23.0	37.9	29.8	5.8	12.7	9.0
1	15.3	17.5	16.3	7.7	14.9	11.0
2	14.6	12.0	13.4	11.7	15.4	13.4
3	12.6	12.3	12.5	13.8	14.8	14.2
4	10.5	7.7	9.2	14.2	13.0	13.6
5	7.1	4.5	5.9	14.3	11.5	13.0
6	5.4	3.0	4.3	10.0	8.1	9.2
7	4.4	1.0	2.8	9.7	5.2	7.6
8	2.1	0.6	1.4	5.6	2.3	4.1
9	1.7	0.7	1.3	3.7	1.1	2.5
10	1.6	0.6	1.1	3.7	1.0	2.5

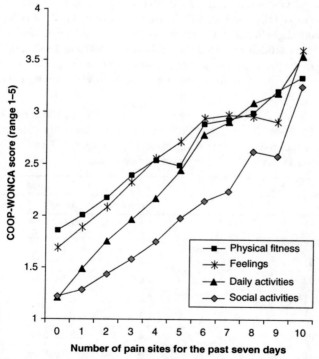

Fig. 7.2 Cross-sectional relationship between number of pain sites during the past 7 days and functional ability. Reproduced from Kamaleri, 2008b. This figure has been reproduced with permission of the International Association for the Study of Pain® (IASP®). The figure may not be reproduced for any other purpose without permission.

number of pain sites, and close linear association of the number of pain sites with worse general health status and poor sleep. We explored these associations further in analyses of Ullensaker III, and showed that single-site pain had little impact on physical fitness, feelings, or daily and social activities [as measured by the Norwegian version of COOP/WONCA (Bentsen et al., 1999)]. Figure 7.2 illustrates a steady increase in problems with increasing number of pain sites for all four aspects of functional status, without any sign of cut-off or levelling out. This strong relationship was maintained after adjusting for age and gender in multivariate linear regression analyses (Kamaleri et al., 2008b).

One implication of these findings is to provide a novel view of regional pain. Using the example of low back pain, we showed, in cross-sectional analysis of Ullensaker I and II, that there were large differences in demographic, lifestyle variables, and functional ability between persons with localized low back pain and persons reporting low back pain as one of a number of other musculoskeletal pains. We launched the hypothesis that localized low back pain and low back pain as part of widespread pain are two different disorders (Natvig et al., 2001).

Prospective analyses

The cross-sectional analyses describing the link between number of pain sites and functional ability cannot disentangle cause and effect. We have, therefore, carried out a series of prospective analyses.

In the first of these, a study of people in Ullensaker I followed up from 1990 to 1994, baseline low back pain as part of widespread pain was a strong predictor for work disability, while localized low back pain did not predict work disability (Natvig et al., 2002).

In the next study, we followed individuals from Ullensaker I to Ullensaker III, a period of 14 years. There was a slight increase in average reported number of pain sites, with a mean of 3.7 sites per person (95% confidence interval (CI): 3.6–3.8) in 1990 and 4.2 sites (95% CI: 4.1–4.4) in 2004. Almost half of the participants reported the same number or one pain site more or less after 14 years. Of those with pain in five or more sites in 1990, 68.8% still reported five or more pain

Table 7.2 Number of pain sites (NPS) (past 12 months) in 1990 and 2004 and stability of reporting (% unchanged, 1990–2004). Reproduced from Kamaleri et al., 2009a. This table has been reproduced with permission of the International Association for the Study of Pain® (IASP®). The table may not be reproduced for any other purpose without permission.

| | 1990 | | | 2004 | | |
NPS	n	%	Mean NPS	95% CI	% unchanged
0	211	13.2	1.9	1.68–2.19	27.0
1	181	11.3	2.7	2.43–3.05	14.4
2	201	12.6	3.6	3.24–3.86	11.4
3	203	12.7	3.8	3.52–4.13	17.2
4	201	12.6	4.2	3.91–4.57	15.9
5	181	11.3	5.2	4.81–5.52	13.8
6	166	10.4	5.4	5.03–5.81	14.5
7	116	7.3	5.9	5.49–6.39	11.2
8	59	3.7	6.4	5.71–7.00	13.6
9	38	2.4	7.1	6.27–8.00	13.2
10	39	2.4	8.3	7.80–8.87	41.0

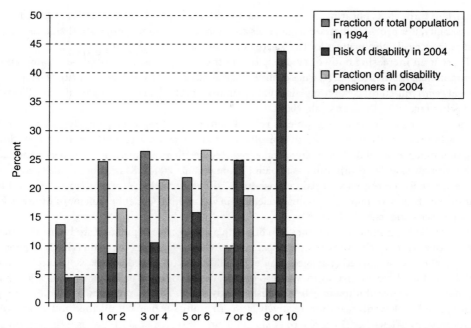

Fig. 7.3 Risk of disability in 2004 based on NPS in 1990, fraction of persons in the population with different NPS in 1990 and fraction of all disability pensioners in 2004 according to NPS in 1990.

sites in 2004 (Kamaleri et al., 2009a). Table 7.2 illustrates substantial stability in NPS over time. An important feature of this finding was that it was consistent across the different age-cohorts, suggesting that the persistence and stability of number of pain sites is set at early ages with a consistent trajectory across the life-course.

About one-third of disability pensioners in Norway has musculoskeletal disorders as their medical cause for disability (Ihlebæk and Lærum, 2004). We have found NPS to be a powerful predictor of disability in longitudinal studies in the Ullensaker population. A high NPS in 1990 predicts more problems with self-reported function measured by COOP-WONCA in 2004 (unpublished results). We have also studied NPS as a predictor for getting disability pension. Among participants of working age in 1990 who participated in 2004 ($n = 1354$), 176 persons (13%) had attained disability pension at the follow-up. The proportion receiving disability pension ranged dramatically from 4.4% to 44% in relation to the number of baseline pain sites reported in 1990 (0 to 9–10). Number of pain sites reported in 1990 was a strong predictor of disability pensioning in 2004 even after adjusting for age and gender (Kamaleri et al., 2009b).

Figure 7.3 illustrates how the risk of pensioned disability in 2004 increases according to NPS reported in 1990. However, even though most people have pain from more than one site, the majority of the population (65%) reports pain in fewer than five sites. This means that most of the risk of pensioned disability linked to NPS is being generated by persons with NPS in the 3–6 pain-site range. About 70% of people being disability pensioned between 1990 and 2004 had NPS <7.

Discussion

The Ullensaker Study has several limitations that raise new research questions. For instance, are all regional pains equally important? In our approach we simply count pains, irrespective of pain intensity and the actual location. Even if we think this simplistic approach has proven to be important through its linear negative relationship with function and its properties as a predictor of disability, it is probable that some pain sites are more important for prognosis than others and that pain intensity also matters for the future of persons with chronic pain.

There is an increasing body of evidence from other studies also that single site pain is less common than multi-site pain (Carnes et al., 2007; Haukka et al., 2006). The majority of people or patients with musculoskeletal complaints have pain from more than just a single pain site (Picavet and Schouten, 2003; Rustoen et al., 2004).

Increasing risk of functional problems related to number of reported pain sites is consistent with a Finnish study illustrating that multi-site pain is associated with reduced function (Saastamoinen et al., 2006). In elderly people, reduced health and impairment has been reported to be strongly associated with multi-site pain (Thomas et al., 2004). Knee pain in older people is more severe in the presence of pain elsewhere (Croft et al., 2005). A recent Norwegian study found that chronic widespread musculoskeletal pain was an independent predictor of future sickness absence (Andersen et al., 2009).

The stability of number of pain sites is in line with a prospective population study that reported a stable prevalence of chronic widespread pain over 7 years, suggesting that pain is likely to persist (or recur) once established (Papageorgiou et al., 2002). As discussed above, we found that the stability in the number of pain sites was also present in the youngest participants, indicating that a pattern of pain distribution may be established early in life. This is supported by studies among children and adolescents that show relatively frequent multi-site pain complaints, both in schoolchildren from Ullensaker (Bruusgaard et al., 2000; Smedbraaten et al., 1998) as well as in other studies from Norway (Haugland et al., 2001; Sjølie, 2004) and UK (McBeth and Jones 2007).

The Ullensaker Study has provided a novel perspective on patterns of pain in the population that could have important implications for research and clinical practice. The number of pain sites is a simple and easily recorded measure that can be applied to general populations. The precise meaning of it, as we point out above, is not yet clear, but it is certainly strongly correlated in cross-sectional studies with important measures of disability in daily life including restricted participation. Even more importantly, this simple measure predicts short- and long-term functional incapacity, including important markers of participation restriction such as long-term absence from work. Whatever the precise causal relationship between the count of pain sites and future disability, it is clear that this could be a useful prognostic marker of risk of poor outcomes.

NPS as a prognostic marker might share some properties with other measures of risk in the population, such as, for instance, blood pressure (BP). Similar to BP measurements, NPS applies to the whole population, it is simple and acts as a marker of risk for future events. The use of BP in population medicine relates to the fact that there is steady increase in risk (e.g. of stroke) across the full distribution of BP measurements. So we can talk about individual risk (e.g. identify those with high risk and target prevention and treatment at that group), but more importantly we can talk about population risk, and a potential to intervene at the population level to shift the average risk in the population in a downward direction.

NPS, like BP, seems to be a simple measure of population risk for future pain-related disability. It can be a marker for interventions if we find ways of reducing the number of pain sites at the individual level or the population level. Better sleep quality, improved physical activity, or reduced obesity are potentially achievable targets, both for society and for the individual, which might reduce NPS and subsequently the risk of reduced function and disability. The high proportion of persons with disability pension from the group with medium high NPS (3–7) (Figure 7.2) calls for population interventions as well as individualized high-risk interventions.

Even though the underlying mechanisms for NPS are less clear than for BP, and it remains possible that the NPS is explained by other factors not yet measured, we think that the Ullensaker

Study results indicate that number of pain sites is a good and useful marker of risk for poor outcome over the short and long term in the general population.

Probably other symptoms than pain, for instance, other subjective health complaints such as fatigue, sleep problems, and gastrointestinal symptoms, also contribute to poor prognosis according to disability and function (Eriksen and Ihlebæk, 2002). Several studies have shown that people reporting musculoskeletal pain also tend to experience other symptoms and complaints such as gastrointestinal discomfort, fatigue, respiratory complaints, depression, and anxiety (Von Korff et al., 2005; Hagen et al., 2006; Ihlebaek et al., 2006; Wiendels et al., 2006). On the other hand, patients with irritable bowel syndrome (Vandvik et al., 2004), neuraesthenia (Stubhaug et al., 2005), and food hypersensitivity (Lind et al., 2005) have a high prevalence of musculoskeletal pain. Approaches to understand and classify such multi-symptom syndromes and illnesses have given rise to a debate about whether the syndromes are truly separate conditions, several conditions with high co-morbidity, or one condition ('the one syndrome hypothesis') (Eriksen and Ursin 2002; Wessely and White 2004; Ursin and Eriksen, 2007). The Ullensaker III offers the opportunity for the next planned step in this continuing story, analysis of how other symptoms influence the linear relationship between number of pain sites and function and disability. The model of prediction described above may then be made more powerful and discriminating with additional information about symptoms other than pain.

Our results do not link population epidemiology to clinical medicine. How are different degrees of widespread pain presented in the clinic, and how are general practitioners and other health professionals in primary care handling the challenge of multi-site pain? It is possible that the emphasis on searching for a diagnosis of regional pain in medical practice may put limitations on how general practitioners might provide more general and helpful treatments for patients with multiple sites of pain or how they focus and prescribe the treatment.

Our approach does not give answers to why and how chronic pain evolves and is maintained. Descriptive epidemiology needs to be supplemented by, and linked to, research about mechanisms. Some form of central hypersensitivity is involved when localized musculoskeletal pain spreads into widespread pain (see Chapter 9) and in the maintenance of pain when acute pain becomes chronic (Clauw, 2007; Yunus, 2008; Ursin and Eriksen, 2007). Descriptive epidemiology about factors associated with the development of central hypersensitivity is one promising line for research in the future (Smith et al., 2007).

Conclusion

Research on chronic pain, in public health and in clinical medicine, that does not include some measure of distribution of other pains, misses an important dimension. A simple count of number of pain sites is linked to future disability, and has potential value as a measure of risk of pain-related disability in a public health approach to pain.

References

Andersen I, Frydenberg H, Maeland JG. 2009: Musculoskeletal disease and sick-leave. (in Norwegian) *Tidsskr Nor Laegeforen* ;**129**:1210–1213.

Bentsen BG, Natvig B, Winnem M. 1999: Questions you didn't ask? COOP/WONCA Charts in clinical work and research. *Fam Pract* ;**16**:190–195.

Bruusgaard D, Smedbraten BK, Natvig B. 2000:Bodily pain, sleep problems and mental distress in schoolchildren. *Acta Paediatr* ;**89**:597–600.

Carnes D, Parsons S, Ashby D, Breen A, Foster NE, Pincus T, et al. 2007:Chronic musculoskeletal pain rarely presents in a single body site: results from a UK population study. *Rheumatology* (Oxford) ; **46**:1168–1170.

Clauw DJ. 2007:Fibromyalgia: Update on mechanisms and management. The ACR criteria for fibromyalgia: The good and the bad. *J Clin Rheum* ;**13**:102–109.

Croft P. 2009:The question is not "have you got it"? But "how much of it have you got"? *Pain* ;**141**:6–7.

Croft P, Dunn KM, Von Korff M. 2007: Chronic pain syndromes: you can't have one without another. *Pain* ;**131**:237–238.

Croft P, Jordan K, Jinks C. 2005: "Pain elsewhere" and the impact of knee pain in older people. *Arthr Rheum* ;**52**:2350–2354.

Croft P, Lewis M, Hannaford P. 2003: Is all chronic pain the same? A 25-year follow-up study. *Pain* ;**105**:309–317.

Croft PR, Dunn KM, Raspe H. 2006: Course and prognosis of back pain in primary care: the epidemiological perspective. *Pain* ;**122**:1–3.

Eriksen HR and Ihlebæk C. 2002: Subjective Health Complaints. *Scandinavian J Psychol* ;**43**:101–103.

Eriksen HR and Ursin H 2002: Sensitization and subjective health complaints. *Scand J Psychol* ;**43**:189–196.

Hagen EM, Svendsen E, Eriksen HR, Ihlebæk C, Ursin H. 2006: Comorbid subjective health complaints in back pain patients. *Spine* ;**31**:1491–1495.

Haugland S, Wold B, Stevenson J, Aaroe LE, Woynarowska B. 2001:Subjective health complaints in adolescence. A cross-national comparison of prevalence and dimensionality. *Eur J Public Health* **11**:4-10.

Haukka E, Leino-Arjas P, Solovieva S, Ranta R, Viikari-Juntura E, Riihimaki H. 2006:Co-occurrence of musculoskeletal pain among female kitchen workers. *Int Arch Occup Environ Health* **80**:141–148.

Ihlebæk, C and Lærum, E. 2004: Bother most – at an expencive cost. Musculoskeletal disorders in Norway. (In Norwegian) Report 01/04 Forskningsenheten/Formidlingsenheten, The Norwegian Back Pain Network.

Ihlebæk C, Ødegaard A, Vikne J, Eriksen HR, Lærum E. 2006: Subjective health complaints in patients with chronic Whiplash Associated Disorder (WAD). Relationships with physical, psychological and collision associated factors. *Norsk Epidemiologi* **16**(2):119–126.

Kamaleri Y, Natvig B, Ihlebaek CM, Benth JS, Bruusgaard D. 2008a: Number of pain sites is associated with demographic, lifestyle, and health-related factors in the general population. *Eur J Pain* **12**: 742–748.

Kamaleri Y, Natvig B, Ihlebaek CM, Bruusgaard D. 2008b:Localized or widespread musculoskeletal pain: does it matter? *Pain* **138**:41–46.

Kamaleri Y, Natvig B, Ihlebaek CM, Benth JS, Bruusgaard D. 2009a:Change in the number of musculoskeletal pain sites: A 14-year prospective study. *Pain* **141**:25–30.

Kamaleri Y, Natvig B, Ihlebaek CM, Bruusgaard D. 2009b: Does the number of musculoskeletal pain sites predict work disability? A 14-year prospective study. *Eur J Pain* **13**:426–430.

McBeth J, Jones K. 2007:Epidemiology of chronic musculoskeletal pain. *Best Pract Res Clin Rheumatol* **21**:403–425.

Kuorinka I, Jonsson B, Kilbom A, Vinterberg H, Biering-Sorensen F, Andersson G, et al. 1987:Standardised Nordic questionnaires for the analysis of musculoskeletal symptoms. *Appl Ergon* **18**:233–237.

Lind R, Arslan G, Eriksen HR, Kahrs G, Haug TT, Florvaag E, et al. 2005: Subjective health complaints and modern health worries in patients with subjective food hypersensitivity. *Digestive Dis Sci* **50**: 1245–1251.

Natvig B, Rutle O, Bruusgaard D, Eriksen WB. 2000:The association between functional status and the number of areas in the body with musculoskeletal symptoms. *Int J Rehabil Res* **23**:49–53.

Natvig B, Bruusgaard D, Eriksen W. 2001:Localized low back pain and low back pain as part of widespread musculoskeletal pain: two different disorders? A cross-sectional population study. *J Rehabil Med* **33**:21–25.

Natvig B, Eriksen W, Bruusgaard D. 2002: Low back pain as a predictor of long-term work disability. *Scand J Public Health* **30**:288–292

Neumann L and Buskila D. 2003: Epidemiology of fibromyalgia. *Curr Pain Headache Rep* **5**:362–368.

Papageorgiou AC, Silman AJ, Macfarlane GJ. 2002: Chronic widespread pain in the population: a seven year follow up study. *Ann Rheum Dis* **61**:1071–1074.

Picavet HS and Schouten JS. 2003: Musculoskeletal pain in the Netherlands: prevalences, consequences and risk groups, the DMC(3)-study. *Pain* **102**:167–178.

Rustoen T, Wahl AK, Hanestad BR, Lerdal A, Paul S, Miaskowski C. 2004: Prevalence and characteristics of chronic pain in the general Norwegian population. *Eur J Pain* **8**:555–565.

Saastamoinen P, Leino-Arjas P, Laaksonen M, Martikainen P, Lahelma E. 2006: Pain and health related functioning among employees. *J Epidemiol Community Health* **60**:793–798.

Sjølie AN. 2004: Persistence and change in nonspecific low back pain among adolescents: a 3-year prospective study. *Spine* **29**:2452–2457.

Smedbraten BK, Natvig B, Rutle O, Bruusgaard D. 1998: Self-reported bodily pain in schoolchildren. *Scand J Rheumatol* **27**:273–276.

Smith BH, Macfarlane GJ, Torrance N. 2007: Epidemiology of chronic pain, from the laboratory to the bus stop: time to add understanding of biological mechanisms to the study of risk factors in population-based research? *Pain* **127**:5–10.

Stubhaug B, Tveito TH, Eriksen HR, Ursin H. 2005: Neurasthenia, subjective health complaints and sensitization. *Psychoneuroendocrinology* **30**(10):1003–1009.

Thomas E, Peat G, Harris L, Wilkie R, Croft PR. 2004: The prevalence of pain and pain interference in a general population of older adults: cross-sectional findings from the North Staffordshire Osteoarthritis Project (NorStOP). *Pain* **110**:361–8.

Ursin H and Eriksen H. 2007: Cognitive activation theory of stress, sensitization, and common health complaints. *Ann N Y Acad Sci* **1113**:304–310.

Vandvik PO, Wilhelmsen I, Ihlebæk C, Farup PG. 2004: Comorbidity of IBS in general practice: A striking feature with clinical implications. *Alimentary Pharmacol Therapeut* **20**:1195–1203.

Von Korff M, Crane P, Lane M, Miglioretti DL, Simon G, Saunders K, et al. 2005: Chronic spinal pain and physical-mental comorbidity in the United States: results from the national comorbidity survey replication. *Pain* **113**:331–339.

Wessely S and White, PD 2004: There is only one functional somatic syndrome. *Br J Psychiatry* **185**:95–6.

Wiendels NJ, van Haestregt A, Knuistingh Neven A, Spinhoven P, Zitman FG, Assendelft WJ, et al. 2006: Chronic frequent headache in the general population: comorbidity and quality of life. *Cephalalgia* **26**(12):1443–1450.

Yunus MB. 2008: Central Sensitivity Syndromes: A new paradigm and group nosology for fibromyalgia and overlapping conditions, and the related issue of disease versus illness. *Semin Arthritis Rheum* **37**:339–352.

Section 3

Mechanisms

Chapter 8

The genetic epidemiology of pain

Alex MacGregor

The pace of gene discovery in human disease is accelerating rapidly. In the last decade, technology has handed researchers the ability to scan the entire human genome, and as a consequence more genes have been discovered for common complex diseases in this time than in the entire period previously (McKusick, 2007). Thus it is understandable that human pain is now being examined from the genetic perspective with as intense scrutiny as is being applied to other human traits. Large-scale collaborative projects are taking place worldwide to identify the genetic contribution to its pathological, clinical, and behavioural components. As with the study of common complex diseases, it is expected that this genetic insight will advance the fundamental understanding of the biological mechanisms of pain and transform its clinical management.

This chapter explores the evidence supporting the notion that variation in pain reporting in human populations has a genetic basis and is amenable to the analytical approaches currently being applied to complex disease. The potential relevance of this genetic knowledge to the wellbeing of individuals suffering pain and also on public health is explored.

Genes as a source of variation in pain perception in human populations

The observation that strain-specific variation for a range of pain behaviours seen in experimental animals can be explained by genetic variation points to the possibility that specific pain-related genes might have sufficient penetrance to influence pain perception in human populations (Mogil and Max, 2006). However, making the step from experimental animals to man is clearly not straightforward. Unlike many physical diseases, pain in itself cannot be considered to be a simple target phenotype. Conceivably, genes might act at a number of levels to influence its expression, from determining the processing of nociceptive stimuli, to influencing behavioural and emotional responses. A distinction may also need to be made according to the nature of the pain, e.g. whether it is acute or chronic, nociceptive or non-nociceptive, and according to the point at which it occurs in the lifetime of an individual. The influence of the wider social and environmental context in which pain is experienced also needs to be taken into account. Thus to demonstrate convincingly that there is a genetic contribution to the perception of pain, and by extension to understand the relevance of any individual genes that might be implicated in pain in man, requires that the net is cast wide.

Influence of ethnicity and gender

The question of whether ethnicity and gender might explain differences in pain perception in different population groups has been a focus of both speculation and controversy over decades (Fillingim, 2004). The existence of significant variation in these groups would provide one possible indication of an influence of genes. However, this is a challenging area to investigate. A particular problem facing studies of gender and ethnicity is their susceptibly to bias. For example, in experimental pain, a range of subtle influences, including the gender differences between the experimenter and their subject, and the nuances of the precise language used in delivering the test and in reporting results, can influence both measurement and the interpretation of data (Zatzick and Dimsdale, 1990). The selection of study subjects also has an important bearing on the way in which pain is reported.

Despite these considerations, consistent evidence of ethnicity and gender differences in pain has emerged. In a review of the more recent literature, Fillingim considered 14 studies that have examined ethno-cultural influences on experimental pain perception (Fillingim, 2004). The strongest comparative data related to differences in pain responses between African Americans and white Americans. Most (although not all) studies demonstrated African Americans to have a lower tolerance for specific painful stimuli including heat pain, ischaemic pain, and cold pressor pain when compared with whites (Rahim-Williams et al., 2007; Campbell et al., 2005). African Americans also showed higher ratings for pain unpleasantness and intensity, and were shown to use passive pain coping strategies more commonly than whites. These reports concur with studies of clinical pain in which African Americans have been recorded as reporting greater levels of pain than whites for a range of conditions including migraine (Stewart et al., 1996), post-operative pain (Faucett et al., 1994), and myofascial pain (Nelson et al., 1996). Systematic differences in clinical and experimental pain have also been reported between other ethnic groups, e.g. Hispanic compared with non-Hispanic American whites (Campbell et al., 2005; Meshack et al., 1998; Bates et al., 1993).

There is an extensive literature that examines the difference in pain reporting between males and females (Wiesenfeld-Hallin, 2005). A number of experimental studies have shown that noxious stimuli are perceived to be more painful by healthy women than healthy men. Women report lower pain thresholds, lower pain tolerance, and greater unpleasantness with pain (Berkley, 1997). Many chronic pain states, including migraine (Bigal and Lipton, 2009), fibromyalgia (Yunus, 2002), and irritable bowel syndrome (Chial and Camilleri, 2002), are also commoner in women. Differences have been reported in analgesic sensitivity to pharmacological agents, in particular to κ-opioids (Gear et al., 1999). There is also evidence of sex differences in analgesic responses to μ-opioids in experimental studies that have been reflected in differences in brain-activation patterns (Zubieta et al., 2002).

Cumulative evidence thus supports the case for gender and ethnicity influencing the variation in pain reporting in human populations. However, understanding the source of this variation presents an additional challenge. Socio-cultural as well as psychological factors are likely to have an important influence; neurochemical and hormonal factors may also account for differences between males and females. Genetic factors may also contribute to this variation. However, to distinguish the influence of genes from other sources of variation requires more targeted epidemiological designs.

Twin and family studies

A classical epidemiological approach to detecting an influence of genes on human traits is to look for an association between the degree of resemblance in traits in family members and their degree of relationship. This is at its most elegant in studies of twins, where a greater similarity (correlation) in traits among monozygotic (MZ) twins (who share all their genetic material) when compared with dizygotic (DZ) twins (who share on average only half their genetic material) can be taken to imply that genetic, as opposed to environmental, factors determine the level of variation in the trait (Spector and MacGregor, 2002). The approach assumes that factors in the family environment of the twins that might influence the trait are shared equally in both types of twin. The extent of genetic influence can be quantified by comparing the numerical value of the correlation coefficient in MZ and DZ twins. This provides an estimate of a quantity termed 'heritability', which can be defined as the proportion of variation in a trait in the population that is attributable to population-level genetic variation (Hopper, 1998).

Insight into the heritability of pain and pain-related traits in recent years has been greatly facilitated by the establishment of a number of large scale twin registers that now constitute a rich source of data on a range of diseases and physical characteristics (Boomsma et al., 2002). A variety of studies now exist with a number of different designs that allow an increasingly detailed picture to be developed of the extent to which genetic variation might explain a range of manifestations of pain.

Diseases characterized by pain

Table 8.1 lists the heritabilities reported from twin and family studies for a range of clinical disease states in which pain is the defining clinical feature. The estimates range from 60% for low back pain to none for facial pain. However, most show a substantial genetic contribution.

An obvious difficulty in interpreting these data is that of separating genetic factors that influence pain from those that cause disease. For example, in low back pain it is not possible to distinguish between genetic factors that might cause a structural lesion in a vertebral disc and the genes that influence the perception of pain relating to the nocicepitive stimulus caused by the disc lesion. Genetic factors that influence the affective component of pain and the ability to recall painful stimuli might also have a contribution.

This problem can be addressed to an extent in multivariate analysis. By considering sets of traits simultaneously among groups of relatives, it is possible to estimate the extent to which the correlation among phenotypic traits in individuals can be explained by a common underlying genetic influence shared between traits (Neale and Cardon., 1992).

This approach has been used in groups of twins with low back pain who have also been studied by magnetic resonance imaging (MRI). Figure 8.1 illustrates the results of a multivariate analysis conducted on data from the UK Twin Registry where MRI scans had been scored for severity of degeneration in 1064 twins (MacGregor et al., 2004). The study participants completed question-naires detailing the severity of back symptoms over their lifetime. Both pain reporting and the degree of disc degeneration were heritable (57% and 71%, respectively). Simultaneously examining the pattern of correlation in the two traits of 'pain reporting' and 'degeneration' in multivariate analysis showed that that the majority of the phenotypic correlation could be accounted for by shared genetic factors but that the level of genetic correlation was only modest (0.2). This suggests that genetic factors influencing degeneration account for only a minority of the genetic variability in low back pain. An analysis of data from the Finnish Twin Cohort reached a similar conclusion (Battie et al., 2007).

The suggestion that 'pain reporting' itself is a heritable phenotype in its own right is also sup-ported by studying the pattern of musculoskeletal pain at different body sites. A questionnaire-based survey conducted in the UK Twin Cohort asked participants to indicate on a diagram whether they had experienced pain of >3 months duration in the neck, back, elbow, knee, thigh, hand, and foot (MacGregor, 2008). The responses at each body site were strongly correlated with a single factor explaining over 95% of the variance. The factor itself showed greater correlation among MZ when compared with DZ twins, corresponding to heritability 40%. Contrastingly, radiographic osteoarthritis is uncorrelated genetically at different body sites in the same twins,

Table 8.1 Examples of heritability values reported for range of clinical, experimental, and behavioural pain-related traits

Heritability scale (%)	Responses to painful experimental stimuli	Diseases characterized by pain	Behavioural traits associated with pain
70			
		Low back pain(4)	
60	Cold pressor pain (1)	Chronic widespread pain (5)	
	Heat pain threshold 32^0C+ (1) (2)	Functional bowel disorder (6)	
	Pinprick hyperalgesia (2)	Neck pain (4)	
		Shoulder and elbow pain (7)	
50		Menstrual pain (8)	
		Migraine (9)	
		Tension headache (10)	
		Gastro-oesophageal reflux pain (11)	Anxiety sensitivity (14)
40		Chronic pelvic pain (12)	
	Pain during burn induction (1;2)		Anxiety (15)
	Brush-evoked allodynia (2)		Depression (15)
	Acid iontophoresis pain (2)		Anger expression (16)
			Distress (17)
30			Pain coping (18)
20	Heat pain threshold 43^0C+ (1)		
	ATP iontophoresis pain (2)		
<20	Pressure pain threshold (3)	Temporomandibular joint pain (13)	
	Post-burn hyperalgesia (2)		

For reference codes please see the end of Table 8.2.

emphasizing the genetic distinction between pain reporting and the degree of joint damage (MacGregor et al., 2009).

Experimental pain

Examining pain responses evoked by standard stimuli might be seen to reflect better the biological processes that underlie the pathophysiological mechanisms of pain. Studies of this type are difficult to carry out in practice for obvious reasons. A more easily standardized approach is through the use of laboratory models of acute and chronic pain.

A study conducted in 2008 in the UK Twin Cohort examined a range of painful stimuli, using well-defined experimental models chosen to reflect both acute and chronic pain (Norbury et al., 2007). The measures studied included an assessment of baseline heat-pain threshold (using a 32-mm probe heated from 32°C at a rate of 0.5 degrees/second until the subject perceived pain) and an assessment of pain during the iontophoresis of adenosine triphosphate (ATP) and

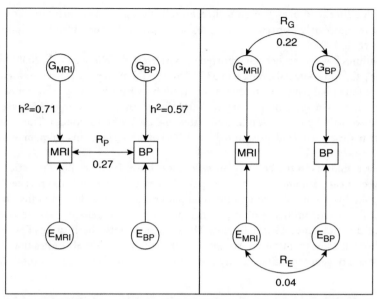

Fig. 8.1 Illustration of multivariate genetic analysis of correlated phenotypes using data from the UK Twin Registry (Macgregor et al., 2004). Lumbar disc degeneration as assessed by magnetic resonance imaging (MRI), and low back pain (BP) have a contribution from genetic (G) and environmental (E) components. The genetic component accounts for heritabilities (h^2) of 0.71 for MRI and 0.57 for BP in these data. MRI and BP have a phenotypic correlation (R_P) of 0.27 among individual in the group as a whole (left-hand panel). By considering the pattern of correlation between lumbar degeneration and low back pain both within individuals, and between members of MZ and DZ twin pairs, multivariate analysis allows the phenotypic correlation among individuals to be split into a genetic (R_G) and an environmental (R_E) component (right hand panel). In this analysis, the genetic correlation accounts for the majority of the phenotypic correlation that is observed between MRI and BP. However, the genetic correlation is relatively low, and genetic factors that are common to disc degeneration and low back pain account for only a small part of the genetic variance of either variable.

hydrochloric acid. Pain was also measured during the induction of a thermal burn and in the 15 minutes following the burn. Measurements were made of the area of post-burn allodynia to brush-stroke (brush-evoked allodynia) and of the area of hyperalgesia (assessed by repeat measurement of the heat-pain threshold at the burn site). These models have direct relevance to clinical pain, e.g. responses in the thermal burn model have been strongly correlated with post-operative pain (Werner et al., 2004).

The study was conducted in 98 (51 MZ and 47 DZ) female–female twin pairs, all of whom were healthy and on no analgesic medication. The experimental setting was rigorously controlled so that the stimuli were applied in a standardized way to all subjects and twins were blinded to their co-twins responses. The design of these experiments is critically important as loss of blinding can substantially bias the within-twin comparison through the well-recognized competitive pressures that exist between members of a twin pair – potentially blunting any distinction between MZ and DZ groups. The results (included in Table 8.1) were that most of the responses showed a genetic contribution. However, the genetic contribution was not uniform, and indeed no heritable contribution was found for post-burn hyperalgesia. An earlier study conducted in the same twin cohort, using a pressure dolorimeter, had also shown little heritability for forehead pressure pain threshold, although the experimental environment had been less rigorously controlled, making a genetic influence more difficult to detect (MacGregor et al., 1997).

Similar findings have recently been reported by Nielsen et al. (Nielsen et al., 2008) in a study of cold-pressor pain and contact-heat pain in 53 MZ and 39 DZ twin pairs from the Norwegian twin registry. Supramaximal pain sensitivity was assessed: heat pain by using a thermode at initially 43°C increasing by 1-degree increments until the Visual Analogue Scale (VAS) exceeded 50%; and cold-pressor pain by immersion in cold water (0–2.5°C for 60 seconds). The results showed that 60% of the variance in cold-pressor pain and 26% of the variance in heat pain was genetically mediated.

Multivariate analysis in the Norwegian twin data showed only modest genetic correlation (0.34) between heat pain and cold-pressor pain. Taken together with the markedly different levels of heritability recorded among individual pain modalities in the UK twins, these finding indicate that the genetic influence on experimental pain is heterogeneous, and accounted for by a number of distinct genetic mechanisms. This contrasts with the findings for clinical pain reporting discussed above, but is consistent with the results of animal studies that have shown independent sets of genes to influence physical response to different painful stimuli (Mogil et al., 1999).

Cognitive, behavioural, and personality traits related to pain

Cognitive, behavioural, and personality factors have an important bearing on the expression of acute and chronic pain. In low back pain, pre-existing psychological distress is one of the strongest predictors of the persistence of pain and disability. Depression, somatization, and maladaptive illness behaviours are among the most important predictors of chronic widespread pain (Gatchel et al., 2007).

As with diseases in which pain forms a major clinical feature, twin and family studies have indicated that there is a genetic influence on many behavioural phenotypes (Table 8.1). Traits that have been studied that are relevant to pain include anxiety and depression, which have been shown to have a heritability of ~50% in diverse population groups (Leonardo and Hen, 2006). Psychological distress as assessed by the General Health Questionnaire (GHQ) is strongly associated with pain reporting and has been shown to have a heritable component (Rijsdijk et al., 2003). Coping strategies relevant to pain have also been examined in a range of age groups and are reported to be heritable (Busjahn et al., 1999). The genetic influence also extends to self-reported fear and fear conditioning, and anger expression (Hettema at al., 2003; Hettema et al., 2007; Wang et al., 2005).

Recognizing that behavioural factors are an important part of pain genetics adds further complexity to the interpretation of the nature of the genetic influence in pain. Again, this is an issue that is beginning to be teased apart with multivariate analysis. In the UK Twin cohort, the twins who were studied for disc degeneration and low back pain were also assessed for psychological distress using the GHQ (MacGregor et al., 2004). Scores on the GHQ were heritable in these data and associated with the report of pain. The relationship between GHQ and pain reporting could be shown in bivariate analysis to be mediated almost entirely genetically, although this only accounted for a small part of the heritability of back pain overall.

Further insight into the complex genetic relationship between cognitive and behavioural traits and pain reporting comes from analyses of data from the Swedish Twin Registry. Kato et al. (Kato et al., 2006; Kato, 2007) conducted a multivariate analysis to examine the common occurrence of chronic widespread pain (CWP), a range of traits associated with CWP (including irritable bowel syndrome and recurrent headache), and self-reported anxiety and depression. The pattern of correlation among all the traits was best explained by two genetically determined latent factors, one loading most heavily on anxiety and depression and the other on CWP and its associated traits. The interpretation is that the variation in CWP has distinct genetically determined affective and somatic components.

Studies of individual genes

Studies of heritability have provided a traditional starting point for more detailed analysis aimed at detecting individual genes. With the advance of genetic technology, and the widespread access to (and reducing cost of) genetic markers spanning the entire genome, it has become practical to look directly for associations with individual genes in an increasingly wide range of clinical, experimental, and behavioural situations. This has also been facilitated by application of efficient case-control study designs that have no requirement for data from pedigrees. In this way many new 'pain phenotypes' have become amenable to this type of enquiry without the need for prior justification from the results of twin and family studies. These new phenotypes have included measures of nociception in clinical settings, the response to analgesic medication, and neuroimaging studies of pain.

Examples showing a selection of reported associations at the time of writing are shown in Table 8.2. This is a rapidly changing field that is increasingly difficult to catalogue because of both its diversity and complexity. However, a number of individual genes have emerged as having particular relevance and merit more detailed consideration.

Catechol-o-methytransferase (COMT)

This enzyme is involved in the regulation of catecholamine and encephalin levels, and polymorphic variation in the COMT gene has been associated with clinical pain processing. In a study of healthy volunteers subjected to intensity-controlled sustained pain induced by the infusion of small amounts of hypertonic saline and studied by positron emission tomography (PET) scanning, Zubieta et al. (2003) showed that a COMT polymorphism altered the downstream cortical responses of μ-opioid neurotransmitters in the thalamus and amygdala. The same variants were associated with the levels of pain reported during the saline infusion. In other studies of experimental pain, COMT polymorphisms have been shown to play a primary role in modulating thermal pain sensitivity and temporal summation to thermal pain (Diatchenko et al., 2006). Further experimental studies have suggested a role for COMT in opiate-induced hyperalgesia (Jensen et al., 2009).

COMT has also been associated with pain traits in other settings. Variants of the COMT gene have been associated with reports of temporomandibular joint pain (Diatchenko et al., 2005), migraine (Park et al., 2007), and fibromyalgia (Gursoy et al., 2007), and with analgesic responses in cancer pain (Rakvag et al., 2008). Associations have also been reported with anxiety and depression (Olsson et al., 2007; Hettema et al., 2008; Burdick et al., 2007), although not consistently (Baekken et al., 2008). In post-operative shoulder pain, an interaction between the COMT genotype and reported level of catastrophizing has also been identified (George et al., 2008).

μ-opioid receptor (OPRM1)

Opioids are the mainstay of pharmacological treatment for pain and polymorphisms of opioid receptor genes have the potential to influence drug efficacy. Polymorphisms of OPRM1 have been

Table 8.2 Examples of candidate-gene associations reported for clinical, experimental, and behavioural pain-related traits

Protein (Gene)	Catechol-O-methyl tyransferase (COMT)	Collagen 9 (COL9A3)	GTP cyclohydrolase (GCH1)	Hypocretin receptor (HCRTR2)	Melanocortin 1 receptor (MC1R)	Monoamine oxidase A (MAOA)	Opioid receptor (OPRM1)	Serotonin receptor (5HTA)	Serotonin transporter (5HTT)	Serotonin transporter regulator (5-HTTLPR)	Transient receptor potential (TRPA1)
Experimental pain											
Heat and cold sensation	◆ (19)				◆ (28)						◆ (19)
Ischaemic pain	◆ (20)		◆ (26)		◆ (28)		◆ (32)				
Pain following hypertonic saline infusion											
Pressure pain	◆ (21)		◆ (26)				◆ (32)				
Thermal pain			◆ (26)				◆ (32)				
Tolerance to electric pulse					◆ (29)						
Painful clinical traits											
Fibromyalgia	◆ (22)							◆ (33)			
Migraine				◆ (27)					◆ (35)		
Pain following discectomy			◆ (26)								
Sciatica		◆ (25)									
Temporomandibular joint pain	◆ (23)										

Behavioural traits

Anger expression ◆ (24)

Anxiety ◆ (30)

Coping strategies ◆ (36)

Depression ◆ (31) ◆ (34) ◆ (37)

Fear processing ◆ (38)

Trait anxiety ◆

1) Nielsen et al. 2007,
2) Norbury et al. 2007,
3) MacGregor et al. 1997,
4) MacGregor et al. 2004,
5) Kato et al. 2006,
6) Morris-Yates et al. 1998,
7) Hakim et al. 2003,
8) Treloar et al. 1998,
9) Mulder et al. 2003,
10) Russell et al. 2007,
11) Mohammed et al. 2003,
12) Zondervan et al. 2005,
13) Michalowicz et al. 2000,
14), Stein et al. 1999,
15) Leonardo et al. 2006,
16) Wang et al. 2005,
17) Rijsdijk et al. 2003,
18) Busjahn et al. 1999,
19) Kim et al. 2006,
20) Zubieta et al. 2003,
21) Diatchenko et al. 2006,
22) Gursoy et al. 2003,
23) Diatchenko et al. 2005,
24) Olsson et al. 2007,
25) Paassilta et al. 2001,
26) Tegeder et al. 2006,
27) Schurks et al. 2007,
28) Mogil et al. 2003,
29) Mogil et al. 2005,
30) Yang et al. 2007,
31) Brummett et al. 2007,
32) Fillingim et al. 2005,
33) Bondy et al. 1999,
34) Albert et al. 2004,
35) Offenbaecher et al. 1999,
36) Wilhelm et al. 2007,
37) Caspi et al. 2003,
38) Brocke et al. 2006,
39) Melke et al. 2001.

shown to influence nociceptive cortical activation (Lötsch et al., 2006). They have an effect on the opioid requirements in patients with pain caused by malignant disease and post-operatively (Klepstad et al., 2004).

GTP cyclohydrolase (GCH1)

This is a rate-limiting enzyme in tetrahydrobiopterin synthesis and essential for regulating catecholamines, serotonin, nitric oxide, and phenylalanine metabolism. In the clinical setting, a haplotype of the GCH1 gene has been associated with persistence of pain after surgical discectomy; and healthy individuals with the pain-protective haplotype have been shown to have a reduced level of pain sensitivity to thermal and ischaemic pain (Tegeder et al., 2006). In rodent models, polymorphic variation in this enzyme has been shown to modulate peripheral neuropathic and inflammatory pain.

Sparteine/debrisoquine oxidase (CYP2D6)

This enzyme is one of the hepatic cytochrome p450 enzymes and is involved in the activation of codeine by o-demethylation to morphine. Over 80 polymorphisms of CYP2D6 are known, resulting in a wide spectrum of metabolic diversity. Homozygotes of inactive alleles of CYP2D6 exhibit deficient hydroxylation of several commonly used drugs, including analgesics and antidepressants. Poor metabolizer status occurs in 10% of whites and 2% of Asians and African Americans. Both in clinical and experimental pain, poor metabolizers show reduced analgesic efficacy to codeine (Poulsen et al., 1996; Sindrup et al., 1990). Basal pain thresholds are also influenced by CYP2D6 status (Sindrup et al., 1993).

Melanocortin 1 receptor (MC1R)

Variants of the melanocortin gene are associated with enhanced analgesia from the κ-opioid antagonist pentazocine in thermal and ischaemic pain (Mogil et al., 2003; Mogil et al., 2005). The association is only seen in women and may in part account for the gender differences in response to analgesia that have been reported. Red hair colour is caused by variants of the melanocortin-1 receptor (MC1R) gene and it is of interest that people with naturally red hair have been reported to be resistant to subcutaneous local anaesthetics and to thermal pain (Liem et al., 2004; Liem et al., 2005). There are also reports that people with red hair are more likely to show higher levels of anxiety related to dental care and fear of dental pain (Binkley et al., 2009).

Limitations of genetic approaches to the study of pain

The foregoing account has highlighted evidence suggesting that genetic factors have an important influence in nociception, pain reporting, and the behavioural response to pain, and has summarized the strengthening data showing an influence of individual genes in various clinical and experimental settings. While this evidence is convincing, there is a need to place these observations in context.

A common interpretation of heritability is that it is a measure of the extent to which an entity is 'genetic'. This is a misconception. Identifying a heritable contribution to a trait in a population is not tantamount to declaring that genes have an overriding deterministic role. This can be illustrated by considering an anthropometric trait such as height. Height in men has a consistent heritability of 90% among different affluent Western European populations (Silventoinen et al., 2003). Despite this, an individual's adult height is quite clearly determined significantly by a range of environmental factors operating through growth and development. Furthermore, the same data that show consistently high heritability also show substantial differences between the mean height of males in different European countries. The reason for this apparent incongruity between the large estimate of heritability for height and the known contribution of the environment can be conceptualized by appreciating that heritability is a measure based on trait variation and not on trait mean. Thus, in populations with a similar level of an environmental exposure (e.g. with similar dietary patterns providing similar levels of nutrition), genetic variation will have the greatest influence in determining differences between individuals. Heritability is also a relative measure of genetic variation. Thus the absolute genetic contribution can only be truly interpreted if the level of environmental variance is known (Hopper, 1992). While the size of a trait's heritability is indicative of the power and likely success of genetic association studies to identify individual genes, it is neither a necessary nor sufficient condition of individual gene action.

It is conceivable that the significance of the overall genetic contribution to pain may have been overestimated in published data. Deriving heritability from classical twin studies relies on the assumption that the shared environments of MZ and DZ twins are equal. If there is an imbalance in environmental sharing, estimates of heritability for traits that are themselves associated with factors in the shared environment may be biased upwards (MacGregor, 2000). Further, the classical twin model itself is recognized to be limited in its power to detect an influence from the shared environment. Failure to take the shared environment into account in statistical models of twin data risks inflating the estimate of the genetic contribution (Hopper, 2000).

The potential for genetic studies to underestimate the contribution of the shared environment is of particular significance for pain. Studies conducted over many years have shown consistently that influences within the family environment have an important bearing on an individual's experience of pain. In two studies published by Turkat et al. in the 1980s, family pain models were shown to exert an influence on pain behaviour in both healthy and diseased individuals (Turkat and Guise, 1983; Turkat and Noskin, 1983). Studies of college students have also shown the number of pain models in the individual's family environment to be associated with the frequency of pain reporting (Lester et al., 1994; Koutantji et al., 1998). Poor models of pain tolerance in family members predict an earlier onset and greater severity of post-operative pain following thoracotomy (Bachiocco et al., 1993). Similarities have also been observed in the way in which children and their mothers describe pain (Campbell, 1975). In the experimental setting, pain tolerance to finger pressure is influenced by a subject's prior exposure to other individuals with either a high or low tolerance to painful stimulation (Turkat and Guise, 1983). Family size and socioeconomic status, an individual's position in the sibship, the quality of their relationships with parents, including early experiences of abuse and early loss of family members, also make a contribution (Payne and Norfleet, 1986).

An influence of shared family or random environment has less of a bearing on the interpretation of genetic association studies. However, these studies have well-recognized limitations of their own (Cardon and Bell, 2001). Spurious genetic associations can arise either through selection bias resulting in confounding through population stratification, or through inadequate statistical correction for multiple testing. To date only a minority of the associations that have been reported with candidate genes have been the subject of the independent replication that is needed to have confidence the findings are real (Hirschhorn et al., 2002).

Interpreting the genetic contribution to pain is further hampered by the complexity of pain itself. It is most likely that future models of pain will need to be extended to reflect this complexity by including the action and interaction of multiple genes and multiple environmental exposures. The differential expression of genes in individual tissues and cells may need to be considered. An indication of the subtlety of gene action that may need to be taken into account in genetic models of pain is hinted at in recent animal studies of the μ-opioid system that have shown neural plasticity to be determined by epigenetic interaction with environmental stimuli (Hwang et al., 2008).

Impact of knowledge of the genetics of pain on individuals and on the population

Genetic knowledge brings with it the expectation that new insight will ultimately improve the lives of people with chronic pain. A tangible benefit would be the discovery of new biological pathways and molecular targets for analgesic action. There is already evidence that this promise is beginning to be realized. Examples of novel analgesic targets, identified in part through genetic studies that have become a focus for drug development, include the sensory neurone transient receptor potential channel (Bevan and Andersson, 2009). Gene-transfer techniques are also under development as an approach to treating neuropathic pain (Kim et al., 2009).

Genetics also brings with it the promise of screening to help target individuals who might be susceptible to pain with a view to prevention, and to help identify those that might benefit optimally from specific therapies. Genetic polymorphisms make a significant contribution to the metabolism of analgesic agents, ranging from opioids to the non-steroidal anti-inflammatory drugs (Desmeules et al., 2004). Knowledge of pain genetics has the potential for personalizing both acute and chronic pain management, and for designing more effective pain medications with improved side-effect profiles.

These practical benefits are unlikely to happen quickly. In a recent study, Lötsch et al. examined the value of genotyping in managing opioid treatment among a cohort of pain patients treated in an outpatient unit. A finite number of gene variants (including OPRM1, COMT, MC1R, and CYP2D6) were examined. All are known to modulate the effects of opioids significantly in controlled homogenous settings (Lötsch et al., 2009). However, in the clinic an individual's genotype profile failed to predict their opioid requirements.

The limited value of single common risk variants for screening in complex disease is well recognized (Holtzman and Marteau, 2000). The performance of genetic testing improves if multiple genes are considered, but it requires hundreds of loci to be included for the discriminative ability of a genetic test to be improved substantially (Janssens et al., 2006). Although this may be attainable with the advent of genome-wide scanning, the complexity of pain, the lack of knowledge of the underlying genetic model, and the need to take into account rare gene variants, gene–gene and gene–environment interactions, all mean that it is likely that this information will only be of value in limited settings.

A more immediate benefit of the new genetic insight into pain is more subtle. An appreciation that a substantial part of the variation in pain perception has a genetic basis has the potential to change attitudes of both patients and their carers towards the nature of the pain itself and the reasons underlying an individual's response to it. The knowledge that pain has a genetic basis may also allow a more precise understanding of the role of the environment in explaining the development of pain in genetically susceptible individuals, opening new avenues for prevention and treatment.

References

Albert PR and Lemonde S. 2004: 5-HT1A receptors, gene repression, and depression: guilt by association. *Neuroscientist* **10**, 575–593.

Bachiocco V, Scesi M, Morselli AM, and Carli G. 1993: Individual pain history and familial pain tolerance models: relationships to post-surgical pain. *Clin.J.Pain* **9**, 266–271.

Baekken PM, Skorpen F, Stordal E, Zwart JA, and Hagen K. 2008: Depression and anxiety in relation to catechol-O-methyltransferase Val158Met genotype in the general population: the Nord-Trondelag Health Study (HUNT). *BMC Psychiatry* **8**, 48.

Bates MS, Edwards WT, and Anderson KO. 1993: Ethnocultural influences on variation in chronic pain perception. *Pain* **52**, 101–112

Battie MC, Videman T, Levalahti E, Gill K, and Kaprio J. 2007: Heritability of low back pain and the role of disc degeneration. *Pain* **131**, 272–280.

Berkley KJ. 1997: Sex differences in pain. *Behav Brain Sci*, **20**, 371–380.

Bevan S and Andersson DA. 2009: TRP channel antagonists for pain--opportunities beyond TRPV1. *Curr Opin Investig Drugs*, **10**, 655–663.

Bigal ME and Lipton RB. 2009: The epidemiology, burden, and comorbidities of migraine. *Neurol Clin*, **27**, 321–334.

Binkley CJ, Beacham A, Neace W, Gregg RG, Liem EB, and Sessler DI. 2009: Genetic variations associated with red hair color and fear of dental pain, anxiety regarding dental care and avoidance of dental care. *J Am Dent Assoc* **140**, 896–905

Bondy B, Spaeth M, Offenbaecher M, Glatzeder K, Stratz T, Schwarz M et al. 1999: The T102C polymorphism of the 5-HT2A-receptor gene in fibromyalgia. *Neurobiol Dis* **6**, 433–439.

Boomsma D, Busjahn A, and Peltonen L. 2002: Classical twin studies and beyond. *Nat Rev Genet* **3**, 872–882.

Brocke B, Armbruster D, Muller J, Hensch T, Jacob CP, Lesch KP et al. 2006: Serotonin transporter gene variation impacts innate fear processing: Acoustic startle response and emotional startle. *Mol Psychiatry* **11**, 1106–1112.

Brummett BH, Krystal AD, Siegler IC, Kuhn C, Surwit RS, Zuchner S et al. 2007: Associations of a regulatory polymorphism of monoamine oxidase-A gene promoter (MAOA-uVNTR) with symptoms of depression and sleep quality. *Psychosom Med* **69**, 396–401.

Burdick KE, Funke B, Goldberg JF, Bates JA, Jaeger J, Kucherlapati R et al. 2007: COMT genotype increases risk for bipolar I disorder and influences neurocognitive performance. *Bipolar Disord* **9**, 370–376

Busjahn A, Faulhaber HD, Freier K, and Luft FC. 1999: Genetic and environmental influences on coping styles: a twin study. *Psychosom.Med* **61**, 469–475.

Campbell CM, Edwards RR, and Fillingim RB. 2005: Ethnic differences in responses to multiple experimental pain stimuli. *Pain* **113**, 20–26

Campbell JD. 1975: Illness is a point of view: the development of childrens' concepts of illness. *Chil Develop* **46**, 92–100.

Cardon LR and Bell JI. 2001: Association study designs for complex diseases. *Nat Rev Genet* **2**, 91–99.

Caspi A, Sugden K, Moffitt TE, Taylor A, Craig IW, Harrington H et al. 2003: Influence of life stress on depression: moderation by a polymorphism in the 5-HTT gene. *Science* 301:386–389.

Chial HJ and Camilleri M. 2002: Gender differences in irritable bowel syndrome. *J Gend Specif Med* **5**, 37–45.

Desmeules JA, Piguet V, Ehret GB, and Dayer P. 2004: Pharmacogenetics and pharmacokinetics, in *The genetics of pain*, JS Mogil, ed., IASP Press, Seattle, pp. 211–237.

Diatchenko L, Slade GD, Nackley AG, Bhalang K, Sigurdsson A, Belfer I et al. 2005: Genetic basis for individual variations in pain perception and the development of a chronic pain condition. *Hum Mol Genet* **14**(1), 135–143.

Diatchenko L, Nackley AG, Slade GD, Bhalang K, Belfer I, Max MB et al. 2006: Catechol-O-methyltransferase gene polymorphisms are associated with multiple pain-evoking stimuli. *Pain* **125**, 216–224.

Faucett J, Gordon N, and Levine J. 1994: Differences in postoperative pain severity among four ethnic groups. *J Pain Symptom Manage* **9**, 383–389.

Fillingim RB. 2004: Social and environmental influences on pain: implications for pain genetics. in *The Genetics of Pain*, JS Mogil, ed., IASP Press, Seattle, pp. 283–303.

Fillingim RB, Kaplan L, Staud R, Ness TJ, Glover TL, Campbell CM, Mogil JS, and Wallace MR. 2005: The A118G single nucleotide polymorphism of the mu-opioid receptor gene (OPRM1) is associated with pressure pain sensitivity in humans. *J Pain*, **6**, 159–167.

Gatchel RJ, Peng YB, Peters ML, Fuchs PN, and Turk DC. 2007: The biopsychosocial approach to chronic pain: scientific advances and future directions. *Psychol Bull* **133**, 4, 581–624.

Gear RW, Miaskowski C, Gordon NC, Paul SM, Heller PH, and Levine JD. 1999: The kappa opioid nalbuphine produces gender- and dose-dependent analgesia and antianalgesia in patients with postoperative pain. *Pain* **83**, 339–345.

George SZ, Wallace MR, Wright TW, Moser MW, Greenfield WH, III, Sack BK, Herbstman DM, and Fillingim RB. 2008: Evidence for a biopsychosocial influence on shoulder pain: Pain catastrophizing and catechol-O-methyltransferase (COMT) diplotype predict clinical pain ratings, *Pain* **136**, 53–61.

Gursoy S, Erdal E, Herken H, Madenci E, Alasehirli B, and Erdal N. 2003: Significance of catechol-O-methyltransferase gene polymorphism in fibromyalgia syndrome. *Rheumatol Int* **23**, 104–107.

Gursoy S, Erdal E, Sezgin M, Barlas IO, Aydeniz A, Alasehirli B, and Sahin G. 2008: Which genotype of MAO gene that the patients have are likely to be most susceptible to the symptoms of fibromyalgia? *Rheumatol Int* **28**, 307–311.

Hakim AJ, Cherkas LF, Spector TD, and MacGregor AJ. 2003: Genetic associations between frozen shoulder and tennis elbow: a female twin study. *Rheumatology* **42**, 739–742.

Hettema JM, Annas P, Neale MC, Kendler KS, and Fredrikson M. 2003: A twin study of the genetics of fear conditioning. *Arch Gen Psychiatry* **60**, 702–728.

Hettema JM, Annas P, Neale MC, Fredrikson M, and Kendler KS. 2007: The Genetic Covariation Between Fear Conditioning and Self-Report Fears. *Biol Psychiatry* **63**, 587–593.

Hettema JM, An SS, Bukszar J, van Den Oord EJ, Neale MC, Kendler KS et al. 2008: Catechol-O-methyltransferase contributes to genetic susceptibility shared among anxiety spectrum phenotypes. *Biol Psychiatry* **64**, 302–310.

Hirschhorn JN, Lohmueller K, Byrne E, and Hirschhorn K. 2002: A comprehensive review of genetic association studies. *Genet Med* **4**, 45–61.

Holtzman NA and Marteau TM. 2000: Will genetics revolutionize medicine? *N Engl J Med* **343**, 141–144.

Hopper JL. 1998: Heritability, in *Encyclopaedia of Biostatistics*, P Armitage and T Colton, eds., Wiley, Chichester, pp. 1905–1906.

Hopper JL. 1992: The epidemiology of genetic epidemiology. *Acta Genet Med Gemellol (Roma)* **41**, 261–273.

Hopper JL. 2000: On why 'common environmental effects' are uncommon in the literature, in *Advances in Twin and Sibpair Analysis*, TD Spector, H Snieder, and AJ MacGregor, eds., Greenwich Medical Media, London, pp. 151–166.

Hwang CK, Song KY, Kim CS, Choi HS, Guo XH, Law PY, Wei LN, and Loh HH. 2008: Epigenetic Programming of Mu Opioid Receptor Gene in Mouse Brain is Regulated by MeCP2 and Brg1 Chromatin Remodeling Factor. *J Cell Mol Med* Oct 13 (epub).

Janssens AC, Aulchenko YS, Elefante S, Borsboom GJ, Steyerberg EW, and van Duijn CM. 2006: Predictive testing for complex diseases using multiple genes: fact or fiction? *Genet Med* **8**, 395–400.

Jensen KB, Lonsdorf TB, Schalling M, Kosek E, and Ingvar M. 2009: Increased sensitivity to thermal pain following a single opiate dose is influenced by the COMT val(158)met polymorphism. *PLoS One* **4**,e6016.

Kato K. 2007: *Genetic Epidemiological Studies of the Functional Somatic Syndromes*. Karolinska Institutet, Stockholm.

Kato K, Sullivan PF, Evengard B, and Pedersen NL. 2006: Importance of genetic influences on chronic widespread pain. *Arthritis Rheum* **54**, 1682–1686.

Kato K, Sullivan PF, Evengard B, and Pedersen NL. 2006: Chronic widespread pain and its comorbidities: a population-based study. *Arch Intern Med* **166**, 1649–1654.

Kim H, Mittal DP, Iadarola MJ, and Dionne RA. 2006: Genetic predictors for acute experimental cold and heat pain sensitivity in humans. *J Med Genet* **43**, e40.

Kim J, Kim SJ, Lee H, and Chang JW. 2009: Effective neuropathic pain relief through sciatic nerve administration of GAD65-expressing rAAV2. *Biochem Biophys Res Commun* **388**, 73–78.

Klepstad P, Rakvag TT, Kaasa S, Holthe M, Dale O, Borchgrevink PC et al. 2004: The 118 A > G polymorphism in the human mu-opioid receptor gene may increase morphine requirements in patients with pain caused by malignant disease. *Acta Anaesthesiol* Scand **48**, 1232–1239.

Koutantji M, Pearce SA, and Oakley DA. 1998: The relationship between gender and family history of pain with current pain experience and awareness of pain in others. *Pain* **77**, 25–31.

Leonardo ED and Hen R. 2006: Genetics of affective and anxiety disorders. *Annu Rev Psychol* **57**, 117–137.

Lester N, Lefebvre JC, and Keefe FJ. 1994: Pain in young adults: I. Relationship to gender and family pain history. *Clin J Pain* **10**, 282–289.

Liem EB, Lin CM, Suleman MI, Doufas AG, Gregg RG, Veauthier JM et al. 2004: Anesthetic requirement is increased in redheads. *Anesthesiology* **101**, 279–283.

Liem EB, Joiner TV, Tsueda K, and Sessler DI. 2005: Increased sensitivity to thermal pain and reduced subcutaneous lidocaine efficacy in redheads. *Anesthesiology* **102**, 509–514.

Lötsch J, Stuck B, and Hummel T. 2006: The human mu-opioid receptor gene polymorphism 118A > G decreases cortical activation in response to specific nociceptive stimulation. *Behav Neurosci* **120**, 1218–1224.

Lötsch J, von Hentig N, Freynhagen R, Griessinger N, Zimmermann M, Doehring A et al. 2009: Cross-sectional analysis of the influence of currently known pharmacogenetic modulators on opioid therapy in outpatient pain centers. *Pharmacogenet Genomics* **19**, 429–436.

MacGregor AJ. 2008: *The genetic determinants of osteoarthritis, spinal degenerative disease and musculoskeletal pain*, PhD, University of London.

MacGregor AJ. 2000: Practical approaches to account for bias and confounding in twin data, in *Advances in Twin and Sib-Pair Analysis*, TD Spector, H Snieder, and AJ MacGregor, eds., Greenwich Medical Media, London, pp. 35–52.

MacGregor AJ, Griffiths GO, Baker J, and Spector TD. 1997: Determinants of pressure pain threshold in adult twins: evidence that shared environmental influences predominate. *Pain*, **73**, 253–257.

MacGregor AJ, Andrew T, Sambrook PN, and Spector TD. 2004: Structural, psychological, and genetic influences on low back and neck pain: a study of adult female twins. *Arthritis Rheum* **51**, 160–167.

MacGregor AJ, Li Q, Spector TD, and Williams FM. 2009: The genetic influence on radiographic osteoarthritis is site specific at the hand, hip and knee. *Rheumatology* **48**, 277–280.

McKusick VA. 2007: Mendelian inheritance in man and its online version, OMIM. *Am J Hum Genet* **80**, 588–604.

Melke J, Landen M, Baghei F, Rosmond R, Holm G, Bjorntorp P et al. 2001: Serotonin transporter gene polymorphisms are associated with anxiety-related personality traits in women. *Am J Med Genet* **105**, 458–463.

Meshack AF, Goff DC, Chan W, Ramsey D, Linares A, Reyna R et al. 1998: Comparison of reported symptoms of acute myocardial infarction in Mexican Americans versus non-Hispanic whites (the Corpus Christi Heart Project). *Am J Cardiol* **82**, 1329–1332.

Michalowicz BS, Pihlstrom BL, Hodges JS, and Bouchard TJ, Jr. 2000: No heritability of temporomandibular joint signs and symptoms. *J Dent Res* **79**, 1573–1578.

Mogil JS. and Max MB. 2006: The genetics of pain, in *Wall and Melzack's Textbook of Pain*, 5th edn, SB McMahon and M Koltzenburg, eds., Elsevier, pp. 159–174.

Mogil JS, Wilson SG, Bon K, Lee SE, Chung K, Raber P et al. 1999: Heritability of nociception II. 'Types' of nociception revealed by genetic correlation analysis. *Pain* **80**, 83–93

Mogil JS, Wilson SG, Chesler EJ, Rankin AL, Nemmani KV, Lariviere WR et al. 2003: The melanocortin-1 receptor gene mediates female-specific mechanisms of analgesia in mice and humans. *Proc Natl Acad Sci USA* **100**, 4867–4872.

Mogil JS, Ritchie J, Smith SB, Strasburg K, Kaplan L, Wallace MR et al. 2005: Melanocortin-1 receptor gene variants affect pain and mu-opioid analgesia in mice and humans. *J Med Genet* **42**, 583–587.

Mohammed I, Cherkas LF, Riley SA, Spector TD, and Trudgill NJ. 2003: Genetic influences in gastro-oesophageal reflux disease: a twin study. *Gut* **52**, 1085–1089.

Morris-Yates A, Talley NJ, Boyce PM, Nandurkar S, Andrews G. 1998: Evidence of a genetic contribution to functional bowel disorder. *Am J Gastroenterol* **93**, 1311–1317.

Mulder EJ, van Baal C, Gaist D, Kallela M, Kaprio J, Svensson DA, Nyholt DR, Martin NG, MacGregor AJ, Cherkas LF, Boomsma DI, and Palotie A. 2003: Genetic and environmental influences on migraine: a twin study across six countries. *Twin Res* **6**, 422–431.

Neale MC and Cardon LR. 1992: *Methodology for Genetic Studies in Twins and Families*. Kluwer Academic Publishers, Dordrecht.

Nelson DV, Novy DM, Averill PM, and BerryLA. 1996: Ethnic comparability of the MMPI in pain patients. *J Clin Psychol* **52**, 485–497.

Nielsen CS, Stubhaug A, Price DD, Vassend O, Czajkowski N, and Harris JR. 2008: Individual differences in pain sensitivity: Genetic and environmental contributions. *Pain* **136**, 21–29.

Norbury TA, MacGregor AJ, Urwin J, Spector TD, and McMahon SB. 2007: Heritability of responses to painful stimuli in women: a classical twin study. *Brain* **130**, 3041–3049.

Offenbaecher M, Bondy B, de Jonge S, Glatzeder K, Kruger M, Schoeps P, and Ackenheil M. 1999: Possible association of fibromyalgia with a polymorphism in the serotonin transporter gene regulatory region. *Arthritis Rheum* **42**, 2482–2848.

Olsson CA, Byrnes GB, Anney RJ, Collins V, Hemphill SA, Williamson R, and Patton GC. 2007: COMT Val(158)Met and 5HTTLPR functional loci interact to predict persistence of anxiety across adolescence: results from the Victorian Adolescent Health Cohort Study. *Genes Brain Behav* **6**, 647–652.

Paassilta P, Lohiniva J, Goring HH, Perala M, Raina SS, Karppinen J et al. 2001: Identification of a novel common genetic risk factor for lumbar disk disease. *JAMA* **285**, 1843–1849.

Park JW, Lee KS, Kim JS, Kim YI, and Shin HE. 2007: Genetic Contribution of Catechol-O-methyltransferase Polymorphism in Patients with Migraine without Aura. *J Clin Neurol* **3**, 24–30.

Payne B and Norfleet MA. 1986: Chronic pain and the family: a review. *Pain* **26**, 1–22.

Poulsen L, Brosen K, Arendt-Nielsen L, Gram LF, Elbaek K, Sindrup SH. 1996: Codeine and morphine in extensive and poor metabolizers of sparteine: pharmacokinetics, analgesic effect and side effects. *Eur J Clin Pharmacol* **51**, 289–295.

Rahim-Williams FB, Riley JL, III, Herrera D, Campbell CM, Hastie BA, Fillingim RB. 2007: Ethnic identity predicts experimental pain sensitivity in African Americans and Hispanics. *Pain* **129**, 177–184.

Rakvag TT, Ross JR, Sato H, Skorpen F, Kaasa S, and Klepstad P. 2008: Genetic variation in the catechol-O-methyltransferase (COMT) gene and morphine requirements in cancer patients with pain. *Mol Pain* **4**, 64.

Rijsdijk FV, Snieder H, Ormel J, Sham P, Goldberg DP, Spector TD. 2003: Genetic and environmental influences on psychological distress in the population: General Health Questionnaire analyses in UK twins. *Psychol Med* **33**, 793–801

Russell MB, Levi N, and Kaprio J. 2007: Genetics of tension-type headache: A population based twin study. *Am J Med Genet B Neuropsychiatr Genet* **144B**, 982–986.

Schurks M, Limmroth V, Geissler I, Tessmann G, Savidou I, Engelbergs J, Kurth T, Diener HC, and Rosskopf D. 2007: Association between migraine and the G1246A polymorphism in the hypocretin receptor 2 gene. *Headache* **47**, 1195–1199.

Silventoinen K, Sammalisto S, Perola M, Boomsma DI, Cornes BK, Davis C et al. 2003: Heritability of adult body height: a comparative study of twin cohorts in eight countries. *Twin Res* **6**, 399–408.

Sindrup SH, Brosen K, Bjerring P, Arendt-Nielsen L, Larsen U, Angelo HR et al. 1990: Codeine increases pain thresholds to copper vapor laser stimuli in extensive but not poor metabolizers of sparteine. *Clin Pharmacol Ther* **48**, 686–693.

Sindrup SH, Poulsen L, Brosen K, Arendt-Nielsen L, and Gram LF. 1993: Are poor metabolisers of sparteine/debrisoquine less pain tolerant than extensive metabolisers? *Pain* **53**, 335–339.

Spector TD and MacGregor AJ. 2002: The St. Thomas' UK Adult Twin Registry. *Twin Res* **5**, 440–443.

Stein MB, Jang KL, and Livesley WJ. 1999: Heritability of anxiety sensitivity: a twin study. *Am J Psychiatry* **156**, 246–251.

Stewart WF, Lipton RB, and Liberman J. 1996: Variation in migraine prevalence by race. *Neurology* **47**, 52–59.

Tegeder I, Costigan M, Griffin RS, Abele A, Belfer I, Schmidt H et al. 2006: GTP cyclohydrolase and tetrahydrobiopterin regulate pain sensitivity and persistence. *Nat Med* **12**, 1269–1277

Treloar SA, Martin NG, and Heath AC. 1998: Longitudinal genetic analysis of menstrual flow, pain, and limitation in a sample of Australian twins. *Behav Genet* **28**, 107–116.

Turkat ID and Guise BJ. 1983: The effects of vicarious experience and stimulus intensity on pain termination and work avoidance. *Behav Res Ther* **21**, 241–245.

Turkat ID and Noskin DE. 1983: Vicarious and operant experiences in the etiology of illness behavior: a replication with healthy individuals. *Behav Res Ther* **21**, 169–172.

Wang X, Trivedi R, Treiber F, Snieder H. 2005: Genetic and environmental influences on anger expression, John Henryism, and stressful life events: the Georgia Cardiovascular Twin Study. *Psychosom Med* **67**, 16–23

Werner MU, Duun P, and Kehlet H. 2004: Prediction of postoperative pain by preoperative nociceptive responses to heat stimulation. *Anesthesiology* **100**, 115–119.

Wiesenfeld-Hallin Z. 2005: Sex differences in pain perception. *Gend Med* **2**, 137–145.

Wilhelm K, Siegel JE, Finch AW, Hadzi-Pavlovic D, Mitchell PB, Parker G, and Schofield PR. 2007: The long and the short of it: associations between 5-HTT genotypes and coping with stress. *Psychosom Med* **69**, 614–620.

Yang JW, Lee SH, Ryu SH, Lee BC, Kim SH, Joe SH, Jung IK, Choi IG, and Ham BJ. 2007: Association between Monoamine Oxidase A Polymorphisms and Anger-Related Personality Traits in Korean Women. *Neuropsychobiology* **56**, 19–23.

Yunus MB. 2002: Gender differences in fibromyalgia and other related syndromes. *J Gend Specif Med* **5**, 42–47.

Zatzick DF and Dimsdale JE. 1990: Cultural variations in response to painful stimuli. *Psychosom Med* **52**, 544–557.

Zondervan KT, Cardon LR, Kennedy SH, Martin NG, and Treloar SA. 2005: Multivariate genetic analysis of chronic pelvic pain and associated phenotypes. *Behav Genet* **35**, 177–188.

Zubieta JK, Smith YR, Bueller JA, Xu Y, Kilbourn MR, Jewett DM, Meyer CR, Koeppe RA, and Stohler CS. 2002: mu-opioid receptor-mediated antinociceptive responses differ in men and women. *J Neurosci* **22**, 5100–5107.

Zubieta JK, Heitzeg MM, Smith YR, Bueller JA, Xu K, Xu Y et al. 2003: COMT val158met genotype affects mu-opioid neurotransmitter responses to a pain stressor. *Science* **299**, 1240–1243.

Chapter 9

The biological response to stress and chronic pain

Anthony K.P. Jones, John McBeth, and Andrea Power

Introduction

The association between stress, stressors, and chronic pain is complex and underpinned by a number of biological, psychological, and social factors and processes that mediate the association. This chapter focuses on the role of the body's innate biochemical responses to stress and their relationship to pain.

Pain often occurs in the absence of peripheral pathology. This observation is particularly relevant when considering how 'stress' may be related to pain. While a stressor may be a traumatic stimulus associated with a peripheral pathology (e.g. fracture, skin abrasion) that directly links to a painful experience, there are numerous other types of stress (including psychological, social, and chemical) where the relationship with pain is less clear. One commonly discussed question is how to determine whether pain in the absence of peripheral pathology is 'real' or not. The same arguments can be applied to all symptoms without measurable peripheral pathologies, such as irritable bowel syndrome and chronic fatigue. What is often implied by this question is whether the symptoms are fabricated as part of malingering or attention-seeking behaviour or whether the pain is imagined. In our experience, evidence for definite malingering is quite rare, but as far as we are aware there are no objective tests for this.

Philosophically, the distinction between imagined pain and 'real pain' is difficult to make. If the pain is real to the patient, then it is real. All aspects of sensory perception are dependent on a delicate balance between what is expected and actual information (e.g. sensory input). Pain is no exception to this. Whether a sensory stimulus is perceived as pain or not is entirely dependent on the context of the stimulus. Non-noxious stimuli presented next to each other in bands of cool and warm will be perceived by most people as painful. This thermal-grill illusion is probably generated by the way the information from warm and cool fibres is summated in the spinal cord (Craig, 1996). At a higher level of processing, the perception of pain can be altered in either direction by manipulating what normal subjects expect from a painful or non-painful stimulus. Distraction from pain by verbal distraction or even white noise can substantially alter the unpleasantness of pain (Boyle et al., 2006). So we are not dealing with a hard-wired system but a system which is dynamically influenced by emotions, motivations, memory, and other sensory and homeostatic input. All these are integrated within a network of structures in the brain called the 'pain matrix'. All types of pain, including imagined pain, are processed within this matrix. Different types of pain appear to demonstrate different patterns of physiological responses within the pain matrix. So it is probably relatively meaningless to categorize pain as 'real' and 'unreal'. A more constructive framework is to think about pain as a common homeostatic response to certain stimuli and stressors that are initiated and maintained by different mechanisms.

In this chapter we outline the ways in which psychological and physical stressors may interact with the pain matrix to generate chronic pain. We then explore how alterations in the molecular response to stress may be associated with chronic pain by examining the role of the neuroendocrine system. Finally, to bring these areas into focus and to explore how both the pain matrix and neuroendocrine function may explain the relationship between stress and chronic pain, we present state-of-the-art data in relation to fibromyalgia, a non-articular rheumatic disorder characterized by chronic widespread pain (CWP).

The pain matrix

Pain is an unpleasant experience resulting from the integration of emotional (how nasty it is), sensory-discriminative (where and when it occurs, its quality and intensity), and motivational components (planned and actual motor responses). Over the last three decades different functional brain-imaging techniques and direct recording during neurosurgery have allowed us to confirm the existence of the pain matrix in the brain (see Figure 9.1) as originally proposed by Melzack (1990) and Bowsher (1957). This matrix is responsible for all types of pain perception during normal and abnormal pain experience.

The pain matrix includes cortical structures such as somatosensory cortical areas S1 and S2, inferior parietal cortex (IPC), the anterior insula, cingulated, and dorsolateral prefrontal

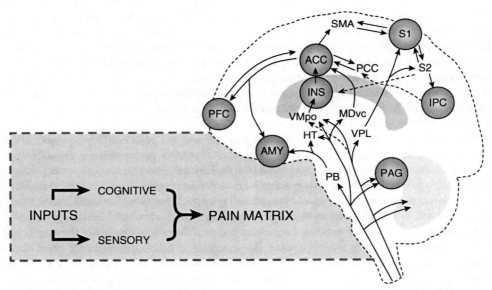

Fig. 9.1 A schematic representation of the complex pathways and structures that form the pain matrix.

These structures are involved in processing pain, and receive top-down (cognitive), bottom-up (sensory), and bilateral inputs.

PAG, periaqueductal gray; PB, parabrachial nucleus of the dorsolateral pons; VMpo, ventromedial part of the posterior nuclear complex; MDvc, ventrocaudal part of the medial dorsal nucleus; VPL, ventroposterior lateral nucleus; ACC, anterior cingulate cortex; PCC, posterior cingulate cortex; HT, hypothalamus; S1 and S2, first and second somatosensory cortical areas; SMA, supplementary motor area; AMY, amygdala; PF, prefrontal cortex; INS, insula cortex; IPC, *inferior* parietal cortex.

cortices (DLPFC) (Derbyshire, 2000; Peyron et al., 2000), and subcortical structures including the amygdala (Derbyshire et al., 1997), striatum, the thalamus, and hypothalamus (Hsieh et al., 1996; Kulkarni et al., 2005; Derbyshire, 1999). The anatomical connections, with their nociceptive inputs to these areas, have been extensively reviewed elsewhere (Peyron et al., 2000; Jones et al., 2003; Jones, 1999; Vogt et al., 1993; Apkarian et al., 1995; Kakigi et al., 2005; Rainville, 2002; Petrovic, 2002; Jones and Derbyshire, 1996; Treede et al., 1999).

One of the main qualities of the pain matrix is the parallel processing. The combination of ascending and descending components suggests an integration of top-down (cognitive) and 'bottom-up' (intensity of nociceptive input) inputs. There are predominantly bilateral nociceptive inputs to most cortical components of the matrix on both anatomical and functional grounds (Schlereth et al., 2003; Youell et al., 2004). This parallel and bilateral processing provides for some physiological redundancy which may be related to species survival. This may explain why ablative surgery to the central nervous system (CNS) is rarely associated with long-term pain ablation.

The change in level and extent of activity within the whole of the pain matrix is proportional to the intensity of pain (Derbyshire et al., 1997; Coghill et al., 1999; Porro et al., 1998), whereas there appears to be some subspecialization of function within the medial and lateral components. The lateral pain system comprises the lateral thalamic nuclei, the somatosensory, and IPC. It is fast and somatotopic (i.e. containing a body map) and may subserve the sensory-discriminative aspects of pain, which include localization, intensity, and duration. The insula cortex (INS) also has some somatotopic nociceptive inputs and may be involved in integrating them with inputs from other sensory modalities (Ostrowsky et al., 2002), such as touch. It has been proposed that the INS cortex may act as an interoceptive cortex, generating an integrated sense of bodily well-being (Craig, 2002). The insular cortex may subserve both medial and lateral pain systems in that, in addition to its somatotopic nociceptive inputs from the ventromedial part of the posterior nuclear complex (VmPO) of the thalamus (Craig, 2003), it also has input from medial thalamic nuclei and reciprocal connections with the amygdala.

The medial pain system is slow (polysynaptic) and non-somatotopic (Rainville, 2002). It includes the midline and intralaminar thalamic nuclei, anterior cingulate and mid-cingulate cortices (ACC and MCC), and DLPFC and possibly structures concerned with the processing of fear and stress responses, such as the amygdale and hypothalamus, respectively.

Evidence for division of function in the pain matrix was based on the effects of selective mid-cingulate lesions in alleviating the affective components of pain (Foltz and White, 1962) and effects of lesions in the region of S1 on the sensory-discriminative components of pain (Ploner et al., 1999; Ploner et al., 2000). Deafferentation of the MCC in patients with chronic intractable pain produces a state where patients still experience pain but it no longer bothers them (Foltz and White, 1962). These effects are quite similar to the clinical observations of the effects of synthetic opiates, which are also rarely pain-ablative, but substantially reduce the unpleasantness of acute and chronic pain. The MCC and ACC also have high concentrations of opioid receptors, whereas there are relatively low concentrations of opioid receptors within the SI (Jones et al., 1991).

Physiological confirmation of this proposed division of function was provided by positron emission tomography (PET) studies, where the only change in instruction prior to a painful or non-painful stimulus was to either attend to the location or to the unpleasantness of pain. These studies suggest that the main division of function is that the lateral system is concerned with localization of pain and that the medial system is predominantly concerned with the affective or emotional components of pain (Kulkarni et al., 2005). In this study, during the attention to unpleasantness, the amygdala and hypothalamus were also activated. It is likely that the amygdala may influence the experience of fear and anxiety associated with the pain experience.

The hypothalamus may act as a common autonomic and neuroendocrine output system for orbitofrontal and amygdala responses to emotions (Bohus et al., 1996). The demonstration of increased hypothalamic activity during attention to unpleasantness is consistent with this hypothesis (Kulkarni et al., 2005). Hsieh et al. (1996) demonstrated hypothalamic responses during severe pain and acupuncture-mediated analgesia (Hsieh et al., 2001). The experiment by Kulkarni and colleagues (2005) also demonstrated the extent to which a change in attentional focus can completely change the pattern of responses within the pain matrix.

Anticipatory responses to pain have been demonstrated throughout the pain matrix (Porro and Carli, 1988). Studies by Brown and colleagues have demonstrated the importance of anticipatory responses to pain in determining amplitude of responses during the actual experience of pain and the corresponding unpleasantness of pain (Brown, 2007). Responses to repeated laser stimuli to the back of the arm were measured by recording both anticipatory and pain-evoked potentials in normal volunteers. There was no correlation between laser energy and pain unpleasantness. However, there was a highly significant correlation between the anticipatory-evoked potential and the pain unpleasantness (Brown, unpublished data). Thus the top-down influences on pain perception would appear to be greater than the bottom-up input. Such shifts in influence of different types of input to the pain matrix are likely to be pivotally influenced by changes in attention.

Placebo analgesia

Placebo analgesia is an example of the positive benefit from top-down effects on the pain matrix. In order to understand the psychological mechanisms, studies have used a technique of experimental placebo to demonstrate that under appropriate conditions 40–60% of normal volunteers can be appropriately induced to experience placebo analgesia (Price et al., 2008; Montgomery and Kirsch, 1997).

Subsequent experiments established that this was a true physiological phenomenon and not due to habituation or increased compliance (i.e. subjects complying with their interpretation of the experimenter's wishes (Watson et al., 2006; Watson et al., 2007). Recent evidence suggests that, under controlled conditions, this placebo response is highly reproducible in individuals and is correlated positively with optimism and negatively with anxiety (Morton et al., 2009). Long-lasting reductions in anticipation for 2–3 weeks after this initial induction suggest enduring cognitive effects of placebo. Functional imaging experiments suggest that the reduction in anticipation that occurs during conditioning and the ensuing placebo analgesia is maintained by a number of brain regions including the DLPFC and orbitofrontal cortex and anterior MCC (aMCC). This would appear to exert a hierarchical effect on some of the main components of the pain matrix during placebo analgesia to maintain a long-term cognitive shift in nociceptive processing. It may, therefore, have the opposite effects to stress. A number of neuromodulators are thought to be involved in the modulation of placebo analgesia including dopamine, endogenous opioid (EO) peptides, and somatostatin (Benedetti and Amanzio, 1997). If placebo analgesia is opioid mediated, it raises the possibility of enhancing placebo analgesic effects by enhancing EO tone in the brain.

In summary there would appear to be potentially opposing effects of stress on placebo. The EO system is likely to be enhancing the placebo responses. As discussed in the following section there is also the possibility that cortisol may increase β-endorphin production. We also know that physical stress during severe exercise increases endogenous opioid activity (Boecker et al., 2008). It is also possible that anxiety *per se*, at least at high levels, may interfere with placebo response by interfering with the positive cognitive processes necessary to maintain placebo response.

Descending control systems, the cingulate cortex and stress

Early studies in animals established the phenomenon of stress-induced analgesia (Watkins et al., 1982) whereby animals subjected to stress such as cold-water swimming exhibited increased pain thresholds that were at least partially reversible by the opioid antagonist naloxone. Direct stimulation of various components of what is now considered part of a descending modulatory system, including the hypothalamus, periaqueductal grey (PAG), and dorsal raphe nuclei in the brainstem, were found to have very similar effects (Willer et al., 1990).

Animal studies suggest that at least part of the descending inhibitory and excitatory responses are opioid and serotonin (5HT) mediated (Willer et al., 1990). We have also shown that 5HT depletion reduces pain threshold and tolerance in human volunteers (Boyle, unpublished data). However, direct evidence of cortical control of these descending control systems in man is relatively sparse (Willer et al., 1981).

We now know this descending modulatory system has substantial input from a number of cortical regions including the ACC (Cummings et al., 1995). The cingulate cortex is involved in integrating emotional and cognitive aspects of brain function and to match these to appropriate motor and autonomic outputs. Descending long afferents exist from the ACC to key sub-cortical structures. These include the hypothalamus, PAG, dorsal raphe nuclei, locus coeruleus noradrenergic (NA) arousal input to most of the brain, midline thalamic nuclei, and amygdala. These provide the means to control most aspects of motor, neuroendocrine, fear, and arousal responses at a cortical to sub-cortical level.

Crucially many of these long afferents from the cingulate cortex in primates and rodents exhibit high levels of opioid receptor binding and are in synaptic contact with opioidergic interneurones. Human studies have shown that both regions of the cingulate cortex have high levels of opioid-receptor binding with the highest levels within the pregenual ACC (pACC) (Cummings et al., 1995), an area particularly involved in affective and autonomic control. We have shown that there was a gradation of increased opioid receptor binding from the executive areas to the affective areas of the cingulate cortex. The pACC has been shown to be involved in affective pain processing in humans (Kulkarni et al., 2005), demonstrates activation of the endogenous opioid system in acute (Zubieta et al., 2001) and chronic pain (Jones, 1999; Jones et al., 1994), and shows a fallout of opioid-receptor binding in post-stroke pain (Jones et al., 2004). In this context it is interesting that maternal deprivation results in long-term changes in brain metabolism in pACC in primates (Rilling et al., 2001). It is also this area together with adjacent orbitofrontal cortex and aMCC which appear to be involved in placebo analgesia (Wager et al., 2004; Bingel et al., 2006). It therefore seems likely that ACC and MCC are involved together with DLPFC to regulate stress, neuroendocrine responses, fear, and motor responses to pain. It is likely that these descending influences are both inhibitory and facilitatory.

Stress, the neuroendocrine response, and chronic pain

When exposed to a stressor the primary stress-response system, the hypothalamic–pituitary–adrenal (HPA) stress axis, is activated. The HPA axis, as part of the neuroendocrine system, is linked to the hypothalamic–pituitary–growth hormone (HPGH) and hypothalamic–pituitary–gonadal (HPG) axes via tightly controlled synthesis and secretion of hormones (see Figure 9.2). For brevity we will focus on the relationship between the HPA axis and pain. On activation of the HPA axis, increased levels of stress products lead to initiation of physiological and behavioural responses, ultimately resulting in allostasis (or achieving stability through change) and adaptive mechanisms. On activation, increased levels of stress products are released which return to

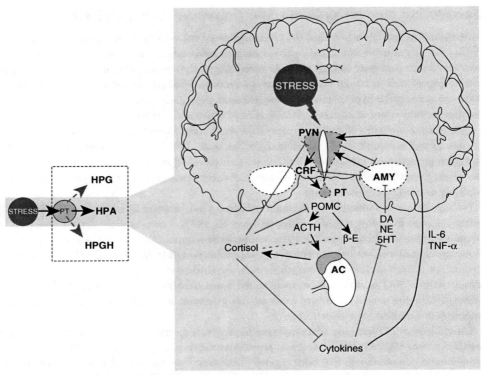

Fig. 9.2 The Hypothalamic–Pituitary–Adrenal Stress Axis

Physical and emotional stress activates three neuroendocrine pathways within the hypothalamus – the hypothalamic–pituitary (PT)-growth hormone (HPGH), the hypothalamic–pituitary–gonadal (HPG), and the hypothalamic–pituitary–adrenal (HPA) axes. The primary stress pathway, the HPA axis (detailed above), is activated by stress-induced-corticotropin releasing factor (CRF) expression within the paraventricular nucleus (PVN), resulting in the sequential release of downstream HPA elements such as pro-opiomelanocortin (POMC), adrenocorticotrophic hormone (ACTH), and cortisol which is secreted from the adrenal cortex (AC). β-endorphin (β-E), an opioid peptide also cleaved from the POMC protein, is temporally coupled to cortisol expression, suggesting a possible regulatory link. Cortisol suppresses HPA function at various points on the axis as well as both up-regulating and inhibiting the production of immune system components, such as interleukins (IL) and tumour necrosis factor-alpha (TNF-α). These components subsequently modulate dopamine (DA), noradrenaline (NE), and serotonin (5HT) metabolism and down-regulates amygdala function. Arrows and bars indicate the positive and negative regulation of downstream components, respectively.

normal levels on removal of the stressor. Failure to do so results in 'allostatic load' (McEwen, 1998), the physiological cost of chronic exposure to stress-response products that has been associated with a number of adverse health outcomes including pain.

As within the pain pathways, the core molecular components of the HPA stress axis are well characterized, and have recently become the focus of much scientific attention. To summarize, stress-activated-release of corticotropin-releasing factor (CRF) from the paraventricular nucleus (PVN) regulates pituitary expression of pro-opiomelanocortin (POMC), its cleavage product adrenocorticotrophic hormone (ACTH), and the subsequent secretion of cortisol from the adrenal cortex (AC). However, cortisol, primarily thought to be a regulator of the stress axis, now appears to be vital in the facilitation of positive and negative stress-induced pain perception, and is responsible for inhibiting a number of components of the pain-response system, such as, hippocampal activity, and cytokine production (Papadimitriou and Priftis, 2009).

Cytokines are crucial to the maintenance of certain chronic pain states such as neuropathic pain in animal models. Indeed, when released in response to activation of inflammatory pathways, these molecules alter the metabolism of key neuropeptides, noradrenaline (NE), 5HT, and dopamine (DA; Millan, 2002), thereby increasing pain sensitivity and shifting the emotional state. For example, pro-inflammatory cytokines, and cytokine modulator substance P (SP), reduce circulating levels of the 5HT precursor, tryptophan (Capuron et al., 2002; Schwarz et al., 1999). Hence, by suppressing cytokine production, cortisol indirectly contributes to increased levels of tryptophan, and to the positive emotional state and pain perception associated with increases in 5HT.

Finally, homeostasis is maintained by concentration-dependant cortisol suppression and cytokine-induced activation at various points in the HPA pathway (Dunn, 2000). In typical situations, this HPA axis activation enables physiological adaptation to short-term stressors. However, chronic exposure to emotional stress results in the alteration and adaptation of the HPA axis to its environment.

Exactly how the function of the HPA axis adapts to change is not fully understood. Animal studies have demonstrated the plasticity of the HPA axis. The stress response, including corticotrophin-releasing factor (CRF) and serum cortisol levels, in pup rats exposed to alcohol *in utero*, was much lower in the first 2 weeks of life compared to a control group of normal rat pups (Angelogianni and Gianoulakis, 1989). The system showed enhanced responsiveness after 2 weeks of postnatal development, although the explanation for this transition is unclear. Maternal deprivation of a pup was found to lead to a hyperactive HPA axis in the adult rat (Plotsky and Meaney, 1993).

Lifetime experiences in humans are thought to affect the HPA-axis response (Crofford, 1998). Adverse events in childhood have been linked to abnormal development of the HPA axis, although the extent of this influence is likely to depend on event-specific factors such as age, type of maltreatment, and parental responsiveness (van Voorhees and Scarpa, 2004). A recent study reported that childhood physical abuse and sexual abuse predicted a flattening of the cortisol rhythm and an increased cortisol response upon wakening. This suggests that childhood abuse acts as a chronic stressor, similar to other chronic stressors (Kunz-Ebrecht et al., 2004), that may be capable of causing dysfunction of the HPA axis in adulthood. However, not all subjects with chronic pain have been exposed to some form of trauma in childhood or later life. It is possible that some people have an innate, genetically determined, poorly functioning axis. Alternatively, other neuroendocrine systems could potentially play a role in the aetiology of chronic pain.

The pathophysiology of fibromyalgia

Fibromyalgia, a disorder characterized by the presence of chronic widespread pain (CWP), affects numerous systems of the human body. In the following review we use the terms fibromyalgia and CWP interchangeably. The pathophysiology of the disorder appears to involve a complex relationship with stress that impacts on a number of physiological and apparently unrelated pathways, such as pain processing, cognition, and sleep. Some of the first studies to examine the relationship between stress and fibromyalgia reported increased rates of mental disorders in fibromyalgia patients (Krag et al., 1994; Yunus et al., 1981) although that association may have been with consultation (Barsky et al., 1986). Population-based epidemiological studies of

CWP have reported that subjects with CWP were 3 times (odds ratio (OR) = 3.2; 95% confidence interval (CI): 2.0–5.1) more likely to have a mental disorder than subjects who were pain-free (Benjamin et al., 2000). Among pain-free subjects, depression (Magni et al., 1994) and markers of the process of somatization (McBeth et al., 2001a; Gupta et al., 2006) predict the onset of pain symptoms.

Occupational and other physical stressors may also be important. However, despite the assertion that widespread pain disorders including fibromyalgia are common sequelae of traumatic road traffic accidents (McLean et al., 2005a), there is a paucity of supporting objective evidence (Buskila et al., 1997a; Tishler et al., 2006; Al-Allaf et al., 2002). These equivocal reports could be explained by the differences in exposure and outcomes measured, and it is very likely that the small sample sizes used in previous studies have hampered analysis and interpretation. Other putative stressors associated with the onset of CWP are workplace injuries (McBeth et al., 2003; Harkness et al., 2004), military deployment (The Iowa Persian Gulf Study Group, 1997; Cherry et al., 2001; Escalante and Fischbach, 1998; Hotopf et al., 2000), chronic viral infections such as Lyme disease, hepatitis C (Buskila et al., 1997b), silicon implants (Wolfe, 1999; McDiarmid et al., 2001), dietary toxins (Smith et al., 2001), cosmetic use (Sverdrup, 2004), and exposure to environmental chemicals (Bell et al., 1998).

A considerable body of evidence suggests that reports of stressful adverse early-life events, such as neglect and physical or sexual abuse, are associated with chronic pain in adulthood (Kopec and Sayre, 2005). Women with fibromyalgia are significantly more likely to report rape and sexual abuse, and physical abuse in adulthood (Ciccone et al., 1996) and childhood (Davis, 1998). Birth factors (low birth weight and neonatal Intensive Care Unit admission) (Mallen et al., 2006), familial and peer-group experiences of pain, and being admitted to hospital during childhood (McBeth et al., 1999) increase the likelihood of having chronic pain in adulthood (Kopec and Sayre, 2005; Ciccone et al., 1996; Davis, 1998; Mallen et al., 2006). There is increasing recognition of the importance of adult attachment style,[1] and its association with hypochondriacal beliefs (Wearden et al., 2006), hypervigilance to pain (McWilliams and Admundson, 2007), increased pain-related fears (McWilliams and Asmundson, 2007), reduced pain threshold (Meredith et al., 2006), poor pain coping (McWilliams and Asmundson, 2007; Meredith et al., 2006; Meredith et al., 2007; Ciechanowski et al., 2003), increased pain perception and disability (McWilliams et al., 2000), and increased psychological distress (Meredith et al., 2007; Ciechanowski et al., 2003). However, it is likely that recall of early-life exposures will be affected by current pain state (McBeth et al., 2001b; Raphael et al., 2001).

Physiologically, fibromyalgia patients display altered HPA function: elevated evening levels of cortisol and lower 24-h urinary free cortisol levels have been noted (Crofford et al., 1994). In addition, Griep and colleagues reported lower basal, urinary free, and plasma free levels of cortisol in fibromyalgia patients when compared to healthy controls (Griep et al., 1998). In response to a CRH challenge test (a dexamethasone suppression test), an exaggerated level of ACTH was noted but without the expected increase in cortisol secretion, suggesting a hypo-responsive adrenal gland in fibromyalgia patients. These alterations in HPA-axis function are not specific to CWP and fibromyalgia; HPA-axis dysfunction has also been noted in other chronic pain syndromes. Following a corticotropin releasing hormone challenge test, patients with

---

[1] An individual's attachment style is determined by early childhood experiences of relationships with primary caregiver(s), based on availability and consistency of care provided. Attachment style is considered to be a stable trait throughout adult life, determines how we relate to others and is linked to our strategies for managing threatening situations.

chronic non-inflammatory low back pain also exhibited an exaggerated ACTH response, but to a lesser extent than fibromyalgia patients (Griep et al., 1998). Abnormalities have also been noted in the HPA axis of rheumatoid arthritis patients (McCain and Tilbe, 1989).

A population-based cross-sectional study considered the independent effects of psychological status and pain on HPA axis function (McBeth et al., 2005). Dysfunction of the axis (low salivary cortisol levels but with an exaggerated response to stress) was reported in subjects with CWP, and those 'at risk' of developing CWP according to their psychological status. This relationship persisted after adjusting for the confounding effects of psychosocial status, including psychological distress. More recently, this group has demonstrated the role of HPA-axis function in moderating the impact of risk factors on the onset of CWP (McBeth et al., 2007). However, these data are equivocal. In a study of 20 fibromyalgia patients and 16 healthy controls, salivary cortisol levels were measured 5 times per day over a 2-day period (McLean et al., 2005b). No differences in 24-h secretion of cortisol were noted, although cortisol levels were associated with early-morning pain symptoms. Subsequently the same group showed that cerebral spinal fluid (CSF) levels of CRF in 26 fibromyalgia patients were associated with sensory and affective aspects of pain, but not fatigue symptoms (McLean et al., 2006). The authors also noted that CSF levels of CRF were lower for female patients who reported a history of sexual or physical abuse ($n = 7$), compared with female patients with no history of abuse ($n = 9$) and a third group of male fibromyalgia patients ($n = 10$).

Such apparently conflicting reports of a hypo- and hyper-responsive HPA axis in subjects with pain are difficult, although not impossible to reconcile. The data would support a morning hypo-responsive and evening hyper-responsive axis, with an exaggerated response to stress testing. Hyper-responsiveness of the HPA axis is associated with the physical and cognitive outcomes observed in individuals with CWP. Increased levels of cortisol are positively associated with levels of pro-inflammatory cytokines (Leonard, 2005) and subsequently with an increased risk of cardiovascular disease that has been noted in this patient group (Rosmond and Bjorntorp, 2000). Increased cortisol production is also associated with decreased production of dehydroepiandrosterone (DHEA) sulphate which, in turn, is associated with the accelerated rate of cognitive decline (Ferrari et al., 2001) that is also evident in patients with fibromyalgia.

Conclusions from these studies support the concept of disturbed HPA-axis function in subjects with chronic pain, and specifically, with fibromyalgia. The focus would appear to be functional deficits in CRF release from the hypothalamus. Enhanced pituitary ACTH responses to ovine CRF, however, may be due to up-regulation of pituitary CRF receptors in response to chronically reduced central CRF release. Central CRF tone itself, therefore, appears to lie at the heart of the interrelationships between stress stimuli and response adaptation. It appears that HPA dysfunction precedes the onset of symptoms. In Figure 9.3 we have summarized these findings in a hypothetical model of the relationship between stress, HPA-axis response, and pain via an immune response mechanism.

It appears that alterations in HPA function directly alter downstream cytokine function (Barnes and Adcock, 2009). Therefore, it is not surprising to learn that fibromyalgia patients display enhanced inflammatory activity. In fact, blood and CSF samples taken from these patients revealed increases in both interleukin (IL)-8, SP (mediator of nociception and cytokine function), and monocyte chemotactic protein-1 (Russell and Vipraio, 1994; Zhang et al., 2008; Wang et al., 2009), while elevated concentrations of pro-inflammatory molecules such as tumour necrosis factor (TNF)-alpha, IL-1, and IL-6 were evident in patient skin samples (Salemi et al., 2003). Furthermore, increases in components such as SP, IL-6, and IL-8 have been linked to symptoms such as sleep disturbance, fatigue, and hyperalgesia (Schwarz et al., 1999; Papanicolaou et al., 1998; Wallace et al., 2001).

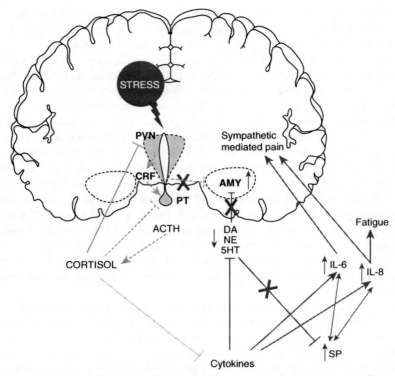

Fig. 9.3 A hypothetical model outlining the proposed impact of a faulty HPA axis in fibromyalgia (FM) syndrome.

FM patients display hypocortisolism and reduced inhibition of amygdala (AMY) and cytokine activity. The production of cytokines such as Interleukin 1 (IL-1), IL-6, and TNF-α results in elevations in circulating levels of substance P (SP) and IL-8, and a consequent reduction in serotonin (5HT) and its precursor, tryptophan. Low levels of 5HT result in increased amygdala activity.

Inhibitory mechanisms are represented by bars, activation is indicated by large arrows. Up- or down-regulation due to hypocortisolism is shown by small adjacent arrows. Black X indicates central inhibitory pathways with reduced function in this fibromyalgia model, resulting in amygdala activation and cytokine up-regulation. PVN, paraventricular nucleus; PT, pituitary gland; CRF, Corticotropin-releasing factor; PVN, paraventricular nucleus; ACTH, adrenocorticotrophic hormone; DA, dopamine; NE, noradrenaline.

Typically, in a stable system, increased cytokine activity maintains monoamine metabolite concentrations and induces CRF expression in the PVN (activating the HPA axis), suppressing cytokine production. However, if this equilibrium is compromised, increases in cytokine concentrations result in the depletion of monoamines such as 5HT, NE, and DA (Dunn and Wang, 1995). Indeed, CSF concentrations of tryptophan, 5HT, NE, and DA are significantly lower in fibromyalgic patients compared to healthy controls (Russell et al., 1992). And as these components are responsible for the regulation of multiple downstream pathways, abnormal concentrations must have a systemic effect. For instance, depletion of tryptophan, the melatonin precursor, results in disruptions to the sleep–wake cycle (Mendlewicz, 2009).

Brain-imaging studies have revealed severe structural and functional abnormalities within a number of brain regions in these patients. Pain-matrix sites, such as the INS, cingulate cortex, supplementary motor area (SMA), S1, and IPC, all display significantly higher levels of activation in patients following the application of a pressure-pain stimulus (Gracely et al., 2002; Burgmer et al., 2009). In addition, the amygdala, a structure critical for the modulation of pain and stress response (Neugebauer et al., 2004), shows a reduction in grey matter volume (Burgmer et al., 2009) and compromised opioid signalling due to a decrease in receptor-binding potential in these patients (Armstrong et al., 2007). Hence, the negative correlation that appears between opioid receptor availability and pain may explain the painful symptoms experienced in fibromyalgia, whilst a reduction in receptor binding may explain the diminished effectiveness of opioid drugs in treating these patients.

Treatment of patients with CWP is unsatisfactory, and individual management strategies are not effective at relieving symptoms. Exercise and cognitive therapies may be beneficial. A Cochrane (Busch et al., 2002) and more recent review (Gowans and deHueck, 2004) concluded that physical exercise improves physical function, reduces tender point pain, and improves pain. The long-term benefits are, however, unknown (Busch et al., 2002). Cognitive behavioural therapy (CBT) is a short-term goal-focused form of psychotherapy. The benefits of CBT as a single treatment modality in fibromyalgia patients have not been demonstrated. Indeed, evidence-based recommendations for the management of fibromyalgia reported that the trials available were 'of insufficient methodological rigour to allow any conclusions to be drawn' (Carville et al., 2008). Multidisciplinary treatment packages are thought to offer the best approach. CBT has been shown to be effective in alleviating pain and reducing tender point pain when used in combination with pharmacological and exercise therapies (Bennett and Nelson, 2006).

Importantly, the bio-mechanisms through which these interventions operate are unclear, although alterations in functioning of the HPA axis offers one plausible mechanism. Exercise has a profound impact on the functioning of the HPA axis (Leal-Cerro et al., 1999) and has been shown to correlate negatively with cortisol levels (Peeters et al., 2007). CBT down-regulates HPA activity among patients with generalized anxiety disorder (Tafet et al., 2005) and human immunodeficiency virus (Antoni et al., 2000). Cortisol response to a psychosocial stressor (the Trier Social Stress Test) is attenuated following a brief cognitive behavioural stress-management course (Gaab et al., 2003), and this effect persists over time (Hammerfald et al., 2006). To date only one study has been published that has investigated HPA function before and after a treatment programme in fibromyalgia patients (Bonifazi et al., 2006). An uncontrolled trial of prescribed exercise and CBT in a small number ($N = 12$) of patients with fibromyalgia reported significant reductions in the number of tender points, reported pain severity, distribution of pain, and levels of depression. These improvements were paralleled by increases in the diurnal variation of salivary free cortisol, marked by increased morning and decreased evening production of cortisol. That study was unable to examine the relationships between treatment modality, HPA function, and outcome. However, the results are consistent with the effects of these therapies being to reverse the alterations in HPA-axis function noted in patients with fibromyalgia.

References

Al-Allaf AW, Dunbar KL, Hallum NS, Nosratzadeh B, Templeton KD, Pullar T. 2002: A case-control study examining the role of physical trauma in the onset of fibromyalgia syndrome. *Rheumatology* **41**:450–453.

Angelogianni P, Gianoulakis C. 1989: Prenatal exposure to ethanol alters the ontogeny of the beta-endorphin response to stress. *Alcohol Clin Exp Res* **13**:564–571.

Antoni MH, Cruess S, Cruess DG, Kumar M, Lutgendorf S, Ironson G, et al. 2000: Cognitive-behavioral stress management reduces distress and 24-hour urinary free cortisol output among symptomatic HIV-infected gay men. *Ann Behav Med* **22**:29–37.

Apkarian P, Bour LJ, Barth PG, Wenniger-Prick L, Verbeeten B, Jr. 1995: Non-decussating retinal-fugal fibre syndrome. An inborn achiasmatic malformation associated with visuotopic misrouting, visual evoked potential ipsilateral asymmetry and nystagmus. *Brain* **118**:1195–1216.

Armstrong T, Strommer L, Ruiz-Jasbon F, Shek FW, Harris SF, Permert J, et al. 2007: Pancreaticoduodenectomy for peri-ampullary neoplasia leads to specific micronutrient deficiencies. *Pancreatology* **7**:37–44.

Barnes PJ and Adcock IM. 2009: Glucocorticoid resistance in inflammatory diseases. *Lancet* **373**:1905–1917.

Barsky AJ, Wyshak G, Klerman GL. 1986: Medical and psychiatric determinanats of outpatient utilization. *Med Care* **24**:548–560.

Bell IR, Baldwin CM, Schwartz GE. 1998: Illness from low levels of environmental chemicals: relevance to chronic fatigue syndrome and fibromyalgia. *Am J Med* **105**(3A):74S–82S.

Benedetti F and Amanzio M. 1997: The neurobiology of placebo analgesia: from endogenous opioids to cholecystokinin. *Prog Neurobiol* **52**:109–125.

Benjamin S, Morris S, McBeth J, Macfarlane GJ, Silman AJ. 2000: The association between chronic widespread pain and mental disorder: A population-based study. *Arthritis Rheum* **43**:561–567.

Bennett R and Nelson D. 2006: Cognitive behavioral therapy for fibromyalgia. *Nat Clin Pract Rheumatol* **2**:416–424.

Bingel U, Lorenz J, Schoell E, Weiller C, Buchel C. 2006: Mechanisms of placebo analgesia: rACC recruitment of a subcortical antinociceptive network. *Pain* **120**:8–15.

Boecker H, Sprenger T, Spilker ME, Henriksen G, Koppenhoefer M, Wagner KJ, et al. 2008: The runner's high: opioidergic mechanisms in the human brain. *Cereb Cortex* **18**:2523–2531.

Bohus B, Koolhaas JM, Korte SM, Roozendaal B, Wiersma A. 1996: Forebrain pathways and their behavioural interactions with neuroendocrine and cardiovascular function in the rat. *Clin Exp Pharmacol Physiol* **23**:177–182.

Bonifazi M, Suman AL, Cambiaggi C, Felici A, Grasso G, Lodi L, et al. 2006: Changes in salivary cortisol and corticosteroid receptor-alpha mRNA expression following a 3-week multidisciplinary treatment program in patients with fibromyalgia. *Psychoneuroendocrinology* **31**:1076–1086.

Bowsher D. 1957: Termination of the central pain pathway in man: the conscious appreciation of pain. *Brain* **80**:606–622.

Boyle Y, Bentley DE, Watson A, Jones AK. 2006: Acoustic noise in functional magnetic resonance imaging reduces pain unpleasantness ratings. *Neuroimage* **31**:1278–1283.

Brown CA. 2007: The role of paradoxical beliefs in chronic pain: a complex adaptive systems perspective. *Scand J Caring Sci* **21**:207–213.

Burgmer M, Gaubitz M, Konrad C, Wrenger M, Hilgart S, Heuft G, et al. 2009: Decreased gray matter volumes in the cingulo-frontal cortex and the amygdala in patients with fibromyalgia 15. *Psychosom Med* **71**:566–573.

Burgmer M, Pogatzki-Zahn E, Gaubitz M, Wessoleck E, Heuft G, Pfleiderer B. 2009: Altered brain activity during pain processing in fibromyalgia. *Neuroimage* **44**:502–508.

Busch A, Schachter CL, Peloso PM, Bombardier C. 2002: Exercise for treating fibromyalgia syndrome. *Cochrane Database Syst Rev* CD003786.

Buskila D, Neumann L, Vaisberg G, Alkalay D, Wolfe F. 1997a: Increased rates of fibromyalgia following cervical spine injury. A controlled study of 161 cases of traumatic injury. *Arthritis Rheum* **40**:446–452.

Buskila D, Shnaider A, Neumann L, Zilberman D, Hilzenrat N, Sikuler E. 1997b: Fibromyalgia in hepatitis C virus infection. Another infectious disease relationship. *Arch Intern Med* **157**:2497–2500.

Capuron L, Ravaud A, Neveu PJ, Miller AH, Maes M, Dantzer R. 2002: Association between decreased serum tryptophan concentrations and depressive symptoms in cancer patients undergoing cytokine therapy. *Mol Psychiatry* **7**:468–473.

Carville SF, rendt-Nielsen S, Bliddal H, Blotman F, Branco JC, Buskila D, et al. 2008: EULAR evidence-based recommendations for the management of fibromyalgia syndrome. *Ann Rheum Dis* **67**:536–541.

Ciccone DS, Just N, Bandilla EB. 1996: Non-organic symptom reporting in patients with chronic non-malignant pain. *Pain* **68**:329–341.

Ciechanowski P, Sullivan M, Jensen M, Romano J, Summers H. 2003: The relationship of attachment style to depression, catastrophizing and health care utilization in patients with chronic pain. *Pain* **104**:627–637.

Cherry N, Creed F, Silman A, Dunn G, Baxter D, Smedley J, et al. 2001: Health and exposures of United Kingdom Gulf War veterans. Part II: The relation of health to exposure. *Occupational & Environmental Med* **58**:299–306.

Coghill RC, Sang CN, Maisog JM, Iadarola MJ. 1999: Pain intensity processing within the human brain: a bilateral, distributed mechanism. *J Neurophysiol* **82**:1934–1943.

Craig AD. 1996: An ascending general homeostatic afferent pathway originating in lamina I7. *Prog Brain Res* **107**:225–242.

Craig AD. 2002: How do you feel? Interoception: the sense of the physiological condition of the body. *Nat Rev Neurosci* **3**:655–666.

Craig AD. 2003: Pain mechanisms: labeled lines versus convergence in central processing. *Annu Rev Neurosci* **26**:1–30.

Crofford LJ, Pillemer SR, Kalogeras KT. 1994: Hypothalamic-pituitary-adrenal axis pertubations in patients with fibromyalgia. *Arthritis Rheum* **37**:1583–1592.

Crofford LJ. 1998: Neuroendocrine abnormalities in fibromyalgia and related disorders. *Am J Med Sci* **315**:359–366.

Cummings SR, Nevitt MC, Browner WS, Fox KM, Ensrud KE, Cauley J, et al. 1995: Risk factors for hip fracture in white women. *N Engl J Med* **332**:767–773.

Davis CG. 1998: Rear-end impacts: vehicle and occupant response. *J Manipulative Physiol Ther* **21**: 629–639

Derbyshire SW, Jones AK, Gyulai F, Clark S, Townsend D, Firestone LL. 1997: Pain processing during three levels of noxious stimulation produces differential patterns of central activity. *Pain* **73**:431–445.

Derbyshire SW. 1999: Locating the beginnings of pain. *Bioethics* **13**:1–31.

Derbyshire SW. 2000: Exploring the pain "neuromatrix". *Curr Rev Pain* **4**:467–477.

Dunn AJ, Wang J. 1995: Cytokine effects on CNS biogenic amines. *Neuroimmunomodulation* **2**:319–328.

Dunn AJ. 2000: Cytokine activation of the HPA axis. *Ann N Y Acad Sci* **917**:608–617.

Escalante A, Fischbach M. 1998: Musculoskeletal manifestations, pain, and quality of life in Persian Gulf War veterans referred for rheumatologic evaluation. *J Rheumatol* **25**:2228–2235.

Ferrari E, Casarotti D, Muzzoni B, Albertelli N, Cravello L, Fioravanti M, et al. 2001: Age-related changes of the adrenal secretory pattern: possible role in pathological brain aging. *Brain Res Brain Res Rev* **37**:294–300.

Foltz EL and White LE, Jr. 1962: Pain "relief" by frontal cingulumotomy. *J Neurosurg* **19**:89–100.

Gaab J, Blattler N, Menzi T, Pabst B, Stoyer S, Ehlert U. 2003: Randomized controlled evaluation of the effects of cognitive-behavioral stress management on cortisol responses to acute stress in healthy subjects. *Psychoneuroendocrinology* **28**:767–779.

Gowans SE, de Hueck A. 2004: Effectiveness of exercise in management of fibromyalgia. *Curr Opin Rheumatol* **16**:138–142.

Gracely RH, Petzke F, Wolf JM, Clauw DJ. 2002: Functional magnetic resonance imaging evidence of augmented pain processing in fibromyalgia. *Arthritis Rheum* **46**:1333–1343.

Griep EN, Boersma JW, Lentjes EGWM, Prins APA, Van der Korst JK, de Kloet ER. 1998: Function of the hypothalamic-pituitary-Adrenal Axis in patients with fibromyalgia and low back pain. *J Rheumatol* **25**:1374–1381.

Gupta A, McBeth J, Macfarlane GJ, Morriss RK, Dickens C, Ray D, et al. 2007: Pressure pain thresholds and tender point counts as predictors of new chronic widespread pain in psychologically distressed subjects. *Ann Rheum Dis* **66**:517–521.

Hammerfald K, Eberle C, Grau M, Kinsperger A, Zimmermann A, Ehlert U, et al. 2006: Persistent effects of cognitive-behavioral stress management on cortisol responses to acute stress in healthy subjects—a randomized controlled trial. *Psychoneuroendocrinology* 31:333–339.

Harkness EF, Macfarlane GJ, Nahit ES, Silman AJ, McBeth J. 2004: Mechanical injury and psychosocial factors in the work place predict the onset of widespread body pain: a two-year prospective study among cohorts of newly employed workers. *Arthritis Rheum* 50:1655–1664.

Hotopf M, David A, Hull L, Ismail K, Unwin C, Wessely S. 2000: Role of vaccinations as risk factors for ill health in veterans of the Gulf War: cross sectional study. *BMJ* 320:1363–1367.

Hsieh JC, Stahle-Backdahl M, Hagermark O, Stone-Elander S, Rosenquist G, Ingvar M. 1996: Traumatic nociceptive pain activates the hypothalamus and the periaqueductal gray: a positron emission tomography study. *Pain* 64:303–314.

Hsieh JC, Tu CH, Chen FP, Chen MC, Yeh TC, Cheng HC, et al. 2001: Activation of the hypothalamus characterizes the acupuncture stimulation at the analgesic point in human: a positron emission tomography study. *Neurosci Lett* 307:105–108.

Jones AK, Liyi Q, Cunningham VV, Brown DW, Ha-Kawa S, Fujiwara T, et al. 1991: Endogenous opiate response to pain in rheumatoid arthritis and cortical and subcortical response to pain in normal volunteers using positron emission tomography. *Int J Clin Pharmacol Res* 11:261–266.

Jones AK, Cunningham VJ, Ha-Kawa S, Fujiwara T, Luthra SK, Silva S, et al. 1994: Changes in central opioid receptor binding in relation to inflammation and pain in patients with rheumatoid arthritis. *Br J Rheumatol* 33:909–916.

Jones AK, Derbyshire SW. 1996: Cerebral mechanisms operating in the presence and absence of inflammatory pain. *Ann Rheum Dis* 55:411–420.

Jones AK. 1999: The contribution of functional imaging techniques to our understanding of rheumatic pain. *Rheum Dis Clin North Am* 25:123–152.

Jones AK, Kulkarni B, Derbyshire SW. 2003: Pain mechanisms and their disorders. *Br Med Bull* 65:83–93.

Jones AK, Watabe H, Cunningham VJ, Jones T. 2004: Cerebral decreases in opioid receptor binding in patients with central neuropathic pain measured by [11C] diprenorphine binding and PET 6. *Eur J Pain* 8:479–485.

Jones AK. Categories of placebo response in the absence of site-specific expectation of analgesia. *Pain* 2006 126:115–122.

Kakigi R, Inui K, Tamura Y. 2005: Electrophysiological studies on human pain perception. *Clin Neurophysiol* 116:743–763.

Kopec JA and Sayre EC. 2005: Stressful experiences in childhood and chronic back pain in the general population. *Clin J Pain* 21:478–483.

Krag NJ, Norregaard J, Larsen JK, Danneskiold-Samsoe B. 1994: A blinded, controlled evaluation of anxiety and depressive symptoms in patients with fibromyalgia, as measured by standardized psychometric interview scales. *Acta Psychiatric Scandinavia* 89:370–375.

Kulkarni B, Bentley DE, Elliott R, Youell P, Watson A, Derbyshire SW, et al. 2005: Attention to pain localization and unpleasantness discriminates the functions of the medial and lateral pain systems. *Eur J Neurosci* 21:3133–3142.

Kunz-Ebrecht SR, Kirschbaum C, Steptoe A. 2004: Work stress, socioeconomic status and neuroendocrine activation over the working day. *Soc Sci Med* 58:1523–1530

Leal-Cerro A, Povedano J, Astorga R, Gonzalez M, Silva H, Garcia-Pesquera F, et al. 1999: The growth hormone (GH)-releasing hormone - GH - insulin-like growth factor-1 axis in patients with fibromyalgia syndrome. *J Clin Endocrin Metab* 84:3378–3381.

Leonard BE. The HPA and immune axes in stress: the involvement of the serotonergic system. *Eur Psychiatry* 2005 20 Suppl 3:S302–S306.

Magni G, Moreschi C, Rigatti-Luchini S, Merskey H. 1994: Prospective study on the relationship between depressive symptoms and chronic musculoskeletal pain. *Pain* 56:289–297.

Mallen CD, Peat G, Thomas E, Croft PR. 2006: Is chronic pain in adulthood related to childhood factors? A population-based case-control study of young adults. *J Rheumatol* **33**:2286–2290.

McBeth J, Macfarlane GJ, Benjamin S, Morris S, Silman AJ. 1999: The association between tender points, psychological distress, and adverse childhood experiences: a community-based study. *Arthritis Rheum* **42**:1397–1404.

McBeth J, Macfarlane GJ, Benjamin S, Silman AJ. 2001a: Features of somatization predict the onset of chronic widespread pain: results of a large population-based study. *Arthritis Rheum* **44**:940–946.

McBeth J, Morris S, Benjamin S, Silman AJ, Macfarlane GJ. 2001b: Associations between adverse events in childhood and chronic widespread pain in adulthood: are they explained by differential recall? *J Rheumatol* **28**:2305–2309.

McBeth J, Harkness EF, Silman AJ, Macfarlane GJ. 2003: Mechanical injury and psychosocial factors in the work-place predict the onset of widespread body pain: a 2-year prospective study amongst cohorts of newly-employed workers. *Arthritis Rheum* **48**(9, Supplement):S237.

McBeth J, Chiu YH, Silman AJ, Ray D, Morriss R, Dickens C, et al. 2005: Hypothalamic-pituitary-adrenal stress axis function and the relationship with chronic widespread pain and its antecedents. *Arthritis Res Ther* **7**:R992–R1000.

McBeth J, Silman AJ, Gupta A, Chiu YH, Ray D, Morriss R, et al. 2007: Moderation of psychosocial risk factors through dysfunction of the hypothalamic-pituitary-adrenal stress axis in the onset of chronic widespread musculoskeletal pain: findings of a population-based prospective cohort study. *Arthritis Rheum* **56**:360–371.

McCain GA, Tilbe KS. 1989: Duirnal hormone variation in fibromyalgia syndrome: a comparison with rheumatoid arthritis. *J Rheumatol* **16** (suppl 19):154–157.

McDiarmid MA, Squibb K, Engelhardt S, Oliver M, Gucer P, Wilson PD, et al. 2001: Surveillance of depleted uranium exposed Gulf War veterans: health effects observed in an enlarged "friendly fire" cohort. *J Occup Environ Med* **43**:991–1000.

McLean SA, Clauw DJ, Abelson JL, Liberzon I. 2005a: The development of persistent pain and psychological morbidity after motor vehicle collision: integrating the potential role of stress response systems into a biopsychosocial model. *Psychosom Med* **67**:783–790.

McLean SA, Williams DA, Harris RE, Kop WJ, Groner KH, Ambrose K, et al. 2005b: Momentary relationship between cortisol secretion and symptoms in patients with fibromyalgia. *Arthritis Rheum* **52**: 3660–3669.

McLean SA, Williams DA, Stein PK, Harris RE, Lyden AK, Whalen G, et al. 2006: Cerebrospinal fluid corticotropin-releasing factor concentration is associated with pain but not fatigue symptoms in patients with fibromyalgia. *Neuropsychopharmacology* **31**:2776–2782.

McEwen BS. Stress, adaptation and disease; Allostasis and allostatic load. *Ann N Y Acad Sci* 1998 **840**:33–44.

McWilliams LA, Cox BJ, Enns MW. 2000: Impact of adult attachment styles on pain and disability associated with arthritis in a nationally representative sample. *Clin J Pain* **16**:360–4.

McWilliams LA and Asmundson GJ. 2007: The relationship of adult attachment dimensions to pain-related fear, hypervigilance, and catastrophizing. *Pain* **127**:27–34.

Melzack R. 1990: Phantom limbs and the concept of a neuromatrix. *Trends Neurosci* **13**:88–92.

Mendlewicz J. 2009: Disruption of the circadian timing systems: molecular mechanisms in mood disorders. *CNS Drugs* **23** Suppl 2:15–26.

Meredith PJ, Strong J, Feeney JA. 2006: The relationship of adult attachment to emotion, catastrophizing, control, threshold and tolerance, in experimentally-induced pain. *Pain* **120**:44–52.

Meredith PJ, Strong J, Feeney JA. 2007: Adult attachment variables predict depression before and after treatment for chronic pain. *Eur J Pain* **11**:164–170.

Millan MJ. 2002: Descending control of pain. *Prog Neurobiol* **66**:355–474.

Morton DL, Watson A, El-Deredy W, Jones AK. 2009: Reproducibility of placebo analgesia: Effect of dispositional optimism. *Pain* **146**:194–8.

Montgomery GH and Kirsch I. 1997: Classical conditioning and the placebo effect. *Pain* **72**:107–113.

Neugebauer V, Li W, Bird GC, Han JS. 2004: The amygdala and persistent pain. *Neuroscientist* **10**:221–234.

Ostrowsky K, Magnin M, Ryvlin P, Isnard J, Guenot M, Mauguiere F. 2002: Representation of pain and somatic sensation in the human insula: a study of responses to direct electrical cortical stimulation. *Cereb Cortex* **12**:376–385.

Papadimitriou A and Priftis KN. 2009: Regulation of the hypothalamic-pituitary-adrenal axis. *Neuroimmunomodulation* **16**:265–271.

Papanicolaou DA, Wilder RL, Manolagas SC, Chrousos GP. 1998: The pathophysiologic roles of interleukin-6 in human disease. *Ann Intern Med* **128**:127–137.

Peeters GM, van Schoor NM, Visser M, Knol DL, Eekhoff EM, De Ronde W, et al. 2007: Relationship between cortisol and physical performance in older persons. *Clin Endocrinol* **67**:398–406.

Petrovic P, Ingvar M. 2002: Imaging cognitive modulation of pain processing. *Pain* **95**:1–5.

Peyron R, Garcia-Larrea L, Gregoire MC, Convers P, Richard A, Lavenne F, et al. 2000: Parietal and cingulate processes in central pain. A combined positron emission tomography (PET) and functional magnetic resonance imaging (fMRI) study of an unusual case. *Pain* **84**:77–87

Ploner M, Schmitz F, Freund HJ, Schnitzler A. 1999: Parallel activation of primary and secondary somatosensory cortices in human pain processing. *J Neurophysiol* **81**:3100–3104.

Ploner M, Schmitz F, Freund HJ, Schnitzler A. 2000: Differential organization of touch and pain in human primary somatosensory cortex. *J Neurophysiol* Mar **83**:1770–1776.

Plotsky PM, Meaney MJ. 1993: Early, postnatal experience alters hypothalamic corticotropin-releasing factor (CRF) mRNA, median eminence CRF content and stress-induced release in adult rats. *Brain Res Mol Brain Res* **18**:195–200.

Porro CA and Carli G. 1988: Immobilization and restraint effects on pain reactions in animals. *Pain* **32**: 289–307.

Porro CA, Cettolo V, Francescato MP, Baraldi P. 1998: Temporal and intensity coding of pain in human cortex. *J Neurophysiol* **80**:3312–3320.

Rainville P. 2002: Brain mechanisms of pain affect and pain modulation. *Curr Opin Neurobiol* **12**: 195–204.

Raphael KG, Widom CS, Lange G. 2001: Childhood victimization and pain in adulthood: a prospective investigation. *Pain* **92**:283–293.

Rilling JK, Winslow JT, O'Brien D, Gutman DA, Hoffman JM, Kilts CD. 2001: Neural correlates of maternal separation in rhesus monkeys. *Biol Psychiatry* **49**:146–157.

Rosmond R, Bjorntorp P. 2000: The hypothalamic-pituitary-adrenal axis activity as a predictor of cardiovascular disease, type 2 diabetes and stroke. *J Intern Med* **247**:188–197.

Russell IJ, Vaeroy H, Javors M, Nyberg F. 1992: Cerebospinal fluid biogenic amine metabolites in fibromyalgia/fibrositis syndrome and rheumatoid arthritis. *Arthritis Rheum* **35**:550–556.

Russell IJ, Vipraio GA. 1994: Serotonin (5HT) in serum and platelets from fibromyalgia patients and normal controls - abstract. *Arthritis Rheum* **37**:S214.

Salemi S, Rethage J, Wollina U, Michel BA, Gay RE, Gay S, et al. 2003: Detection of interleukin 1beta (IL-1beta), IL-6, and tumor necrosis factor-alpha in skin of patients with fibromyalgia. *J Rheumatol* **30**: 146–150.

Schlereth T, Baumgartner U, Magerl W, Stoeter P, Treede RD. 2003: Left-hemisphere dominance in early nociceptive processing in the human parasylvian cortex. *Neuroimage* **20**:441–454.

Schwarz MJ, Spath M, Muller-Bardorff H, Pongratz DE, Bondy B, Ackenheil M. 1999: Relationship of substance P, 5-hydroxyindole acetic acid and tryptophan in serum of fibromyalgia patients. *Neurosci Lett* **15** 259:196–188.

Smith JD, Terpening CM, Schmidt SO, Gums JG. 2001: Relief of fibromyalgia symptoms following discontinuation of dietary excitotoxins. *Ann Pharmacother* **35**:702–706.

Sverdrup B. 2004: Use less cosmetics--suffer less from fibromyalgia? *J Womens Health* **13**:187–194.

Tafet GE, Feder DJ, Abulafia DP, Roffman SS. 2005: Regulation of hypothalamic-pituitary-adrenal activity in response to cognitive therapy in patients with generalized anxiety disorder. *Cogn Affect Behav Neurosci* **5**:37–40.

The Iowa Persian Gulf Study Group. 1997: Self-reported illness and health status among Gulf War veterans. A population-based study. *JAMA* **277**:238–245.

Tishler M, Levy O, Maslakov I, Bar-Chaim S, mit-Vazina M. 2006: Neck injury and fibromyalgia—are they really associated? *J Rheumatol* **33**:1183–1185.

Treede RD, Kenshalo DR, Gracely RH, Jones AK. 1999: The cortical representation of pain. *Pain* **79**:105–11.

van Voorhees E, Scarpa A. 2004: The effects of child maltreatment on the hypothalamic-pituitary-adrenal axis. *Trauma Violence Abuse* **5**:333–352.

Vogt MJ, Heffner JE, Sahn SA. 1993: Vomiting, abdominal pain, and visual disturbances in a 31-year-old man. *Chest* **103**:262–263.

Wager TD, Rilling JK, Smith EE, Sokolik A, Casey KL, Davidson RJ, et al. 2004: Placebo-induced changes in FMRI in the anticipation and experience of pain. *Science* 20 **303**:1162–1167.

Wallace DJ, Linker-Israeli M, Hallegua D, Silverman S, Silver D, Weisman MH. 2001: Cytokines play an aetiopathogenetic role in fibromyalgia: a hypothesis and pilot study. *Rheumatology* **40**:743–749.

Wang H, Buchner M, Moser MT, Daniel V, Schiltenwolf M. 2009: The role of IL-8 in patients with fibromyalgia: a prospective longitudinal study of 6 months. *Clin J Pain* **25**:1–4.

Watkins LR, Cobelli DA, Mayer DJ. 1982: Classical conditioning of front paw and hind paw footshock induced analgesia (FSIA): naloxone reversibility and descending pathways. *Brain Res* **243**:119–132.

Watson A, El-Deredy W, Vogt BA, Jones AK. 2007: Placebo analgesia is not due to compliance or habituation: EEG and behavioural evidence. *Neuroreport* **18**:771–775.

Wearden A, Perryman K, Ward V. 2006: Adult attachment, reassurance seeking and hypochondriacal concerns in college students. *J Health Psychol* **11**:877–886.

Willer JC, Dehen H, Bourea F, Cambier J, Albe-Fessard D. 1981: Nociceptive reflexes and pain sensation in man. *Pain* **10**:405–410.

Willer JC, Le Bars D, De Broucker T. 1990: Diffuse noxious inhibitory controls in man: involvement of an opioidergic link. *Eur J Pharmacol* **182**:347–355.

Wolfe F. 1999: "Silicone related symptoms" are common in patients with fibromyalgia: No evidence for a new disease. *J Rheumatol* **26**:1172–1175.

Youell PD, Wise RG, Bentley DE, Dickinson MR, King TA, Tracey I, et al. 2004: Lateralisation of nociceptive processing in the human brain: a functional magnetic resonance imaging study. *Neuroimage* **23**:1068–1077.

Yunus M, Masi AT, Calabro JJ, Miller KA, Feigenbaum SL. 1981: Primary fibromyalgia (fibrositis): clinical study of 50 patients with matched normal controls. *Semin Arthritis Rheum* **11**:151–171.

Zhang Z, Cherryholmes G, Mao A, Marek C, Longmate J, Kalos M, et al. 2008: High plasma levels of MCP-1 and eotaxin provide evidence for an immunological basis of fibromyalgia. *Exp Biol Med* **233**: 1171–1180.

Zubieta JK, Smith YR, Bueller JA, Xu Y, Kilbourn MR, Jewett DM, et al. 2001: Regional mu opioid receptor regulation of sensory and affective dimensions of pain. *Science* **293**:311–315.

Glossary

Ablative surgery – It is the irreversible surgical removal, by burning or freezing, of brain tissue

Afferent nerve – Nerve fibres that carry electrical impulses towards the central nervous system

Allostatic load – The physiological adaptive response to maintain homeostasis in responses to external stressors

Anticipatory-evoked potential – An electrical response in the brain due to the anticipation of a stimulus

Deafferentation – Interruption of sensory nerve impulses by destroying or injuring the sensory nerve fibres

Dexamethasone suppression test – A clinical test that measures the ability of dexamethasone to suppress ACTH and cortisol secretion by the adrenal gland

Hyperalgesia – An increased sensitivity to pain, caused by damage to nociceptors or peripheral nerves

Interoceptive – Relating to sensations originating inside the body

Neuropathic pain – Pain due to injury to the nervous system

Nociceptive – Relating to activation of nerve fibres that are specialized to respond to damaging or potentially damaging stimuli that may be perceived as painful

Pain-evoked potentials – An electrical response in the brainstem or cerebral cortex that is elicited by a pain stimulus

Placebo analgesia – Pain relief as a result of exposure to an inert substance or procedure (pill, cream, or injection) that has no direct physiological effect

Pro-inflammatory cytokines – Secreted proteins that regulate the inflammatory response

Somatization – Disorders of psychological origin

Chapter 10

Musculoskeletal pain complaints from a sex and gender perspective

H. Susan J. Picavet[1]

Summary

Musculoskeletal pain is a major public health problem because of high prevalence rates and the considerable burden in terms of work disability and health care use.

Prevalence rates of musculoskeletal pain are higher in women than in men. There are three explanations for this:

1 the 'gender-role' theory assumes that it is socially more accepted for women to report pain than for men;

2 the 'exposure' theory states that women are more exposed than men to risk factors for musculoskeletal pain; and

3 the 'vulnerability' theory proposes that women are more vulnerable to developing musculoskeletal pain than men.

Scientific evidence for the 'gender-role' and 'exposure' theories is scarce. Most evidence points in the direction of the 'vulnerability' theory. Sex hormones seem to play a role in explaining the higher prevalence of musculoskeletal pain in women.

Further insights into the pathophysiology of sex differences may – in the future – provide clues for improvement of prevention and treatment of musculoskeletal pain and chronic pain more generally.

Epidemiology

Women report musculoskeletal pain complaints more often than men.(5) For instance, 39% of the Dutch men between 25 and 64 years of age reported chronic musculoskeletal pain (>6 months) compared to 45% of the women in a population-based survey (Dutch population-based Musculoskeletal Complaints and Consequences Cohort (DMC3) study). This 6% difference paints a rosy picture because it is a sum of several anatomical locations of pain, and women have pain relatively more frequently at more than one location: multiple pain is reported by 23% of the women versus 17% of the men.

---

[1] This text is a revised translation of the following Dutch paper and presented here with permission of the co-authors and the Dutch Journal of Physiotherapy:

Wijnhoven HAH, de Vet HCW, Hooftman WE, van der Beek AJ, de Heer K, Picavet HSJ. Waarom rapporteren vrouwen vaker pijnklachten van het bewegingsapparaat dan mannen? [Why do women report more often musculoskeletal pain than men?] Ned Tijdschrift voor Fysiotherapie [Dutch Journal of Physiotherapy] 2008;118:109-112

Table 10.1 Range of female/male prevalence ratios for musculoskeletal pain in several studies in the general or working population*

Anatomical site of pain	Lower RR**	Upper RR
Neck	1.26	2.68
Shoulders	1.21	2.61
Higher back	1.20	3.45
Elbow	0.91	1.72
Wrist/hand	0.96	2.35
Lower back	0.96	2.04
Hip	1.31	2.48
Knee	0.89	1.16
Ankle	1.13	2.25
Foot	1.21	2.47

*based on review of Wijnhoven et al. 2006(6)

**RR = relative risk

The sex differences are found for pain in the neck, shoulder, higher back, elbow, wrist/hand, hip, and ankle/foot. For the wrist/hand region the reported pain among women is twice as high as it is among men. For low back pain and knee pain the sex difference is almost absent. Sex differences in musculoskeletal pain are found in most prevalence studies in all Western countries.(5) Table 10.1 presents the range of female–male prevalence ratios for musculoskeletal pain at different body sites found in the literature up to 2005. More recent studies also suggest that the higher prevalence of pain in women is pretty consistent across countries and cultures elsewhere in the world. A population-based survey among adults aged 20 years and older in Brazil showed that 48.4% of the women reported chronic pain versus 32.8% of the men.(10) In a study in Japan among 1017 and 1209 pain-free men and women, respectively, 40% of the men and 54% of the women developed incident pain during the 1-month follow-up. The predominance of women was especially found for neck and knee pain.(11) Chronic pain was also systematically higher in adult women compared to adult men in all age categories in eight developing and 10 developed countries which participated in the World Mental Health Surveys.(12)

For health care the differences between men and women are even more distinct because women are more inclined to seek health care.(13) Among those with chronic musculoskeletal pain 55% of the men and 61% of the women reported contact with a general practitioner, medical specialist and/or physiotherapist, as shown by the earlier mentioned population-based survey.(6)

Mechanisms

There are three possible explanations for the observed sex differences in musculoskeletal pain: first, the 'gender-role' theory assumes that it is more socially acceptable for women to report pain than for men; second, the 'exposure' theory states that women are more exposed than men to risk factors for musculoskeletal pain; and, third, the 'vulnerability' theory hypothesises that women are more prone to developing musculoskeletal pain than men.

Gender-role theory

The gender-role theory refers to socially learned behaviour: big boys don't cry. This might explain the lower prevalence of pain reporting among men. The idea is that women and men experience the same pain but react to it differently. Experiments using standard pain stimuli, such as pressure pain, electrical pain, and heat or cold pain, were performed to determine whether women experience more pain, or only report more pain. These experiments show that healthy women report more intense pain compared to men, and that men have a higher pain threshold and a higher tolerance compared to women.(14–18) Along with self-reported pain, dilatation of the pupil can be used as a measure of pain experience in an experimental setting. Pupil dilatation may be a more 'objective' measure of the actual experience and intensity of pain than self-reported pain, but this is still debated. One study, which used tonic pressure of the fingers as the pain stimulus,(14) showed that women not only report more, and more intense, pain given the same stimulus, but also that they had greater pupil reaction than men. The reaction of the pupil was highly correlated with both the intensity of pain and the pain reporting. Such studies suggest that women do experience more pain than men given the same pain stimulus, which supports the vulnerability rather than the gender-role theory.

Another experiment provides support for the gender-role theory. There is some evidence that men have a higher pain threshold. An experiment using cold-water stimuli showed that women report pain sooner than men after such provocation.(15) In this particular study also, the effect of different instructions was studied. If, just before the experiment, it was said that a typical man or woman (referring to the participant's own gender) can hold their hand in cold water for 30 s (or longer periods – up to 90 s), there were no differences in the time to reporting pain between men and women. The participants appeared to react according to expectations linked to their gender, which supports the gender-role theory in explaining sex differences in pain reporting.

Further research on whether the gender role affects the prevalence of musculoskeletal pain could usefully draw on cross-cultural studies. An interesting question is whether the sex differences in pain reporting are the same in different cultures, for which there is accumulating evidence from crude prevalence studies reviewed above, or whether this varies between cultures with different sex-related social roles.

Exposure theory

If women in general have higher exposure than men to risk factors for musculoskeletal pain, this would also affect the prevalence of pain. Within the workforce, men and women are not equally distributed across professions and type of work. Even if they have the same profession, men and women may be carrying out different activities (19) or perform the same tasks in a very different way.(20) These results suggest that there are sex differences in exposure to work-related factors, such as physical load and stress, which are important risks for musculoskeletal pain complaints.(21) Besides differences in workload in paid work and employment, sex differences are also apparent in leisure-time and household activities: women often play the largest part in household activities and care of children.

The Study on Musculoskeletal disorders, Absenteeism Stress and Health (SMASH) study (see Box 10.1) showed that sex differences in exposure to work-related physical and psychosocial risk factors varies for different jobs or professions.(22) Male construction workers reported risk factors for back pain more often than their female colleagues, while exposure to risk factors for upper extremity pain was more often reported by female than male clerks. Work-related psychosocial risk factors were measured using the 'Demand-Control-Support' model of Karasek, and a question on satisfaction with the job completed.(23) Three sources of stress are distinguished in Karasek's model: too high task demands, too little autonomy and lack of social support. Women reported relatively less autonomy and higher task demands, but were also more satisfied with the job.(22)

Another part of the SMASH study focused on sex differences in the performance of the same tasks. Duration and frequency of physical load was assessed by video recording and analysed.

Box 10.1 Dutch epidemiological research on sex differences in musculoskeletal pain

This chapter is an English version of a Dutch paper (1), which summarizes findings from two Dutch research projects on sex differences in musculoskeletal pain.

One project was a PhD-project (2) using data from the

◆ Study on Musculoskeletal disorders, Absenteeism Stress and Health (SMASH), a longitudinal study focused on determining risk factors for musculoskeletal complaints, which recruited nearly 1800 employees in 34 companies.

At the 1994 baseline measurements, participants filled out a questionnaire, which included questions on both physical and psychosocial exposures at work. A more detailed description of the study design can be found elsewhere. (3,4) The study also included an assessment of the physical load by video recording.

The second project (5–8) was based on data from two population-based surveys:

◆ the Dutch population-based Musculoskeletal Complaints and Consequences cohort study (DMC$_3$-studie),(9) with a baseline measurement and one follow-up after 6 months, of around 3500 men and women aged ≥25 years, and the Monitoring study on Risk Factors and Health in the Netherlands (MoRGen-study) (5) with >20 000 men and women in the age range of 20–60 years.

No differences between men and women were found, which suggests that, if there are differences in exposure between men and women, this is not because they perform the same tasks differently but because they carry out different tasks.(24)

If the exposure theory were the major explanation for women reporting more musculoskeletal pain than men, then sex differences found in a statistical model would disappear after taking the relevant risk factors into account. In the Dutch studies, the sex differences in incident musculoskeletal pain in fact remained the same in the univariate as in the multivariate analyses, adjusting for exposure to different risk factors. This was found for both the working population of the SMASH study (25) and for the general population of the DMC3-study.(8) The model in the SMASH study included many risk factors measured a year before incident pain complaints: socio-demographic factors, physical and psychosocial work-related facors, and physical and psychosocial non-work-related factors. The DMC3-study showed that the sex difference in chronic musculoskeletal pain also did not disappear after adding exposures, such as smoking, overweight, and physical activities.

In sum it can be concluded that there is little indication that sex differences in musculoskeletal pain can be explained by the exposure theory.

Vulnerability theory

Women and men differ in anatomy and physiology, and these differences might be the basis for a greater vulnerability to developing musculoskeletal pain among women compared with men. This was also suggested by experimental studies discussed above, which showed women report more pain than men given the same pain stimulus. The vulnerability theory refers to sex-specific effects of common risk factors, or sex-specific risk factors affecting pain experiences and pain perception.

For work-related risk factors, both physical and psychosocial, no proof has been found for there being sex-specific associations between established risk factors and musculoskeletal pain. This was shown in a systematic review and in analyses of the SMASH study.(26,27) Moreover, where a sex-specific effect size was found, the association was usually stronger for men than for women. The DMC3 population-based survey showed one exception to this: overweight was more strongly related to musculoskeletal pain among women than among men.(8) This sex-specific effect of overweight was also found in a study among the elderly,(28) although there are conflicting studies not finding this effect.(29)

The role of sex hormones

One major theme in considering sex-specific risk factors refers to sex hormones. Although the effect of sex hormones on pain is a popular research theme – especially in experimental research – their exact role is not yet clear.(30) Hormones and reproduction-related characteristics were associated with low back pain in a sample of >11 000 Dutch women in the age range of 20–60 years from the population-based MoRGeN (the monitoring project on risk factors and health in The Netherlands) study.(7) The factors were: parity, a young age at first childbirth, long duration of pill use, oestrogen supplementation during menopause, an early menarche, an unusual menstruation cycle (irregular or very long), and hysterectomy. These findings suggest an effect of hormones and reproduction-related characteristics on musculoskeletal pain.

Some proposed underlying explanations for the role of hormones in pain are as follows. One is that relaxine, the 'pregnancy hormone', stimulates laxity of the ligaments of the pelvis which can result in back pain.(7) Pill use might also contribute to higher concentrations of relaxine. Another explanation is that a decreasing or fluctuating level of oestrogen is associated with pain experience. This was shown in a study on temporomandibular pain focusing on the role of oestrogen use, the menstrual cycle, pregnancy, and puberty.(31–34) There is also a pathophysiologic explanation for this: oestradiol affects some forms of neurotransmission, the system of information exchange between nerves. In particular, a low oestrogen level is associated with a lower activity of opioid-mediated neurotransmission and a lower level of pain reporting.(35)

In sum, sex hormones probably have an effect on pain nociception. This can, at least in part, explain sex differences in musculoskeletal pain via the vulnerability theory.

The role of psychology

Besides biological differences, there are also sex-related psychological differences that may affect pain. A psychological premise is that women have a more emotionally focused coping strategy for increased pain sensations – and men a more problem-oriented coping strategy.(36) One example of negative emotionally focused coping is pain catastrophizing: having extreme negative thoughts and behaviour concerning pain experience. There is some indication that pain catastrophizing is more often seen among women than men.(8) A higher prevalence of pain catastrophizing among women does not necessary explain their higher prevalence of musculoskeletal pain. For pain catastropizing, the association with pain is stronger in men than in women.(8,37,38) This could mean that, although pain catastrophizing is more frequently found among women, it is a stronger risk in men for the continuation of pain. The consequence might be that psychological interventions such as cognitive behavioural therapy are more effective among men than among women.

Public health consequences of sex differences

One of the reasons for investigating the exact mechanisms of higher pain prevalence in women is that they may reveal potentially preventable components of the gender difference which would be valuable to tackle from a public health perspective. One reason that gender differences are so important to the public health perspective is that, by definition, the 'exposure' to the risk factor of gender is common, basically ~50% of any population, and the disease conditions (painful musculoskeletal syndromes) are also universally common.

If we accept the consistency of the findings presented above about painful muscloskeletal syndromes in women as representing a conservative overall relative risk estimate of 1.2 (i.e. 20% higher risk than men), and that 60% of chronic pain worldwide is musculoskeletal in origin, then a conservative estimate of the proportion of all chronic pain that can be attributed to gender or to some characteristic related to gender is

$$\{60 \times (0.50 \times (1.2-1))/(0.50 \times (1.2-1)+1))\} = 5\%$$

(This is probably an underestimate to the extent that painful conditions other than musculoskeletal conditions are more common in women also, but allows for the substantial concurrence of these other conditions with musculoskeletal pan).

This means that, very crudely and approximately, 5% of chronic pain in the world is attributable to female gender or a characteristic linked to female gender.

Final reflections

Sex differences in musculoskeletal pain are clear but this does not hold for the explanation of sex differences. The explanation is probably not to be found in the difference in exposures. The vulnerability theory might be true because, for instance, sex hormones might affect musculoskeletal pain. It is largely unknown how sex-specific social roles and expectations affect pain reporting and pain perception.

Musculoskeletal pain represents a large public health problem due to its high prevalence, and its relation to work leave, work disability, and health care utilization. The fact that women have a higher frequency of pain than men should alone justify increased attention being paid to the prevention of pain among women. However, more research on the mechanisms behind sex differences in musculoskeletal pain may contribute more generally to the further development of effective preventive interventions and treatments.

Finally, the mechanisms reviewed in this chapter might conribute both to the onset of musculoskeletal pain and to the likelihood that it will persist. Specific evidence, that being a man or woman can also affect long-term outcome of musculoskeletal pain even after intense interventions, is provided by a study on prognostic factors for the 1-year outcome of 283 patients with sciatica (including ~60% having surgery) showing that female gender was a strong predictor of unsatisfactory outcome at 1 year.(39)

References

1 Wijnhoven HAH, de Vet HCW, Hooftman WE, van der Beek AJ, de Heer K, Picavet HSJ. 2008: Waarom rapporteren vrouwen vaker pijnklachten van het bewegingsapparaat dan mannen? Ned Tijdschrift voor Fysiotherapie 118:109–112

2 Hooftman WE. 2006: *Gender differences in work-related risk factors for musculoskeletal symptoms and absenteeism* [PhD thesis]. Amsterdam: VU Amsterdam.

3 Hoogendoorn WE, Bongers PM, de Vet HCW, et al. 2000: Flexion and rotation of the trunk and lifting at work are risk factors for low back pain: results of a prospective cohort study. Spine. 25:3087–3092

4 Ariëns GAM, Bongers PM, Douwes M, Miedema M, Hoogendoorn WE, Wal G van der, et al. 2001: Are neck flexion, neck rotation and sitting at work risk factors for neck pain? Results of a prospective cohort study. Occup Environ Med **58**:200–207.

5 Wijnhoven HAH, Vet HCW de, Picavet HSJ. 2006: Prevalence of musculoskeletal disorders is systematically higher in women than in men. Clin J Pain 22:717–724.

6 Wijnhoven HAH, de Vet HCW, Picavet HSJ. 2007: Sex differences in consequences of musculoskeletal pain. Spine 32:1360–1367.

7 Wijnhoven HAH, Vet HCW de, Smit HA, Picavet HSJ. 2006: Hormonal and reproductive factors are associated with chronic low back pain and chronic upper extremity pain in women – the MORGEN study. Spine 13:1496–1502.

8 Wijnhoven HAH, Vet HCW de, Picavet HSJ. 2006: Explaining sex differences in chronic musculoskeletal pain in a general population. Pain 124:158–166.

9 Picavet HSJ, Schouten JSAG. 2003: Musculoskeletal pain in the Netherlands: prevalences, consequences and risk groups, the DMC3-study. Pain 102:167–178.

10 Sa KN, Baptista AF, Matos MA, Lessa I. 2008: Chronic pain and gender in Salvador population, Brazil. Pain 139:498–506.

11 Tokuda Y, Ohde A, Takahashi O, Shakudo M, Yanai H, Shimbo T, et al. 2007: Musculoskeletal pain in Japan: prospective health diary study. Rheumatol Int 28:7–14.

12 Tsang A, Von Korff M, Lee S, Alonso J, Karam E, Angermeyer MC, et al. 2008: Common chronic pain conditions in developed and developing countries: gender and age differences and comorbidity with depression-anxiety disorders. J Pain 9:883–891.

13 Picavet HSJ, Struijs JN, Westert GP. 2008: Utilization of health resources due to low back pain – survey and registered data compared. Spine 33:436–444.

14 Ellermeier W, Westphal W. 1995: Gender differences in pain ratings and pupil reactions to painful pressure stimuli. Pain 61:435–439.

15 Robinson ME, Gagnon CM, Riley JL, Price DD. 2003: Altering gender role expectations: effects on pain tolerance, pain treshold, and pain ratings. J Pain 4:284–288.

16 Riley JL, Robinson ME, Wise EA, Myers CD, Fillingim RB. 1998: Sex differences in the perception of noxious experimental stimuli: a meta-analysis. Pain 74:181–188.

17 Wiesenfeld-Hallin Z. 2005: Sex differences in pain perception. Gender Medicine. 2:137–145.

18 Fillingim RB, King CD, Ribeiro-Dasilva MC, Rahim-Williams B, Riley III JL. 2009: Sex, gender and pain: a review of recent clinical and experimental findings. J Pain 10:447–485.

19 Messing K, Dumais L, Courville J, Seifert AM, Boucher M. 1994: Evaluation of exposure data from men and women with the same job title. J Occup Med 36:913–917.

20 Beek AJ van der, Kluver BDR, Frings-Dresen MHW, Hoozemans MJM. 2000: Gender differences in exerted forces and physiological load during pushing and pulling of wheeled cages by postal workers. Ergonomics 43:269–281.

21 Waters TR, Dick RB, Davis-Barkley J, Krieg EF. 2007: A cross-sectional study of risk factors for musculoskeletal symptoms in the workplace using data from the General Social Survey (GSS). J Occup Environ Med 49:172–184.

22 Hooftman WE, Beek AJ van der, Bongers PM, Mechelen W van. 2005: Gender differences in self-reported physical and psychosocial exposures in jobs with both female and male workers. J Occup Environ Med 47:244–252.

23 Karasek R, Brisson C, Kawakami N, Houtman ILD, Bongers PM, Amick B. 1998: The job content questionnaire (JCQ): an instrument for internationally comparative assessments of psychosocial job characteristics. J Occup Health Psychol 3:322–355.

24 Hooftman WE, Beek AJ van der, Wal BG van der, Knol DL, Bongers PM, Burdorf A, Mechelen W van. 2009: Equal task, equal exposure? Are men and women with the same tasks equally exposed to physical risk facors for work-related musculoskeletal disorders? Ergonomics 52:1079–1086.

25 Hooftman WE, Beek AJ van der, Bongers PM, Punnett L, van Mechelen W. 2006: Gender differences in the prevalence of musculoskeletal symptoms are not explained by exposure differences. In: Hooftman WE ed. Gender differences in work-related risk factors for musculoskeletal symptoms and absenteeism. [PhD thesis]. Amsterdam: VU Amsterdam.

26 Hooftman WE, Poppel MNM van, Beek AJ van der, Bongers PM, Mechelen W van. 2004: Gender differences in the relations between work-related physical and psychosocial risk factors and musculoskeletal complaints. Scand J Work Environ Health **30**:261–278.

27 Hooftman WE, Beek AJ van der, Bongers PM, Mechelen W van. 2006: Physical and psychosocial risk factors at work in relation to (sickness absence due to) musculoskeletal symptoms; is there a gender difference? In: Hooftman WE ed. *Gender differences in work-related risk factors for musculoskeletal symptoms and absenteeism* [PhD thesis]. Amsterdam: VU Amsterdam.

28 Leveille SG, Zhang Y, McMullen W, Kelley-Hayes M, Felson DT. 2005: Sex differences in musculoskeletal pain in older adults. Pain **116**:332–338.

29 Leboeuf-Yde C. 2000: Body weight and low back pain. A systematic literature review of 56 journal articles reporting on 65 epidemiologic studies. Spine **25**:226–237.

30 Aloisi AM, Bonifazi M. 2006: Sex hormones, central nervous system and pain. Horm Behav **50**:1–7.

31 LeResche L, Saunders K, Korff MR von, Barlow W, Dworkin SF. 1997: Use of exogenous hormones and risk of temporomandibular disorder pain. Pain **69**:153–160.

32 LeResche L, Mancl LA, Drangsholt MT, Saunders K, Korff M von. 2005: Relationship of pain and symptoms to pubertal development in adolescents. Pain **118**:201–209.

33 LeResche L, Mancl L, Sherman JJ, Gandara B, Dworkin SF. 2003: Changes in temporomandibular pain and other symptoms across the menstrual cycle. Pain **106**:253–261.

34 LeResche L, Sherman JJ, Huggins K, Saunders K, Mancl LA, Lentz G, et al. 2005: Musculoskeletal orofacial pain and other signs and symptoms of temporomandibular disorders during pregnancy: a prospective study. J Orofac Pain **19**:193–201.

35 Smith YR, Stohler CS, Nichols TE, Bueller JA, Koeppe RA, Zubieta J. 2006: Pronociceptive and antinociceptive effects of estradiol through endogenous opioid neurotransmission in women. J Neurosci **26**:5777–5785.

36 Tamres LK, Janicki D, Helgeson VS. 2002: Sex differences in coping behavior: a meta-analytic review and an examination of relative coping. Pers Soc Psychol Rev **6**:2–30.

37 Keefe FJ, G Affleck, France CR, Emery CF, Waters S, Caldwell DS, et al. 2004: Gender differences in pain, coping, and mood in individuals having osteoarthritic knee pain: a within-day analysis. Pain **110**:571–577.

38 Jones A, Elkit A. 2007: The association between gender, coping style and whiplash related symptoms in sufferers of whiplash associated disorder. Scand J Psychol **48**:75–80.

39 Peul WC, Brand R, Thomeer RTWM, Koes BW. 2008: Influence of gender and other prognostic factors on outcome of sciatica. Pain **138**:180–191.

Section 4

Common pain syndromes

Chapter 11

Introduction

Peter Croft, Fiona M. Blyth, and Danielle var der Windt

The chapters in this section are designed to give empirical flesh to the concepts, ideas, and methods of the previous sections. They each convey similar messages about the prevalence of pain in populations:-

- The most common pains overall are musculoskeletal pain and headache.
- Patterns vary with age.
- Pain is generally commoner in women.
- Multi-site pain is the most common 'phenotype' in populations, with chronic widespread pain sitting at one end of the spectrum.

In Chapter 12, van der Windt introduces and discusses the idea that all regional pains (i.e. pain at different body sites – neck or back or knee, for example) are similar in their natural history, prognosis, and associated characteristics. The most frequent risk factor for a new episode of pain in a particular body site is a prior history of pain in that same site or a prior history of pain in another site. Studies in children (Chapter 14), older adults (Chapter 16), and across the life-course (Chapter 15) add to this picture of chronic pain tracking across time in individuals, and provide evidence for the idea of a 'propensity' for chronic pain that may emerge early in life.

Because multi-site pain is the commonest phenotype, and since chronic regional pains have similar characteristics, the focus on site-specific pain in the literature may be unhelpful. Most persons who report chronic back pain have pains elsewhere in their body, and most persons with chronic widespread pain have chronic back pain.

One of the reasons for not attempting coverage of all chronic pain syndromes is that it would have been a book of repetition, the epidemiological equivalent of a John Adams symphony. The disadvantage is that the reader's syndrome of interest may not be found here. We have selected headache as an example for a chapter (Chapter 13), written exclusively from the point of view of one pain syndrome. From a population perspective, however, all chronic pain is here in this section, if the principle is accepted that the person in pain, rather than the specific pain site or trigger, is the crucial issue of interest. This is how to make sense of the epidemiology summarized above.

Therefore, the chapters in this section provide overviews and examples as evidence for the chronic pain syndrome as an amplified symptom complex, with psychosocial, behavioural, and cultural associations, and determinants that track throughout the life-course.

Chapter 12

The symptom of pain in populations

Danielle van der Windt

Introduction

Everyone will have an episode of pain sometime in their life. Such sensations are normal, but there is great variation between individuals. Some people go through life with few episodes of pain, whereas others seem to be more easily injured or frequently experience pain problems without a clear precipitating cause. This results in a continuum of pain from common pain problems to the rarer chronic pain syndromes, e.g. from incidental headache to chronic tension-type headache; from an episode of regional musculoskeletal pain to chronic widespread pain (CWP) or fibromyalgia; or from occasional abdominal symptoms to irritable bowel syndrome (IBS). People interpret changes in their body subjectively, and this varies across individuals; pain or other symptoms may cause concern or distress in some, resulting in presentation of their symptoms to a health care professional, whereas others might wait longer or do not seek help at all (Wessely et al., 1999).

This chapter aims to explore similarities and differences across different types of pain. The chapter hopes to shed some light on the following questions: Do different people report different types of pain or do different symptoms co-occur in the same individuals? What are the characteristics of people with multiple pains? Are different symptoms all expressions of the same syndrome, or do they represent separate entities? What are the possibilities for preventing the onset of chronic pain, or its long-term consequences in daily life?

Pain in the community

Occurrence of pain problems

The results of a survey conducted among a random sample of 4771 adults in the Netherlands showed that an episode of musculoskeletal pain, headache, or abdominal pain in the past month (lasting at least 24 h) was reported by 17% (ankle/foot problems) to 39% (back pain) of all responders ($n = 2447$, Table 12.1; van der Windt et al., 2008a). These rates are very similar to other community-based surveys carried out in the UK, (Boardman et al., 2003; Papageorgiou et al., 1995; Pope et al., 1997), Norway (Kamaleri et al., 2008), the USA (Kroenke and Price, 1993; Koloski et al., 2002), and the Netherlands (Picavet and Schouten, 2003).

Although the prevalence of these different types of pain varied, the duration, frequency and impact on daily activities were more consistent, especially musculoskeletal pain in different locations of the body (van der Windt et al., 2008a). Responders with musculoskeletal pain had often been affected for more than 3 months (from 77% for shoulder pain to 83% for hip or knee pain), and pain impacted on daily activities on more than half of all days in 32% (back or neck pain) to 42% (foot problems). Frequency and impact of the pain problem was higher for musculoskeletal pain than for headache or abdominal pain (Table 12.1).

Table 12.1 Pain in the community: frequency, duration, and impact on daily activities of different types of pain (n = 2447)

	Prevalence N (%)	Duration >3 months %	Frequency (very often) * %	Impact on daily activities (very often) %
Headache	991 (40.4)	66.3	16.0	10.9
Abdominal problems	572 (23.4)	67.3	29.5	18.1
Back pain	960 (39.2)	80.6	45.0	32.4
Neck pain	754 (30.8)	80.9	46.6	31.5
Shoulder pain	710 (29.0)	79.3	50.9	33.1
Hand/wrist problems	563 (23.0)	76.6	52.2	37.3
Hip/knee pain	693 (28.3)	82.9	54.7	39.8
Ankle/foot problems	428 (17.4)	80.0	61.0	42.3

*on more than half of all days

Reproduced from van der Windt et al., 2008a, with permission.

These prevalence rates represent people reporting an occasional episode of musculoskeletal pain as well as persons suffering from chronic pain syndromes. A recent review (Creavin, 2008) identified nine studies that investigated the prevalence of CWP in the general population. The prevalence of CWP was consistently estimated between 9% and 14%, using the criteria proposed by the American College of Rheumatology (ACR).

Most population-based studies have asked responders about specific types of pain, or pain in different regions of the body. Studies asking about chronic pain more generally give an overall picture of prevalence and impact whilst avoiding the complexities of aggregating reports of pain in multiple body sites. Elliott et al (1999) carried out a large survey among a random sample of 5036 people ≥25 years of age attending participating general practices in Scotland. Out of 3605 responders 50.4% reported chronic pain or discomfort that started at least 3 months ago, with prevalence increasing with age from 32% in the youngest to 62% in the oldest age group (Elliott et al., 1999). Female sex, rented rather than owned housing, and being retired or unable to work was associated with increased prevalence of chronic pain. In 14.1% of responders the pain problem was associated with use of pain medication and presentation to health care, in 6.3% chronic pain was classified as severe and resulting in high disability and severe limitation in daily activities (Smith et al., 2001). In a 4-year follow-up of this study, the annual incidence of new-onset chronic pain was estimated at 8.3%, with annual recovery rate of 5.4%. This means that chronic pain was persistent in most people, with 78.5% of individuals at baseline still reporting chronic pain after 4 years (Elliott et al., 2002).

Pain in children and adolescents

Although population-based research has mostly addressed pain problems in adults, chronic pain is common in children and adolescents, with prevalence rates approaching those among adults. For example, the prevalence of back pain in children was reported to be low (1–6%), but rapidly increasing in the adolescent years to 18–50%, similar to adults (Taimela et al., 1997; McMeeken et al., 2001; Leboeuf-Yde and Kyvik, 1998; Mathers and Penm, 1999). In a Canadian study, trajectories of headache, abdominal pain, and back pain were studied repeatedly over an 8-year assessment period. A considerable proportion of children and adolescents in the age range of 12–19 years reported weekly or more frequent headaches (26–32%), abdominal pain (14–22%), or musculoskeletal pain (18–26%; Stanford et al., 2008). Jones et al. (2003) conducted a population-based prospective cohort study among 1440 children in the age range of 11–14 years. Prevalence of widespread pain was 14.6%. Children with widespread pain also reported more headaches, sore throat, stomach ache, or tiredness. These cross-sectional studies seem to indicate that pain problems develop quite early in adolescent years, regardless of the type or location of pain, and that even generalized pain problems are already common in adolescence.

Pain in older people

The prevalence of chronic pain has been estimated between 45% and 80% among older people in the community and in institutionalized settings (Maxwell et al., 2008). In the majority of older people, pain is caused by musculoskeletal conditions (mainly osteoarthritis in multiple joints). The impact of chronic pain also is particularly high in this age group. The presence of pain in older people has been associated with depression, sleep problems, limitations in activity and participation, and increased health care-resource use (Maxwell et al., 2008). Research shows that pain in older people is not always recognized or managed adequately. For example, pain medication is less frequently prescribed in older people even when pain in quite severe (Landi et al., 2001; Sawyer et al., 2006; Shega et al., 2006; Smalbrugge et al., 2007; Chodosh et al., 2004). Several explanations have been offered for the inadequate management of pain in the elderly: (1) physicians may be reluctant to prescribe medication in older people given the higher risk of adverse reactions especially in those already taking multiple drugs; (2) other chronic conditions (e.g. diabetes, pulmonary, or cardiovascular conditions) may receive attention and more continuous care; (3) identifying pain may not be easy in the presence of cognitive decline; and (4) older people themselves may consider pain to be a natural consequence of getting older, and something they just have to deal with. However, pain in older people is common, and often results in activity limitations and loss of independence, requiring specific attention from health care providers.

Limitation in activities and health care-resource use

As mentioned above, individuals will interpret physical symptoms differently and not all will be equally concerned by pain problems. This also means that not everyone consults health care services for their pain problem. Several studies show that ~20–30% of those reporting pain problems consult their primary care or general practitioner regardless of the type of pain (van der Windt, 2008a; Picavet, 2004), and that ~70% of those with chronic pain consult (Picavet and Hoeymans, 2004). Users of health services generally have more severe pain, more symptoms of anxiety or depression, and poorer general health (Elliott et al., 2004; Hagen et al., 2000; van der Windt et al., 2002; Jordan et al., 2006).

Using data from the Dutch community-based study (2447 adults), Fig. 12.1 demonstrates the impact of chronic pain (duration of at least 3 months) for different types of pain on a population level. As a result of a relatively high prevalence (39.2%, Table 12.1), back pain was associated with the largest impact on limitations in activities, and highest consultation rate in general practice: 9% of all responders had consulted a general practitioner for their back problem. Musculoskeletal pain, in general, was associated with considerable limitations in activities in the population. Abdominal pains and headache, although less often reported to cause limitations in activities, were a relatively frequent reason to consult a health care practitioner. The results of other population-based surveys confirm the impact of pain problems on daily activities and participation. The Scottish survey showed a low prevalence of inability to work in persons with no pain (1.3%), but high frequency in people with pain, increasing to 61.1% in those with severe chronic pain (Smith et al., 2001).

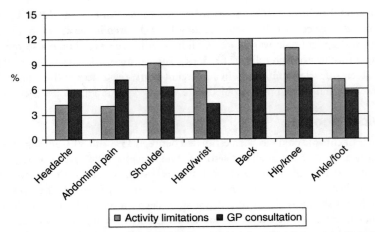

Fig. 12.1 Population burden (*n* = 2447) of different types of chronic pain: activity limitations (on more than half of all days, %), and GP consultation (%). Reproduced from van der Windt, 2008a, with permission.

Similarities and differences in characteristics of people with different pain problems

As summarized above, different types of pain seem to have similar characteristics in terms of duration, frequency, impact on daily activities, and health care-resource use. Table 12.2 presents the characteristics of responders to the Dutch survey who reported isolated headache, abdominal pain, or regional musculoskeletal pain (either a hand/wrist problem or back pain). These were mutually exclusive groups, although they could have other co-occurring symptoms. Compared with responders reporting no pain, responders reporting any regional pain problem were less physically active, and reported more negative health experiences during childhood, more symptoms of anxiety and depression, more sleeping problems, and less positive health perceptions. Responders with different types of pain varied in demographic characteristics: responders with headache were younger, had a higher education level, and more often paid work, especially compared with those with hand problems.

Most responders in this study, however, did not have pain confined to one area and reported more than one pain problem; 332 of these were classified (based on American College of Rheumatology criteria) as having CWP. Table 12.2 shows that individuals with widespread pain were more likely to be female, least active, had the highest body mass index, lowest educational level, poorest childhood health experiences, and highest scores for psychological problems.

Multiple pains

This chapter so far indicates that, although there is some variation in characteristics of subgroups with different types of pain, there are many similarities between the groups. Localized single-site pain is relatively rare and most people report multiple pains. A Norwegian survey showed that only 16.8% of responders (*n* = 3179) reported localized musculoskeletal pain, whereas 53% reported pain in more than one site (Kamaleri et al., 2008). Using data from a national co-morbidity survey (*n* = 5692), Von Korff et al. (2005) found that the prevalence of chronic

Table 12.2 Characteristics of people with different types of pain in a Dutch community sample

	No pain* (n = 346)	Headache* (n = 287)	Abdominal pain* (n = 96)	Hand pain* (n = 129)	Back pain* (n = 256)	CWP (n = 332)
Demographic variables						
Sex (% female)	42.5	67.6	47.9	65.1	46.1	71.1
Age (years), mean (SD)	52.6 (17.5)	44.5 (13.1)	50.3 (16.6)	56.4 (16.6)	53.1 (16.3)	54.1 (14.4)
Educational level (%)						
- primary	27.2	19.9	19.8	34.1	29.7	42.4
- secondary	34.5	39.4	39.6	36.4	34.4	38.8
- college/university	38.3	40.8	40.6	29.5	35.9	18.8
Paid work (%)	73.7	88.4	65.3	55.7	61.8	51.6
Body mass index, mean (SD)	25.1 (3.8)	25.4 (11.6)	25.7 (4.2)	26.8 (8.2)	26.0 (5.3)	27.1 (11.2)
Physically active (%) at least 3 times/week	20.8	13.2	18.1	11.2	15.8	13.5
Childhood experiences						
More often ill than other children (%)	5.2	11.2	14.6	13.2	7.8	19.3
Admitted to hospital as a child (%)	21.5	31.2	33.3	25.6	25.5	32.2
Family members with chronic illness (%)	17.4	26.2	34.4	32.0	27.8	40.2
Psychological problems						
Anxiety (HADS, %)						
- no (score 0–7)	95.7	76.8	76.6	80.6	84.3	57.5
- possible anxiety (score 8–10)	3.5	13.9	19.1	11.6	8.3	18.0
- probable anxiety (score > 10)	0.9	9.3	4.3	7.8	7.5	24.5
Depressive symptoms (HADS, %)						
- no (score 0-7)	95.0	85.3	84.2	83.7	87.0	66.2
- possible depression (score 8-10)	3.5	8.6	11.6	7.0	7.5	18.6
- probable depression (>10)	1.5	6.1	4.2	9.3	5.5	15.2
Sleeping problems (>50% of nights, %)	4.3	9.8	7.3	10.1	12.9	34.0
Health perceptions: not able to influence health (%)	5.6	7.3	4.3	12.6	6.8	16.3

*mutually exclusive groups: e.g. responders with headache, did not report back, hand or abdominal pain

spinal pain was >3 times as high among persons who reported other chronic pain conditions as those without these conditions: 34.1 versus 9.6%. In a population-based survey (2504 responders), Macfarlane et al. (2002) showed that the number of people with both orofacial pain and CWP (4%) was larger than expected based on prevalence of CWP (6%) and orofacial pain (23%) alone. Co-occurrence of symptoms not only holds for musculoskeletal pain. In a study among Swedish twins (33 190 pair-wise respondents, and 11707 single respondents), Kato et al (2006) reported that people with CWP more often reported chronic fatigue or IBS.

Similarly, migraine has been shown to co-occur with musculoskeletal pain, with 39% of people with migraine reporting chronic musculoskeletal pain compared with 25% of those without migraine (Terwindt et al., 2000).

Several studies have demonstrated that the number of pain problems or the number of physical symptoms is associated with reduced physical functioning, feelings of anxiety and depression, and sleeping problems (van der Windt et al., 2008a; Kamaleri et al., 2008; Von Korff et al., 2005; Kato et al., 2006; Terwindt et al., 2000). Experiencing a single pain had little impact on physical fitness, emotions, or daily and social activities; functional consequences largely depended on how widespread the pain was or how many co-morbidities were reported. Von Korff et al. showed that after adjusting for demographic factors, the odds of mood disorders or anxiety was 2.5 times as high in those with chronic spinal pain compared with those without chronic pain (Von Korff et al., 2005). Co-morbidity also negatively affects health care utilization and costs. For example, the number of concurrent conditions among patients with fibromyalgia was the strongest predictor of total health care costs in a 7-year prospective study in the USA (Wolfe et al., 1997).

Overlap between pain syndromes

If population-based surveys show that most people report multiple symptoms of pain, co-occurrence of pain problems may also be expected at the other end of the continuum: in patients diagnosed with a chronic pain syndrome. Researchers have shown considerable overlap in symptoms between patients diagnosed with different chronic somatic or painful syndromes, such as chronic fatigue syndrome, fibromyalgia, temporomandibular disorder (TMD), and IBS (Deary, 1999; Aaron et al., 2000; Aaron and Buchwald, 2001; Ciccone and Natelson, 2003). For example, 13–18% of patients with TMD also meet criteria for fibromyalgia, while conversely, 75% of those with fibromyalgia meet criteria for TMD (Aaron and Buchwald, 2001). Overlap was especially prominent for muscle and abdominal pain and sleep and concentration difficulties.

More formal methods to analyse clustering of symptoms have been applied by a few researchers. Schur et al. (2007) studied interrelationships between symptoms related to different functional syndromes in 3982 twins, and demonstrated that co-morbidity of nine syndromes exceeded chance expectations. Latent class analysis yielded a 4-class solution as follows: a small cluster (2% of responders) showed high frequencies of each of the nine conditions; another group (8%) showed multiple psychiatric diagnoses; the largest group (apart from the generally healthy twins) reported high proportions of major depression, chronic low back pain, and chronic tension-type headache. Nimnuan et al. (2001) studied 550 patients with a functional somatic syndrome referred to secondary care, and used factor analysis to investigate clustering of symptoms. About half of all patients (53.6%) met the criteria for more than one syndrome, and a one-factor model explained 30% of variance. A two-factor model offered an optimal solution, with pain and fatigue syndromes loading on the first factor: IBS, TMD, facial pain, dyspepsia, pelvic pain, tension headache, fibromyalgia, and fatigue. The second factor mainly represented cardio-respiratory symptoms.

Part of the clustering of syndromes within individuals can be explained by similarities in the clinical definitions of functional syndromes. The studies confirm that patients with chronic pain report many additional physical and mental health problems, which may complicate management of these patients. Individual syndromes are often managed separately; physicians instinctively seek, diagnose, and treat conditions they know well, and coexisting other problems may be ignored. This narrow focus may also result in over-investigation when patients consult different specialists for different types of health problems (Nimnuan et al., 2001).

Trajectories of pain over time

Given the similarities and clustering between different pain or pain-related syndromes, there may also be overlap in the trajectories of pain over time. Figure 12.2 shows the results of several studies investigating the prognosis of musculoskeletal pain in primary care populations (Bot et al., 2005; van der Waal et al., 2005; Spies-Dorgelo et al., 2008; van Tulder et al., 1998; Hay et al., 2005). The course of pain, presented here as mean pain-intensity scores, was quite similar over a period of 12 months following consultation in primary care for either neck/shoulder pain, hand/wrist problems, or hip pain/knee problems. The duration of pain at presentation is commonly found to be an important predictor of the course of pain, and this is confirmed by the much more favourable trajectory of acute back pain (duration <6 weeks) compared with that of chronic low back pain (>3 months at presentation), both presented in Fig. 12.2.

Most prospective cohort studies have investigated the course of pain by measuring pain intensity or recovery of pain at a few specific moments in time. However, this may not reflect the recurrent, episodic nature of pain. Dunn et al. (2006) used latent class analysis to demonstrate that primary care patients with back pain can be classified into four distinct groups with different pathways in the course of back pain over time: persistent mild pain, recovering pain, fluctuating pain, or severe chronic back pain. These clusters of patients also showed significant differences in a range of other factors, such as disability, work status, and psychological variables. Although such sophisticated analyses have not been carried out for many other pain problems, research has clearly shown that pain, regardless of type or location, is often recurrent and characterized by episodes of exacerbating pain and disability, followed by periods of no or little pain interference.

We still do not have a very clear picture of how episodes of pain are related. We do know that many people report multiple pains, but what are the patterns of these pain problems over time? The findings by Kamaleri et al. (2009) indicate that the number of pain sites can remain fairly constant over time, with a mean increase of only 0.5 sites over a period of 14 years. The most important predictor of the number of pain sites at follow-up was the number of pains at baseline. Repeated episodes of pain and disability may be manifestations of the same underlying condition

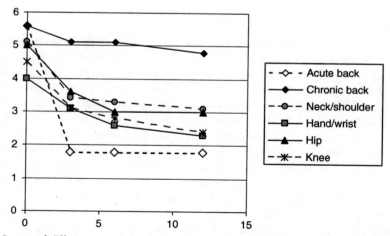

Fig. 12.2 Course of different types of pain (scale 0-10) over 12 months follow-up in primary care attenders. (Bot et al., 2005; Van der Waal et al., 2005; Spies-Dorgelo et al., 2008; van Tulder et al., 1998; Hay et al., 2005)

that is being repeatedly aggravated. Alternatively, each episode may be truly distinct, and other factors in a person's life may increase the risk of new pain problems (Linton et al., 2005). Some of these factors may be closely related to the specific pain problem (e.g. physical load at work), whereas other factors may be more generic, and similar across patients reporting different types of pain.

Few researchers have looked at the temporal associations between the onset of pain episodes within individuals. Croft et al. (2003) investigated information from surveys on pain problems linked with general practice records over a period of 25 years, and showed that regional pain syndromes seem to track distinctively over time. Back pain was most strongly predicted by earlier episodes of back pain; abdominal pain by earlier episodes of gastrointestinal problems. However, there was some evidence of earlier occurrence of anxiety and depression with all regional musculoskeletal pain problems and especially with CWP, which provides some evidence of a common mechanism associated with different types of pain.

Risk factors

As many pain problems are already quite common in children and adolescents, it is hardly possible to study the onset of first-ever episodes of pain. Yet, many studies have investigated factors that may predict the onset of new episodes of pain, or risk factors for the persistence of a pain episode (prognostic factors). Mallen et al. (2007) conducted a systematic review of prospective cohort studies in populations with different types of pain, and identified a wide range of potential risk factors for persistence. Regardless of the type of pain syndrome, older age, female sex, previous episodes of pain, and psychological factors predicted onset of new episodes or persistence of a chronic pain problem. Macfarlane (1999) also noted that both regional and generalized pain syndromes seem to have similar risk factors. The effects of mechanical factors (including heavy workloads, vibration, and incorrect posture), were mostly investigated in regional pain syndromes and often showed very specific associations with the particular regional syndrome, but by contrast, psychological factors were common to the likelihood of persistence across different regional syndromes.

The role of psychological factors

The relation between psychological factors and pain has been widely studied, but studies have examined different sets of psychological factors and used different statistical approaches to analyse associations with pain. This makes it difficult to tease out those factors that are consistently associated with onset or persistence of pain. Strong predictors, however, seem to be anxiety, depression and catastrophizing beliefs about pain. Catastrophizing is an exaggerated orientation towards pain stimuli and is considered to be an inadequate coping strategy (Sullivan et al., 1995). People worry excessively about their pain problem and have poor expectations of outcome. These perceptions have been shown to be associated with a poor prognosis in people with back pain (Boersma and Linton, 2006; van der Windt et al., 2007), shoulder pain (Bot et al., 2005; van der Windt et al., 2007), hand or wrist problems (Spies-Dorgelo et al., 2008), hip problems (van der Waal et al., 2005), knee pain (Botha-Scheepers et al., 2006) and chronic fatigue (Nijrolder et al., 2009).

McBeth and Silman (1999) commented that mental disorders may not be an intrinsic element of the chronic pain syndrome, but rather reflect the influence of mental disorders on health care-seeking behaviour. They emphasized that temporal relations between chronic pain and mental health problems remain unclear. A systematic review examined the temporal relations between pain and depression using the results of 83 studies. There was greater support for the consequence and scar hypothesis (depression as a result of chronic pain) than for the antecedent hypothesis (depression precedes onset of chronic pain), but both directions of the association were reported (Fishbain et al., 1997). In a systematic review of 244 studies on the relationship between unexplained physical symptoms and mental health problems, Henningsen et al. (2003) also showed that depression and anxiety are a regular, although not universal, accompanying problem of different types of symptoms. Gureje et al. (2008) analysed data from population samples in 17 countries around the globe (World Mental Health Surveys) on the presence of multiple pain and mental disorders. The results consistently show that as the number of pain problems increases, the prevalence of depressive illness also increases. This relationship also applied to various anxiety disorders (Gureje et al., 2008).

Risk factors in childhood

The association between psychological factors and pain has also been confirmed in childhood. The strongest predictors of high or increasing levels of different types of pain in children were anxiety and depression (Stanford et al., 2008). Jones et al. (2003) investigated onset and persistence of CWP in school-aged children. Multivariable analyses revealed three significant predictors of new-onset CWP: psychosocial difficulties, level of sports activity, and headaches. The finding that spending the most time on active sports doubled the risk of CWP suggested that part of the pain may be the result of injury. Other risk factors seemed to indicate that processes found in adults may already be part of the development of chronic pain in children.

Furthermore, adverse childhood experiences and parental modelling of illness behaviour have been shown to be associated with increased adult vulnerability to the development of chronic pain or other functional syndromes (Hotopf et al., 1999; Mallen et al., 2006). Mallen et al. (2006) found that recalled childhood experiences of pain or illness were associated with current pain status in young adulthood. Young adults with pain remembered themselves as being comparatively ill as a child, and aware of family members with pain. Families may have illnesses that are inherited, which may explain trends within family groups. However, the results could equally be related to learned behaviour and modelling, which is particularly potent in childhood. In a prospective birth cohort established in 1946, Hotopf et al. (1999) showed a strong relationship between poor reported health of parents in 15-year-old children and symptoms later in adulthood. Unexplained symptoms during adulthood were also associated with abdominal pain in childhood but not with specific childhood disease. These results seemed to indicate that unexplained symptoms can be related to prior experience of family illness and previous unexplained symptoms in the individual, reflecting a learned process whereby illness experience leads to more symptom awareness.

Jones et al. (2007) used data from the 1958 British Birth Cohort Study (>10 000 subjects) and also showed that multiple symptoms in childhood are associated with increased risk of CWP in adulthood. The magnitude of the risk was modest, however (adjusted relative risk: 1.3), and the number of children with multiple problems at childhood appeared to be small, resulting in a population attributable risk of only 0.64% (i.e. the proportion of all CWP in the population that might be attributable to multiple problems in childhood was <1%). Therefore, the early pain pathway may apply, but only in a small proportion of individuals with CWP in adulthood (Jones et al., 2007). Other potential influences (triggers) may play a role later in life, including psychological problems, life events, and social circumstances.

Social and occupational factors

The role of social factors, including personal factors (e.g. education, income, and social support) or factors on a population level (e.g. deprivation or environmental factors) has only recently caught the attention of researchers. Using data from a community-based survey, Jordan et al. (2008) showed that neighbourhood deprivation, no further education, and (perceived) income inequalities were associated with onset of pain interfering with daily activities, although these effects were less strong compared with those of multiple pains, higher age, and high scores for anxiety or depression. Results of the Scottish survey on chronic pain also show that living in council-rented accommodation, being retired or unable to work, and lower educational level were related to the presence of severe or significant chronic pain (Smith et al., 2001).

A review by Shaw et al. evaluating occupational risk factors for the onset or persistence of low back pain emphasized the potential influence of poor job control, expectations for return-to-work, and fear of re-injury (Shaw et al., 2006a). Compared with psychological factors, however, less is known about the effects of social and occupational factors on pain. The occurrence of pain or the extent to which pain interferes with life may be influenced by partner or family responses to pain, demands and control at work, employer and co-worker reactions to pain, or even by broader issues such as the job market. This is an important area for further study; if causal associations can be established for important risk factors, and these factors are potentially modifiable, it may be important to develop and evaluate population-based interventions addressing these factors.

The one-syndrome hypothesis

The epidemiology of regional and generalized pain seems to indicate that these may not be distinct entities. Patients with different chronic pain syndromes have similar characteristics, show similar trajectories over time, similar risk factors, and may even respond to similar treatments. Some authors have suggested that the similarities outweigh the differences, and have proposed to abandon the use of different case definitions in favour of more broadly defined clusters of symptoms (Wessely et al., 1999). Some authors have even hypothesized that pain and other unexplained physical symptoms may be expressions of one underlying syndrome, and several mechanisms have been proposed which include psychological as well as physiological processes.

Evidence summarized in the previous sections suggested that poor illness perceptions (e.g. catastrophizing thoughts), anxiety, and depressive disorders play important roles in the persistence of pain. Poor perceptions about health and illness may increase attention to bodily symptoms, and strengthen the attribution of such sensations to physical illness. These processes are a normal response to signs of illness in many people, but can reach disabling proportions in some, resulting in (undifferentiated) somatization disorder (Brown, 2004; Kirmayer and Looper, 2006). Responses of family members, employers, and physicians may reinforce these processes, leading to exacerbation or persistence of pain (Barsky and Norus, 1999). Some people, e.g. those with a history of trauma, adverse childhood experiences, psychiatric conditions, or those undergoing life stress may also be more vulnerable to this process of increased bodily awareness and symptom amplification (Barsky and Borus, 1999).

Several studies have demonstrated altered pain perception and abnormal pain processing in individuals with widespread pain. In a community-based study, McBeth et al. (2005) demonstrated that CWP was associated with altered hypothalamic–pituitary–adrenal (HPA) axis function. The presence of CWP was associated with lower levels of salivary cortisol and higher levels of post-stressor serum cortisol. This indicates a failure to mount an adequate stress response to psychological insult, which seems to predispose to the development of CWP. Alterations in the HPA axis and the autonomic nervous system are assumed to result in sensitization of the central nervous system, which explains the changes in pain perception and pain processing in people with chronic pain (Buskila and Press, 2001). Traumatic or distressing events have been suggested to initiate such changes, but many triggers have been described, all of which fall into the category of 'stressors', including various emotional, immune, and physical traumata. Prospective data are needed to confirm these hypotheses.

It has also been suggested that there may be a genetic predisposition to develop chronic pain and that these triggers can either initiate or aggravate the condition (Buskila and Press, 2001). Kato et al. (2006) studied >33 000 twins and showed that the co-occurrence between CWP, IBS, chronic fatigue, or other functional syndromes was partly mediated by unmeasured genetic or family environmental factors. Associations between CWP and psychiatric disorders mostly disappeared in monozygotic analyses, indicating a contributing role of genetic factors. The extent to which these associations were explained by familial or genetic factors was syndrome-specific. For example, the association between CWP and migraine or tension-type headache could not be attributed to genetic or family environmental factors, indicating that this co-morbidity may be mediated through other, exogenous factors, such as stress (Kato et al., 2006).

Further investigation of the interactions between neurophysiological, psychological, and social processes may help to explain disposition, onset, and prognosis of chronic pain syndromes (Henningsen et al., 2003). Division into different syndromes is not always helpful, and a scheme using a multiaxial approach, including the number of symptoms, duration, associated mood disturbance, patients' attributions, and identifiable physiological processes, may be more useful to understand the development and outcome of pain syndromes.

Potential for prevention

Pain problems are very common in the population. Most of these problems may not cause long-term interference with daily life, and may simply represent variations in normal health. Chronic pain, however, was shown to result in considerable disability and health care-resource use in a large number of people, emphasizing the importance of preventing chronic pain and its consequences.

The fact that similar risk factors seem to be important across different types of pain holds promise for intervention at population level. Since both individual-level risk factors and population-level risk factors are associated with onset or persistence of pain, this suggests that opportunities for intervention exist at more than one level (Blyth, 2008). Ignoring population-level factors and intervening exclusively on high-risk individuals could limit options for reducing the overall community burden of chronic pain. A larger number of people at lower increased risk may contribute more to this overall burden than a smaller number of people at high increased risk of chronic, disabling pain, even though the latter group is often easier to identify (Blyth, 2008; Rose, 1985). This section discusses three possibilities for intervention, in which different approaches are used to target populations or make decisions regarding intervention.

Population-based prevention

Given the general nature and favourable course of many pain episodes, several authors have argued that there is limited scope for primary prevention of episodes of musculoskeletal pain (Burton et al., 2005; Tveito et al., 2004; Linton and van Tulder, 2001). However, a multimedia campaign in Australia (Buchbinder et al., 2001) providing simple messages about back pain (i.e. to stay active and exercise, not to rest for prolonged period, and to remain at work) resulted in improvements in population beliefs about back pain, and had a sustained effect on physician's beliefs and stated management up until 4.5 years after cessation of the campaign. This seems to indicate that a population-based intervention addressing not only people with back pain, but also employers, care providers, and policy-makers, may be effective in shifting individual and societal attitudes towards pain and disability, perhaps leading to changes in ways of dealing with pain.

Other authors have also underlined the potential of population-based interventions for chronic pain. Blyth et al. (2005) showed that passive coping strategies (e.g. taking medication, resting, or hot or cold packs) were reported nearly twice as often as active strategies (e.g. exercise), and that the use of passive strategies was associated with a threefold risk of a high number of health care visits, and 2 times higher levels of disability. The authors suggest that, in order to achieve a greater use of effective self-management of pain in the community, specific measures are required, varying from training health care professionals to public health campaigns. Lorig et al. (2002) investigated the use of a Web-based self-management intervention for people with chronic back pain, including e-mail discussions, a back-pain help book, and videotape. The website hosting the intervention was accessed >46 000 times, demonstrating the accessibility of the intervention. Of the 580 people who met the eligibility criteria, 475 completed data collection at 6 months. Drop-out was mainly the result of an overload of e-mails distributed to participants in the first few days of the intervention. Final results showed significant improvements of pain, disability, role function, and health distress, as well as enhanced levels of self-efficacy and self-orientation. Potential pitfalls of population-based self-management approaches, as identified by Smith and Elliott (2005), are that indiscriminate application may prevent or delay presentation of serious disease to health care, or could encourage people to self-medicate inappropriately. They also emphasize, however, the multiple potential benefits of population-based interventions for preventing chronic pain and disability in the community.

Population-based interventions may not only be targeted at people with pain, but also at employers. The importance of employer's attitudes has been shown in a recent cohort study of workers with back pain; workers' satisfaction with their employer's treatment of their disability claim was more important in explaining return to work than satisfaction with health care providers or their expectations of recovery (Butler et al., 2007). Optimization of the response of supervisors to work injuries through training seems to be a promising approach (Shaw et al., 2006b; 2006c), and may complement or optimize the effectiveness of interventions aimed at individual patients. This seems to support a public health approach to managing pain problems, rather than a curative approach only.

Target populations may also include children, and their parents, teachers, or schools, as pain problems are certainly not limited to the adult population. Lifestyle interventions for children, positioned in primary and secondary schools, are increasingly being developed, and may result in health gains that could be worthwhile on a population level. So far, most of these interventions have focused on inactivity and overweight, showing modest reductions in body mass index or activity behaviours (e.g. Plachta-Danielzik et al., 2007; Taylor et al., 2007; Haerens et al., 2007). The sustainability of these effects and their long-term benefits (possibly also in the prevention of chronic pain and disability in adulthood) still need to be demonstrated.

Risk stratification

Rather than targeting whole populations, researchers have proposed to identify and target vulnerable subgroups of people who are at increased risk to develop chronic, interfering pain problems. This approach departs from the viewpoint that there may be more scope for preventing the consequences of pain (rather than the onset of pain), and that interventions may be more effective early in the course of an episode of pain.

Using information about risk factors for the persistence of pain problems (i.e. prognostic factors), a variety of screening tools have been developed to identify vulnerable subgroups.

Examples of these screening tools include the Örebro Musculoskeletal Pain Screening Questionnaire (ÖMPSQ; Linton and Hallden, 1998), which was one of the first questionnaires designed to identify people at high risk of long-term disability due to musculoskeletal pain. More recently, Kuijpers et al. (2006) developed a prediction rule to estimate the risk of persisting symptoms in primary care patients with shoulder pain; and Dionne et al. (2005) developed a tool for early identification of workers presenting with back pain who are at high risk of adverse occupational outcome.

These tools may help health care practitioners when making decisions about the management of pain in individual patients A stepped-care approach seems to match up well with a system using risk stratification. Von Korff and Moore (2001) proposed a stepped-care approach for managing back pain in primary care. The approach includes three levels of care of increasing intensity and complexity: step 1 can be targeted at all patients with pain and mainly consists of self-care and educational materials; step 2 is targeted at patients who still report activity limitations after 6–8 weeks and includes identification of individual difficulties, functional goal setting, and reactivation; step 3 is reserved for patients with substantial disability in work or family roles and includes interventions to restore role functions, an exercise programme, and management of psychological problems. Stepped care is based on the principle of starting with low-intensity, low-cost interventions, 'stepping up' to more intense and more costly interventions in patients who show inadequate responses to previous steps. However, individualization based on initial evaluation (e.g. risk stratification) is possible, facilitating early targeting of more intensive interventions at those with an increased risk of poor outcome (Von Korff and Moore, 2001).

Screening and targeting

Screening tools have also been designed to identify and subsequently target specific risk factors. For example, the Pain-Disability Prevention (PDP) Program is a community-based intervention programme that offers packages of structured activity schedules and graded activity involvement to target specific risk factors (such as fear of movement) in individual patients with elevated scores on these risk factors (Sullivan and Stanish, 2003). This approach allows interventions to be tailored to the needs of individual patients, rather than to offer the same intervention to all patients in a specific risk category. The PDP programme has been translated to a community-based intervention, and shows encouraging results with higher rates of return to work compared with usual care. So far, these programmes have mainly focused on general psychological factors such as pain catastrophizing, fear of re-injury, and depressive symptoms, but similar strategies could perhaps also address work-related or social factors, including perceptions of poor social support, high job demands, or poor expectations of return to work, and may include elements of stress management, problem-solving therapy, effective reassurance, and improvement of communication between supervisors and injured workers (Shaw et al., 2006a; Faucett et al., 2002). Delivery of such strategies will require additional training of public health, occupational, and health care professionals to acquire the necessary skills and competencies, and to make sure that consistent messages are delivered across care providers (Sullivan et al., 2005; Jellema et al., 2005; van der Windt et al., 2008b).

Finally, it is important to recognize that the external validity of screening tools can be disappointing and that testing of the performances of a screening tool in other populations, and particularly in clinical practice, is necessary before implementation of these tools can be considered. Furthermore, the use of screening tools is only of value if they provide additional information that assist care providers in making adequate decisions regarding referral or treatment (Reilly and Evans, 2006). Consequently, research needs to determine whether screening and targeting approaches actually lead to better patient outcomes or more efficient (cost-effective) care for chronic pain.

Conclusions and directions for future research

This chapter shows that pain and especially multiple pains are very common in the population. If chronic pain affects about half the population, as the results of the Scottish survey suggested (Smith et al., 2001), this also means that in many people the pain can be denoted as mild, and not intrusive enough to cause activity limitations or require medical attention. However, severe chronic disabling pain affects ~6% of the population, and is associated with increased health care-resource use and productivity losses. The perception, impact, and prognosis of pain varies widely between individuals and across different groups of people, and seems to depend on a variety of factors. Some of these factors are specific to the type of pain (e.g. age and gender), but most are generically important across different types of pain, and include an individual's history of pain, presence of multiple pains or other physical symptoms, and several psychological and social factors. This seems to imply that – regardless of the type of pain or medical diagnosis, and whether or not symptoms can be explained by physiological processes – the impact of pain can be described on a continuum from infrequent localized mild pain to chronic widespread disabling pain, along with associated psychosocial characteristics.

Future research may need to determine the direction and causality of associations between risk factors and outcome, and unravel the interactions among somatic, psychological, and social factors in the development and consequences of pain in the community. There seems to be scope for the development and evaluation of individual and population-based interventions that may use either stepwise approaches or specifically address important risk factors. Screening tools may need to be developed and tested in order to identify appropriate target populations for promising interventions. Challenges for the future (summarized in Table 12.3) also include investigation of

Table 12.3 Challenges for future research

- Design longitudinal studies to investigate how episodes of mild localized pain develop into chronic pain syndromes. These studies may include research into physiological, psychological, as well as social processes

- Investigate the effect of multiple pains or other physical symptoms in determining consequences and prognosis of pain

- Investigate the effects of social and family factors on the development, consequences, and prognosis of chronic pain

- Identify which factors (at individual or population level) are likely to be causally associated with the consequences of pain and to what extent these may be modifiable

- To develop and test individual as well as population-based interventions that focus on risk factors for the development of chronic pain or the consequences of pain

- To develop screening tools for identification of appropriate target populations for promising interventions

- To investigate the effects, feasibility, and costs of individual and population-based interventions for chronic pain

- To use a public health perspective for estimating relative costs and health gains of individual and population-based interventions for chronic pain, that vary in terms of target population, intensity, expected effects, and costs

---

the effects and costs of interventions for chronic pain that use a public health perspective. This may help to estimate the relative costs and health gains of individual and population-based interventions, which can range from extensive pain management programmes targeted at small groups of chronic pain patients to simple educational interventions targeted at whole populations.

References

Aaron, L.A. and Buchwald, D. 2001: A review of the evidence for overlap among unexplained clinical conditions. *Ann Intern Med* **134**, 868–881.

Aaron, L.A., Burke, M.M., Buchwald, D. 2000: Overlapping conditions among patients with chronic fatigue syndrome, fibromyalgia, and temporomandibular disorder. *Arch Intern Med* **160**, 221–227.

Barsky, A.J. and Borus, J.F. 1999: Functional somatic syndromes. *Ann Intern Med* **130**, 910–921.

Blyth, F.M. 2008: Chronic pain—is it a public health problem? *Pain* **137**, 465–466.

Blyth, F.M., March, L.M., Nicholas, M.K., Cousins, M.J. 2005: Self-management of chronic pain: a population-based study. *Pain* **113**, 285–292.

Boardman, H.F., Thomas, E., Croft, P.R., Millson, D.S. 2003: Epidemiology of headache in an English district. *Cephalalgia* **23**, 129–137.

Boersma, K. and Linton, S.J. 2006: Expectancy, fear and pain in the prediction of chronic pain and disability: a prospective analysis. *Eur J Pain* **10**, 551–557.

Bot, S.D., van der Waal, J.M., Terwee, C.B., van der Windt, D.A., Scholten, R.J., Bouter, L.M. et al. 2005: Predictors of outcome in neck and shoulder symptoms: a cohort study in general practice. *Spine* **30**, E459–E470.

Botha-Scheepers, S., Riyazi, N., Kroon, H.M., Scharloo, M., Houwing-Duistermaat, J.J., Slagboom, E. et al. 2006: Activity limitations in the lower extremities in patients with osteoarthritis: the modifying effects of illness perceptions and mental health. *Osteoarthritis Cartilage* **14**, 1104–1110.

Brown, R.J. 2004: Psychological mechanisms of medically unexplained symptoms: an integrative conceptual model. *Psychol Bull* **130**, 793–812.

Buchbinder, R., Jolley, D., Wyatt, M. 2001: 2001 Volvo Award Winner in Clinical Studies: Effects of a media campaign on back pain beliefs and its potential influence on management of low back pain in general practice. *Spine* **26**, 2535–2542.

Burton, A.K., Balague, F., Cardon, G., Eriksen, H.R., Henrotin, Y., Lahad, A. et al. 2005: How to prevent low back pain. *Best Pract Res Clin Rheumatol* **19**, 541–555.

Buskila, D., and Press, J. 2001: Neuroendocrine mechanisms in fibromyalgia-chronic fatigue. *Best Pract Res Clin Rheumatol* **15**, 747–758.

Butler, R.J., Johnson, W.G., Cote, P. 2007: It pays to be nice: employer-worker relationships and the management of back pain claims. *J Occup Environ Med* **49**, 214–225.

Chodosh, J., Solomon, D.H., Roth, C.P., Chang, J.T., MacLean, C.H., Ferrell, B.A. et al. 2004: The quality of medical care provided to vulnerable older patients with chronic pain. *J Am Geriatr Soc* **52**, 756–761.

Ciccone, D.S. and Natelson, B.H. 2003: Comorbid illness in women with chronic fatigue syndrome: a test of the single syndrome hypothesis. *Psychosom Med* **65**, 268–275.

Creavin, S.T. 2008: *Prevalence and characteristics of pain, fatigue, and combinations of these symptoms: a cross-sectional survey and follow-up study* [thesis]. Keele University, UK

Croft, P., Lewis, M., Hannaford, P. 2003: Is all chronic pain the same? A 25-year follow-up study. *Pain* **105**, 309–317.

Deary, I.J. 1999: A taxonomy of medically unexplained symptoms. *J Psychosom Res* **47**, 51–59.

Dionne, C.E., Bourbonnais, R., Fremont, P., Rossignol, M., Stock, S.R., Larocque, I. 2005: A clinical return-to-work rule for patients with back pain. *CMAJ* **172**, 1559–1567.

Dunn, K.M., Jordan, K.P., Croft, P.R. 2006: Characterising the course of low back pain: a latent class analysis. *Am J Epidemiol* **163**, 754–761.

Elliott, A.M., Smith, B.H., Hannaford, P.C. 2004: Chronic pain and health status: how do those not using healthcare services fare? *Br J Gen Pract* **54**, 614–616.

Elliott, A.M., Smith, B.H., Hannaford, P.C., Smith, W.C., Chambers, W.A. 2002: The course of chronic pain in the community: results of a 4-year follow-up study. *Pain* **99**, 299–307.

Elliott, A.M., Smith, B.H., Penny, K.I.,Smith, W.C., Chambers, W.A. 1999: The epidemiology of chronic pain in the community. *Lancet* **354**, 1248–1252.

Faucett, J., Garry, M., Nadler, D., Ettare, D. 2002: A test of two training interventions to prevent work-related musculoskeletal disorders of the upper extremity. *Appl Ergon* **33**, 337–347.

Fishbain, D.A., Cutler, R., Rosomoff, H.L., Rosomoff, R.S. 1997: Chronic pain-associated depression: antecedent or consequence of chronic pain? A review. *Clin J Pain* **13**, 116–137.

Gureje, O., Von Korff, M., Kola, L., Demyttenaere, K., He, Y., Posada-Villa, J. et al. 2008: The relation between multiple pains and mental disorders: results from the World Mental Health Surveys. *Pain* **135**, 82–91.

Haerens, L., De, B.I., Maes, L., Cardon, G., Deforche, B. 2007: School-based randomized controlled trial of a physical activity intervention among adolescents. *J Adoles Health* **40**, 258–265.

Hagen, K.B., Bjorndal, A., Uhlig, T., Kvien, T.K. 2000: A population study of factors associated with general practitioner consultation for non-inflammatory musculoskeletal pain. *Ann Rheum Dis* **59**, 788–793.

Hay, E.M., Mullis, R., Lewis, M., Vohora, K., Main, C.J., Watson, P. et al 2005: Comparison of physical treatments versus a brief pain-management programme for back pain in primary care: a randomised clinical trial in physiotherapy practice. *Lancet* **365**, 2024–2030.

Henningsen, P., Zimmermann, T., Sattel, H. 2003: Medically unexplained physical symptoms, anxiety, and depression: a meta-analytic review. *Psychosom Med* **65**, 528–533.

Hotopf, M., Mayou, R., Wadsworth, M., Wessely, S. 1999: Childhood risk factors for adults with medically unexplained symptoms: results from a national birth cohort study. *Am J Psychiatr* **156**, 1796–1800.

Jellema, P., van der Windt, D.A., van der Horst, H.E., Blankenstein, A.H., Bouter, L.M., Stalman, W.A. 2005: Why is a treatment aimed at psychosocial factors not effective in patients with (sub) acute low back pain? *Pain* **118**, 350–359.

Jones, G.T., Silman, A.J., Macfarlane, G.J. 2003: Predicting the onset of widespread body pain among children. *Arthritis Rheum* **48**, 2615–2621.

Jones, G.T., Silman, A.J., Power, C., Macfarlane, G.J. 2007: Are common symptoms in childhood associated with chronic widespread body pain in adulthood? Results from the 1958 British Birth Cohort Study. *Arthritis Rheum* **56**, 1669–1675.

Jordan, K., Jinks, C., Croft, P. 2006: A prospective study of the consulting behaviour of older people with knee pain. *Br J Gen Pract* **56**, 269–276.

Jordan, K.P., Thomas, E., Peat, G., Wilkie, R., Croft, P. 2008: Social risks for disabling pain in older people: a prospective study of individual and area characteristics. *Pain* **137**, 652–661.

Kamaleri, Y., Natvig, B., Ihlebaek, C.M., Benth, J.S., Bruusgaard, D. 2008: Number of pain sites is associated with demographic, lifestyle, and health-related factors in the general population. *Eur J Pain* **12**, 742–748.

Kamaleri, Y., Natvig, B., Ihlebaek, C.M., Benth, J.S., Bruusgaard, D. 2009: Change in the number of musculoskeletal pain sites: A 14-year prospective study. *Pain* **141**, 25–30.

Kato, K., Sullivan, P.F., Evengard, B., Pedersen, N.L. 2006: Chronic widespread pain and its comorbidities: a population-based study. *Arch Intern Med* **166**, 1649–1654.

Kirmayer, L.J. and Looper, K.J. 2006: Abnormal illness behaviour: physiological, psychological and social dimensions of coping with distress. *Curr Opin Psychiatry* **19**, 54–60.

Koloski, N.A., Talley, N.J., Boyce, P.M. 2002: Epidemiology and health care seeking in the functional GI disorders: a population-based study. *Am J Gastroenterol* **97**, 290–299.

Kroenke, K. and Price, R.K. 1993: Symptoms in the community. Prevalence, classification, and psychiatric comorbidity. *Arch Intern Med* **153**, 2474–2480.

Kuijpers, T., van der Windt, D.A., Boeke, A.J., Twisk, J.W., Vergouwe, Y., Bouter, L.M. et al. 2006: Clinical prediction rules for the prognosis of shoulder pain in general practice. *Pain* **120**, 276–285.

Landi, F., Onder, G., Cesari, M., Gambassi, G., Steel, K., Russo, A. et al. 2001: Pain management in frail, community-living elderly patients. *Arch Intern Med* **161**, 2721–2724.

Leboeuf-Yde, C. and Kyvik, K. 1998: At what age does low back pain become a common problem? *Spine* **23**, 228–234.

Linton, S.J., Gross, D., Schultz, I.Z., Main, C., Cote, P., Pransky, G. et al. 2005: Prognosis and the identification of workers risking disability: research issues and directions for future research. *J Occup Rehabil* **15**, 459–474.

Linton, S.J. and Hallden, K. 1998: Can we screen for problematic back pain? A screening questionnaire for predicting outcome in acute and subacute back pain. *Clin J Pain* **14**, 209–215.

Linton, S.J. and van Tulder, M.W. 2001: Preventive interventions for back and neck pain problems: what is the evidence? *Spine* **26**, 778–787.

Lorig, K.R., Laurent, D.D., Deyo, R.A., Marnell, M.E., Minor, M.A., Ritter, P.L. 2002: Can a Back Pain E-mail Discussion Group improve health status and lower health care costs?: A randomized study. *Arch Intern Med* **162**, 792–796.

Macfarlane, G.J. 1999: Generalized pain, fibromyalgia and regional pain: an epidemiological view. *Baillieres Best Pract Res Clin Rheumatol* **13**, 403–414.

Macfarlane, T.V., Blinkhorn, A.S., Davies, R.M., Ryan, P., Worthington, H.V., Macfarlane, G.J. 2002: Orofacial pain: just another chronic pain? Results from a population-based survey. *Pain* **99**, 453–458.

Mallen, C.D., Peat, G., Thomas, E., Croft, P.R. 2006: Is chronic pain in adulthood related to childhood factors? A population-based case-control study of young adults. *J Rheumatol* **33**, 2286–2290.

Mallen, C.D., Peat, G., Thomas, E., Dunn, K.M., Croft, P.R. 2007: Prognostic factors for musculoskeletal pain in primary care: a systematic review. *Br J Gen Pract* **57**, 655–661.

Mathers, C. and Penm, R. 1999: *Health system costs of injury, poisoning and musculoskeletal disorders in Australia 1993-94*. Canberra, University of Sydney and the Australian Institute of Health and Welfare, Australia

Maxwell, C.J., Dalby, D.M., Slater, M., Patten, S.B., Hogan, D.B., Eliasziw, M. et al. 2008: The prevalence and management of current daily pain among older home care clients. *Pain* **138**, 208–216.

McBeth, J., Chiu, Y.H., Silman, A.J., Ray, D., Morriss, R., Dickens, C. et al. 2005: Hypothalamic-pituitary-adrenal stress axis function and the relationship with chronic widespread pain and its antecedents. *Arthritis Res Ther* **7**, R992–R1000.

McBeth, J. and Silman, A.J. 1999: Unraveling the association between chronic widespread pain and psychological distress: an epidemiological approach. *J Psychosom Res* **47**, 109–114.

McMeeken, J., Tully, E., Stillman, B., Nattrass, C.L., Bygott, I.L., Story, I. 2001: The experience of back pain in young Australians. *Manual Therapy* **6**, 213–220.

Nijrolder, I., van der Windt, D.A., van der Horst, H.E. 2009: Prediction of outcome in patients presenting with fatigue in primary care. *Br J Gen Pract* **59**, e101–e109.

Nimnuan, C., Rabe-Hesketh, S., Wessely, S., Hotopf, M. 2001: How many functional somatic syndromes? *J Psychosom Res* **51**, 549–557.

Papageorgiou, A.C., Croft, P.R., Ferry, S., Jayson, M.I., Silman, A.J. 1995: Estimating the prevalence of low back pain in the general population: evidence from the South Manchester Back Pain Survey. *Spine* **20**, 1889–1894.

Picavet, H.S. and Hoeymans, N. 2004: Health related quality of life in multiple musculoskeletal diseases: SF-36 and EQ-5D in the DMC3 study. *Ann Rheum Dis* **63**, 723–729.

Picavet, H.S. and Schouten, J.S. 2003: Musculoskeletal pain in the Netherlands: prevalences, consequences and risk groups, the DMC(3)-study. *Pain* **102**, 167–178.

Plachta-Danielzik, S., Pust, S., Asbeck, I., Czerwinski-Mast, M., Langnase, K., Fischer, C. et al. 2007: Four-year follow-up of school-based intervention on overweight children: the KOPS study. *Obesity* 15, 3159–3169.

Pope, D.P., Croft, P.R., Pritchard, C.M., Silman, A.J. 1997: Prevalence of shoulder pain in the community: the influence of case definition. *Ann Rheum Dis* 56, 308–312.

Reilly, B.M. and Evans, A.T. 2006: Translating clinical research into clinical practice: impact of using prediction rules to make decisions. *Ann Intern Med* 144, 201–209.

Rose, G. 1985: Sick individuals and sick populations. *Int J Epidemiol* 14, 32–38.

Sawyer, P., Bodner, E.V., Ritchie, C.S., Allman, R.M. 2006: Pain and pain medication use in community-dwelling older adults. *Am J Geriatr Pharmacother* 4, 316–324.

Schur, E.A., Afari, N., Furberg, H., Olarte, M., Goldberg, J., Sullivan, P.F. et al. 2007: Feeling bad in more ways than one: comorbidity patterns of medically unexplained and psychiatric conditions. *J Gen Intern Med* 22, 818–821.

Shaw, W.S., Linton, S.J., Pransky, G. 2006a: Reducing sickness absence from work due to low back pain: how well do intervention strategies match modifiable risk factors? *J Occup Rehabil* 16, 591–605.

Shaw, W.S., Robertson, M.M., McLellan, R.K., Verma, S., Pransky, G. 2006b: A controlled case study of supervisor training to optimize response to injury in the food processing industry. *Work* 26, 107–114.

Shaw, W.S., Robertson, M.M., Pransky, G., McLellan, R.K. 2006c: Training to optimize the response of supervisors to work injuries--needs assessment, design, and evaluation. *AAOHNJ* 54, 226–235.

Shega, J.W., Hougham, G.W., Stocking, C.B., Cox-Hayley, D., Sachs, G.A. 2006: Management of noncancer pain in community-dwelling persons with dementia. *J Am Geriatr Soc* 54, 1892–1897.

Smalbrugge, M., Jongenelis, L.K., Pot, A.M., Beekman, A.T., Eefsting, J.A. 2007: Pain among nursing home patients in the Netherlands: prevalence, course, clinical correlates, recognition and analgesic treatment--an observational cohort study. *BMC Geriatr* 7, 3.

Smith, B.H. and Elliott, A.M. 2005: Active self-management of chronic pain in the community. *Pain* 113, 249–250.

Smith, B.H., Elliott, A.M., Chambers, W.A., Smith, W.C., Hannaford, P.C., Penny, K. 2001: The impact of chronic pain in the community. *Fam Pract* 18, 292–299.

Spies-Dorgelo, M.N., van der Windt, D.A., Prins, A.P., Dziedzic, K.S., van der Horst, H.E. 2008: Clinical course and prognosis of hand and wrist problems in primary care. *Arthritis Rheum* 59, 1349–1357.

Stanford, E.A., Chambers, C.T., Biesanz, J.C., Chen, E. 2008: The frequency, trajectories and predictors of adolescent recurrent pain: a population-based approach. *Pain* 138, 11–21.

Sullivan, M.J.L., Bishop, S., Pivik, J. 1995: The pain catastrophising scale: development and validation. *Psychol Assessment* 7, 524–532.

Sullivan, M.J., Feuerstein, M., Gatchel, R., Linton, S.J., Pransky, G. 2005: Integrating psychosocial and behavioral interventions to achieve optimal rehabilitation outcomes. *J Occup Rehabil* 15, 475–489.

Sullivan, M.J. and Stanish, W.D. 2003: Psychologically based occupational rehabilitation: the Pain-Disability Prevention Program. *Clin J Pain* 19, 97–104.

Taimela, S., Kujala, U.M., Salminen, J.J., Viljanen, T. 1997: The prevalence of low back pain among children and adolescents. A nationwide, cohort-based questionnaire survey in Finland. *Spine* 22, 1132–1136.

Taylor, R.W., McAuley, K.A., Barbezat, W., Strong, A., Williams, S.M., Mann, J.I. 2007: APPLE Project: 2-y findings of a community-based obesity prevention program in primary school age children. *Am J Clin Nutr* 86, 735–742.

Terwindt, G.M., Ferrari, M.D., Tijhuis, M., Groenen, S.M., Picavet, H.S., Launer, L.J. 2000: The impact of migraine on quality of life in the general population: the GEM study. *Neurology* 55, 624–629.

Tveito, T.H., Hysing, M., Eriksen, H.R. 2004: Low back pain interventions at the workplace: a systematic literature review. *Occup Med (Lond)* 54, 3–13.

van der Waal, J.M., Bot, S.D., Terwee, C.B., van der Windt, D.A., Scholten, R.J., Bouter, L.M. et al. 2005: Course and prognosis of knee complaints in general practice. *Arthritis Rheum* 53, 920–930.

van der Windt, D., Croft, P., Penninx, B. 2002: Neck and upper limb pain: more pain is associated with psychological distress and consultation rate in primary care. *J Rheumatol* 29, 564–569.

van der Windt, D.A., Dunn, L.M., Spies, M.N., Mallen, C.D., Blankenstein, A.H., Stalman, W.A.B. 2008a: Impact of physical symptoms on perceived health in the community. *Psychosom Res* 64, 265–274.

van der Windt, D., Hay, E., Jellema, P., Main, C. 2008b: Psychosocial interventions for low back pain in primary care: lessons learned from recent trials. *Spine* 33, 81–89.

van der Windt, D.A., Kuijpers, T., Jellema, P., van der Heijden, G.J., Bouter, L.M. 2007: Do psychological factors predict outcome in both low-back pain and shoulder pain? *Ann Rheum Dis* 66, 313–319.

van Tulder, M.W., Koes, B.W., Metsemakers, J.F., Bouter, L.M. 1998: Chronic low back pain in primary care: a prospective study on the management and course. *Fam Pract* 15, 126–132.

Von Korff, M., Crane, P., Lane, M., Miglioretti, D.L., Simon, G., Saunders, K. et al. 2005: Chronic spinal pain and physical-mental comorbidity in the United States: results from the national comorbidity survey replication. *Pain* 113, 331–339.

Von Korff, M. and Moore, J.C. 2001: Stepped care for back pain: activating approaches for primary care. *Ann Intern Med* 134, 911–917.

Wessely, S., Nimnuan, C., Sharpe, M. 1999: Functional somatic syndromes: one or many? *Lancet* 354, 936–939.

Wolfe, F., Anderson, J., Harkness, D., Bennett, R.M., Caro, X.J., Goldenberg, D.L. et al. 1997: A prospective, longitudinal, multicenter study of service utilization and costs in fibromyalgia. *Arthritis Rheum* 40, 1560–1570.

Chapter 13

Headache

Helen Boardman

Headache is not one condition but describes a wide range of head pains of various origins and impacts on the lives of sufferers. Headache is often considered to be a relatively minor event with minimal effect on the sufferer, but for some it can be a disabling condition with a substantial impact on work and social life, and rarely, it is the symptom of serious illness such as a tumour. Headache differs from many other pain syndromes in its episodic nature – with only a small number of sufferers reporting chronic headache. However, for most sufferers, episodic headache is a recurrent event and so it is 'persistent' in a rather different sense to the experience of chronic pain. The high period prevalence of headache means that the population impact of its effects is large.

Definitions and pathophysiology

Similarly to other pain, headache is unseen by others and we rely on individuals' subjective reports of the frequency, duration, and severity of their pain. In order to better understand and research headache, the International Headache Society has developed classification criteria for all headaches – these are widely adopted for both research and clinical use (International Headache Society, 2008). The criteria are designed to classify all individual types of headache in each patient, rather than classifying the patient. The classification divides headaches into three major categories: primary headaches, secondary headaches, and cranial neuralgias and other facial pain. The classification provides a detailed guide to symptomology of each headache type, of which the major types are briefly described below.

Primary headaches

Primary headaches principally consist of migraine, tension-type headache, and cluster headache. The mechanisms of primary headaches are not fully understood, although there are many factors associated with their occurrence, including those considered to 'trigger' individual attacks.

Migraine describes a unilateral headache of moderate to severe intensity which lasts 4–72 h, characterized by accompanying symptoms which include nausea and vomiting and/or photophobia and phonophobia. For some sufferers, migraine also has prodromal effects which include visual and other sensory phenomena – the migraine aura (International Headache Society, 2008). During migraine both neurological and vascular changes have been observed. A cortical spreading depression (short-lived, reversible depression of electrical activity which moves from the rear to the front of the brain) has been observed in migraine sufferers and is thought to contribute to migraine aura and pain through the resulting effects on cerebral blood flow and meningeal trigeminal nerve fibres. There is much debate on the cause of migraine (Rothrock, 2008; Cutrer and Charles, 2008), and the relative contribution of vascular and neural changes to the onset and duration of attacks is not fully understood.

Cluster headache is an intense unilateral headache with an orbital or supraorbital location which, whilst having the shortest duration of the primary headaches (from 15 to 180 min), has pain that is severe or very severe with accompanying same-side symptoms in the face, eye, and nose. Cluster headache is so named as the headache attacks tend to occur in clusters of up to eight per day over a period of time, followed by headache-free intervals (International Headache Society, 2008). The timing of cluster headaches, shortly after falling asleep and early morning, has led to investigations about the role of the hypothalamus in generating cluster headaches. Current thinking suggests that activation of the hypothalamus leads to stimulation of the trigeminal nerve, resulting in the generation of cluster headaches (May, 2005).

Tension-type headache is a bilateral mild-to-moderate headache with pain described as having a tightening or pressing quality and lasting from 30 min to 7 days (International Headache Society, 2008). Increased responsiveness (sensitization) of myofascial tissues occurs in patients with tension-type headache, and this is thought to occur alongside sensitization to the pain stimuli in the brain. The relative contributions of peripheral and central mechanisms are thought to differ between episodic and chronic tension-type headache, with the degree of central nervous sensitization being linked to increasingly frequent headaches (Fumal and Schoenen, 2008).

Secondary headaches

Secondary headaches can be attributed to many causes, from substance withdrawal, such as those occurring after use of alcohol and caffeine, to headaches resulting from head or neck injury or those resulting from underlying illness. Prevention of these headaches lies generally with prevention of the underlying cause, and treatment may include treating both the headache and the cause.

Chronic headaches

Headache is rarely continuous and 'chronic headache' is defined as a headache which is present on ≥15 days per month for at least 3 months. Chronic headache can represent progression of episodic variants of both tension-type headache and migraine (International Headache Society, 2008). Chronic headache has been found to affect ~3–4% of general populations, and is thought to arise from both the progression of episodic headache and overuse of analgesics.

Headache occurrence, significance, and impact on populations

Headache affects almost everyone at some time in their lives with lifetime headache prevalence estimated at >90% for most age-groups. In a UK survey, more than two-thirds of the population report a headache in the previous 3 months (Boardman et al., 2003). People can experience different headache types during the same time period, and different headaches may affect them at different times during their life. Additionally headache symptoms may vary for a headache type within an individual over time.

Most headaches do not result from underlying disease and are episodic in nature; however this does not, for some sufferers, lessen the impact on their lives. Migraine is one of the biggest contributors to disability – e.g. in women in the age range of 15–44 years it is rated by the World Health Organization in the top 15 global causes of disease burden (World Health Organization, 2004).

Lost and reduced-ability work-days are perhaps the biggest public health impact of headache. In a UK population survey, 14% of the population reported at least moderate headache-related disability (minimum of 6 days in 3 months where work, home, or social life were affected; Boardman et al., 2003). From this survey it was estimated that 1327 work days per 1000 workers are lost per year to headache, with another 5213 work days per 1000 workers per year in which ability to work is reduced by half or more due to headache. Of the primary headaches, migraine has the biggest impact on the individual sufferer, in that they usually need to stop their activity and this can lead to absence from work. However, the higher prevalence of tension-type headache means that overall (in public health terms) this headache type contributes more to lost work time through both absence and reduced ability at work due to headache (Jensen, 2003).

Sufferers reporting more severe headaches are unsurprisingly more likely to ask for advice about their headaches; those reporting more frequent, more painful, longer duration, and more disabling headaches are more likely to consult a health care professional, as are women and younger people. Health care practitioners consulted (in the UK system) are principally general practitioners, but opticians, pharmacists, and hospital specialists are also consulted about headache (Thomas et al., 2004). Studies in other health care systems of migraine and severe headache sufferers find similarly that general practitioners are the main professionals consulted, with neurologists being the main source of specialist care (Lipton et al., 1998; Radtke and Neuhauser, 2009). The use of the emergency department for headache care has been reported in the USA (Friedman et al., 2009), with unbearable pain and the lack of access to primary care physicians being the main reason reported for using the emergency department – whether a similar pattern of use is seen in other health care systems is unknown. However, professionals are not the only source of advice about headaches; lay networks also play a key role, with the high prevalence of headache meaning friends and family are likely to have experienced not only headache, but similar headache types (Thomas et al., 2004). Whilst headache is a familiar and normal symptom for many people, it still raises considerable concern for individuals as demonstrated in the high volume of advice sought from the free-of-charge direct access telephonic advice service provided by the National Health Services (NHS) in the UK (NHS Direct) – headache is the second most common symptom for which advice is sought for adults and the eighth for children (Office for National Statistics, 1999).

Most headache sufferers will treat their headache with medicines. Even in the UK, this primarily occurs outside the state health care system through direct over-the-counter (OTC) sales of medicines in pharmacies and supermarkets (Boardman et al., 2004), which means the impact of headache on health care system costs can seem relatively small. A similar pattern is seen in other Western countries with different health care systems, and even amongst those with more severe headache around half use only OTC medicines to treat their headaches (Radtke and Neuhauser, 2009; Lipton et al., 2003). Again, women and those reporting more severe headache characteristics are more likely to report using medicine to treat their headaches. In the UK, headache is primarily treated with simple analgesics, with a small number being prescribed migraine-specific treatments such as triptans (Boardman et al., 2004). There is limited evidence suggesting that those who treat a headache early, before the pain is unbearable, find that treatment is more effective (Boardman et al., 2004; Goadsby, 2008).

Studies investigating specific headache types similarly report that more severe headaches increase the likelihood of physician consultation and medicine use. Migraine has been shown to be more likely to result in both general practitioner and specialist consultation and prescription medicine use compared with frequent tension-type headache (Lyngberg et al., 2005). In the UK, use of migraine-specific drugs such as triptans has been shown to be associated with referral to specialists, suggesting that those prescribed triptans have more severe migraine (Becker et al., 2008). The availability of an over-the-counter triptan (sumatriptan) has yet to be evaluated but may result in fewer general practitioner consultations; although in the UK its high price, when directly purchased, compared with the standard price of an NHS prescription, and the restriction of over-the-counter availability to low strength (50 mg tablets), may limit the effects of the reclassification.

The impact and health care utilization related to headache have been shown to be higher in individuals who experience more than one headache type during a time period. A Danish population study found people who experienced both migraine and tension-type headache had increased work absences, higher medication use, and were more likely to consult a doctor compared with those experiencing only one type of headache (Lyngberg et al., 2005).

Descriptive epidemiology

Headache occurrence varies with age and headache type – overall headache prevalence is highest in younger adults and declines with increasing age. Women report a higher prevalence of headache compared with men and they also report more severe headache – higher frequency, longer duration, and more painful. People reporting one of these characteristics as severe are more likely to report other severe headache characteristics (Boardman et al., 2003). For nearly all headache types, women have a higher prevalence compared with men. Migraine prevalence peaks in the late 30s and 40s, whilst tension-type headache is most prevalent in the 20s and 30s (Scher et al., 1999; Speciali et al., 2008).

Headache varies in different populations. For example, African populations report lower levels of headache. Studies in the USA suggest that, in people of African origin, prevalence of migraine is higher than that reported in African countries, but lower than the Caucasian population in the USA (Stewart et al., 1996). Headache prevalence appears to be stable over time with overall prevalence estimates in UK surveys finding similar results in the 1970s and 2001 (Thomas et al., 2005).

Whilst the effects of missed work and reduced work-ability are clear at a population level, the impact on the individual can also be significant in terms of the effects on their work, home and social life. In a Canadian study the majority of headache sufferers reported that their headaches affected decisions about work and their relationships with both family members and friends. (Edmeads et al., 1993). In the same study, migraine sufferers also reported opting not to attend social and family events because of worries that they may experience a headache (Edmeads et al., 1993). It has been suggested that the higher prevalence of migraine in those with lower incomes is a result of the impact of headache on the sufferers' daily lives – frequent disruption to daily activities of sufferers impedes their ability to study or carry out a challenging job role (Stewart et al., 1992). However, the relationship is not clear and other studies have suggested that the causal pathway lies in the other direction. For example, a prospective study in Norway suggested that low socioeconomic status predicted future frequent headache, although the measure of headache presence or absence at baseline depended on reports of analgesic use or not (Hagen et al., 2002).

Migraine co-morbidity has been investigated and shown for conditions such as stroke and depression (Carolei et al., 1996; Breslau et al., 1994) – there is less evidence for co-morbidity related to other headache types. Associations with all headaches have been less widely studied, although a number of important links have been found. Headache has been shown to be associated with anxiety and depression, other painful conditions, and sleep problems. Additionally, it has been demonstrated that the strength of such associations increases with increasing headache frequency and severity (Boardman et al., 2005; Zwart et al., 2003; Hagen et al., 2002; Rains and Poceta, 2006). Co-morbidity is of concern as it appears to increase the impact of headache on sufferers (Saunders et al., 2008).

Risk factors for onset and persistence

Risk factors for first-ever headache are difficult to establish – most people will experience their first headache as a child and establishing the first occurrence of a new headache type in children or young adults can be difficult. However, headache occurrence is a common experience for most people during their life-time, and the episodic nature of headache has to be interpreted in the light of the fact that episodes recur, often persistently, over time. A follow-up study of a UK population survey found that, over a 1-year period, recovery from headache was low – ~6% of those with a headache in the previous 3 months at baseline reported being headache-free during the follow-up year (Boardman et al., 2005). Around one-third of those free of headache at baseline reported headache during the follow-up year. Women and younger respondents were more likely to report both headache persistence and new headache, which contributes to the general finding that cross-sectional prevalence estimates are higher in women and younger age groups.

The same population study investigated predictors of onset and recovery from headache. The risk of developing a new headache, in persons free of headache at baseline, was higher in those with baseline characteristics of previous headache, sleep problems, the presence of other pain, and caffeine consumption. Complementary to this, less severe headache characteristics increase the likelihood of recovery from headache, as do the absence of other problems – notably pain, sleep problems, and anxiety (Boardman et al., 2006).

Risk factors for the development of chronic headache have also been investigated and reflect some of the areas that increase the risk of new and persistent headache. More severe headache characteristics, snoring, caffeine, stressful life events, and co-morbid pain, alongside obesity and medication overuse, are all risk factors for the development of chronic headache (Bigal and Lipton, 2006; Scher et al., 2008).

Sufferers themselves attribute their headaches to a range of other factors including stress, tiredness, disruption to sleeping and eating patterns, and the consumption of alcohol, caffeine, and other foods (Boardman et al., 2005). They thus have an awareness of some of the factors contributing to their headaches, which may explain in part why headache decreases with increasing age – people learn what, for them, increases the risk of headache, and they develop strategies to reduce their exposure to these risks and the likelihood of a resultant headache.

Potential for prevention

Whilst individuals can influence some headaches, such as hangovers or caffeine-related headaches, primary headaches may be more difficult to prevent. Individuals do adopt strategies to reduce the risk of headache, using their past experience of headache, and the factors they believe are related, by trying to eliminate such factors from their lives. However, this is not always possible.

Potentially, the best prevention strategy to reduce both occurrence and impact of headache is to provide sufferers with ways to reduce or change factors associated with new onset and persistence of headache. The research evidence suggests that addressing sleep problems might have the largest impact as they are associated with onset of new headache, persistence of existing headache, and the development of chronic headache. Methods to achieve this include providing information about sleep hygiene so that people can adopt such strategies to minimize the risks. Anxiety is another area where a public health campaign aimed at the general population could improve the general wellbeing of the population as well as reducing the impact of headaches. There are very few studies of interventions to reduce the impact of headache. The two studies in workplaces did not report about rates of headache occurrence, but were able to show short-term reductions in pain intensity in a workplace exercise programme (Sjogren et al., 2005) and disability associated with headaches following a presentation about headaches and their management (Mannix et al., 1999). A more intensive behavioural intervention in migraine sufferers was able to demonstrate a reduction in headache frequency but this would not be suitable for the general population (Nicholson et al., 2005). The failure of a pharmacist-led intervention to change headache frequency or pain may have been a result of it concentrating on effective medicines use in headache rather than combining this with other methods to reduce the occurrence and impact of headache (Hoffman et al., 2008).

Tackling risk factors for both persistence and chronicity in existing headache sufferers has the potential to not only improve the life of the sufferer but also reduce the impact of lost work potential and sickness absence. Again, tackling sleep problems is an important area for intervention. Strategies need to both reduce the impact of headache through effective treatment and prevention, but also nullify influences, such as stressful life events, by providing methods to tackle stress and anxiety. Encouragement to lead a healthy lifestyle, including reducing weight, if needed, and avoiding known problematic foods is also likely to reduce the impact of headache. Health care professionals need to consider the wider issues in headache care, rather than merely concentrating on effective pain relief.

Pharmacotherapy for most headaches comprises simple analgesics, but these may not be sufficient for migraine and other more severe headaches. The British Association for the Study of Headache (BASH) recommends a stepwise approach to migraine therapy (British Association for the Study of Headache, 2007). Some international data challenges this with the view that stratified care is more appropriate, i.e. assess a sufferer's disability from headaches and commence therapy based on this assessment (Lipton et al., 2000). However, the BASH guidelines suggest, whilst this is the ideal, there is insufficient evidence for the efficacy of many acute migraine treatments, other than the triptans and aspirin/metoclopramide combination, or for the superiority of any individual treatment. There is also a call to use therapy early in a headache, rather than waiting until the pain is intolerable (Goadsby, 2008). Whilst this may be more effective, care needs to be taken in encouraging the early use of analgesics when medication overuse is implicated in the development of chronic daily headache. Where sufferers are using analgesics nearly daily, other strategies to treat headaches need to be adopted. Preventative therapy has been shown to be effective in reducing the frequency of migraine (Holroyd et al., 1991; Bussone et al., 2005), although some sufferers might be reluctant to embark on daily medication or find the side effects of preventative regimens are intolerable, others will be keen to reduce the impact of headache on their lives.

Research direction

Not enough is yet known about why headache persists and what strategies might be adopted that may result in recovery from headache. Further investigation of the decline in headache prevalence with age may provide some insights and potential areas for intervention in young adults.

In terms of primary prevention, intervention studies are needed to test whether strategies to prevent and reduce the impact of headache are effective. Given that work is impacted by headache, the workplace may be an appropriate place to start particularly for general health campaigns aimed at reducing sleep problems and anxiety levels.

In terms of secondary prevention, as most sufferers use OTC medicines purchased from pharmacies to treat their headaches, we need to better understand how sufferers select and use medicine to treat headache and any advice they request or receive in the pharmacy. This would enable the development of an intervention delivered in pharmacies that would aim to reduce both the occurrence and impact of headache.

There have been many studies looking at the effectiveness of newer medicines in migraine and this needs to be extended to all medicines and to tension-type headaches, so that sufferers can be better advised about which medicine to use. In addition, further studies are needed to determine if early treatment of headache really is more effective in reducing the impact of headache, without increasing the development of medication overuse headache. Whilst pharmacotherapy has its place, other methods to reduce the occurrence of headache in those who are missing work and social events through headache need to be found. Such strategies might usefully link to primary prevention of other pain syndromes discussed elsewhere in this book.

References

Becker, C., Brobert, G.P., Almqvist, P.M., Johanson, S., Jick, S.S., Meier, C.R. 2008: Migraine incidence, comorbidity and health resource utilization in the UK. *Cephalalgia* **28**, 57–64.

Bigal, M.E. and Lipton, R.B. 2006: Modifiable risk factors for migraine progression. *Headache* **46**, 1334–1343.

Boardman, H.F., Thomas, E., Croft, P.R., Millson, D.S. 2003: Epidemiology of headache in an English district. *Cephalalgia* **23**, 129–137.

Boardman, H.F., Thomas, E., Millson, D.S., Croft, P.R. 2004: Cross-sectional survey of medication used for headache in a general population. *Int J Pharm Pract* **12**, 91–99.

Boardman, H.F., Thomas, E., Millson, D.S., Croft, P.R. 2005: Psychological, sleep, lifestyle and co-morbid associations with headache in a cross-sectional survey of a UK adult population sample. *Headache* **45**, 657–669.

Boardman, H.F., Thomas, E., Millson, D.S., Croft, P.R. 2005: One-year follow-up of headache in an adult general population. *Headache* **45**, 337–345.

Boardman, H.F., Thomas, E., Millson, D.S., Croft, P.R. 2006: The natural history of headache: predictors of onset and recovery. *Cephalalgia* **26**, 1080–1088.

Breslau, N., Merikangas, K., Bowden, C.L. 1994: Comorbidity of migraine and major affective disorders. *Neurology* **44**(suppl 7), S17–S22.

British Association for the Study of Headache. 2007: Guidelines for All Healthcare Professionals in the Diagnosis and Management of Migraine, Tension-Type, Cluster and Medication-Overuse Headache. 3rd edition. Available at: http://216.25.88.43/upload/NS_BASH/BASH_guidelines_2007.pdf.

Bussone, G., Diener, H-C., Pfeil, J., Schwalen, S. 2005: Topiramate 100mg/day in migraine prevention: a pooled analysis of double-blind randomised controlled trials. *Int J Clin Pract* **59**, 961–968.

Carolei, A., Marini, C., De Matteis, G., 1996: Italian National Research Council Study Group on Stroke in the Young. 1996: History of migraine and risk of cerebral ischaemia in young adults. *Lancet* **347**, 1503–1506.

Cutrer, F.M, Charles, A. 2008: The neurogenic basis of migraine. *Headache* **48**, 1411–1414.

Edmeads, J., Findlay, H., Tugwell, P., Pryse-Philips, W., Nelson, R.F., Murray, T.J. 1993: Impact of migraine and tension-type headache on life-style, consulting behaviour, and medication use: a Canadian population survey. *Can J Neuro Sci* **20**, 131–137.

Friedman, B.W., Serrano, D., Reed, M., Diamond, M., Lipton, R.B. 2009: Use of the emergency department for severe headache. A population-based study survey. *Headache* **49**, 21–30.

Fumal, A. and Schoenen, J. 2008: Tension-type headache: current research and clinical management. *Lancet Neurol* **7**, 70–83.

Goadsby, P.J. 2008: The 'Act when Mild' (AwM) study: a step forward in our understanding of early treatment in the acute treatment of migraine. *Cephalalgia* **28**, 36–41.

Hagen, K., Einarsen, C., Zwart, J-A., Svebak, S., Bovim, G. 2002: The co-occurrence of headache and musculoskeletal symptoms amongst 51050 adults in Norway. *Eur J Neurol* **9**, 527–533.

Hagen, K., Vatten, L., Stovner, L.J., Zwart, J-A., Krokstad, S., Bovim, G. 2002: Low socio-economic status is associated with increased risk of frequent headache: a prospective study of 22718 adults in Norway. *Cephalalgia* **22**, 672–679.

Hoffman, W., Herzog, B., Mühlig, S., Kayser, H., Fabian, R., Thomsen, M., Cramer, M., Fiß, T., Gresselmeyer, D., Janhsen, K. 2008: Pharmaceutical care for migraine and headache patients: a community-based, randomized intervention. *Ann Pharmacother* **42**, 1804–1803.

Holroyd, K.A., Penzien, D.B., Cordingley, G.E. 1991: Propranolol in the management of recurrent migraine: a meta-analytic review. *Headache* **31**, 333–340.

International Headache Society. 2008: The International Classification of Headache Disorders. 2nd edn. Available at: http://ihs-classification.org/en/.

Jensen, R. 2003: Diagnosis, epidemiology and impact of tension-type headache. *Current Headache Reports* **2**, 455–459.

Lipton, R.B., Scher, A.I., Steiner, T.J., Bigal, M.E., Kolodner, K., Liberman, J.N., Stewart, W.F. 2003: Patterns of health care utilization for migraine in England and in the United States. *Neurology* **60**, 441–448.

Lipton, R.B., Stewart, W.F., Simon, D. 1998: Medical consultation for migraine: results from the American Migraine Study. *Headache* **38**, 87–96.

Lipton, R.B., Stewart, W.F., Stone, A.M., Láinez, M.J.A., Sawyer, J.P.C. 2000: Stratified care vs step care strategies for migraine. The disabilities in strategies of care (DISC) study: a randomized trial. *JAMA* **284**, 2599–2605.

`Lyngberg, A.C., Rasmussen, B.K., Jørgensen, T. and Jensen, R. 2005: Secular changes in health care utilization and work absence for migraine and tension-type headache: A population based study. *Eur J Epidemiol* **20**, 1007–1014.

Mannix, L.K., Solomon, G.D., Kippes, C.M., Kunkel, R.S. 1999: Impact of headache education program in the workplace. *Neurology* **53**, 868–871.

May, A. 2005: Cluster headache: pathogenesis, diagnosis, and management. *Lancet* **366**, 843–855.

Nicholson, R., Nash, J., Andrasik, F. 2005: A self-administered behavioural intervention using tailored messages for migraine. *Headache* **45**, 1124–1139.

Office for National Statistics. 1999: Ten most common symptoms on which advice is sought from NHS Direct, *Social Trends 30*. Available at: http://www.statistics.gov.uk/StatBase/xsdataset.asp?vlnk=673&Pos=1&ColRank=2&Rank=256.

Radtke, A. Neuhauser, H. 2009: Prevalence and burden of headache and migraine in Germany. *Headache* **49**, 79–89.

Rains, J.C. and Poceta, J.S. 2006: Headache and sleep disorders: review and clinical implications for headache management. *Headache* **46**, 1344–1363.

Rothrock, J.F. 2008: "Outside-in" vs "inside-out": revisiting migraine's vascular hypothesis. *Headache* **48**, 1409–1410.

Saunders, K., Merikangas, K., Low, N.C.P., Von Korff, M., Kessler, R.C. 2008: Impact of comorbidity on headache-related disability. *Neurology* **70**, 538–547.

Scher, A.I., Midgette, L.A., Lipton, R.B. 2008: Risk factors for headache chronification. *Headache* **48**, 16–25.

Scher, A.I. Stewart, W.F., Lipton, R.B. 1999: Migraine and headache: a meta-analytic approach. In: Crombie, I.K. (editor). *Epidemiology of pain*. Seattle: IASP Press.

Sjögren, T., Nissinen, K.J., Järvenpää, S.K., Ojasen, M.T., Vanharanta, H., Mälkiä, E.A. 2005: Effects of a workplace physical exercise intervention on the intensity of headache and neck and shoulder symptoms and upper extremity muscular strength of office workers: a cluster randomised controlled cross-over trial. *Pain* **116**, 119–128.

Speciali, J.G., Eckeli, A.L., Dach, F. 2008: Tension-type headache. *Expert Rev Neurother* **8**, 839–53.

Stewart, W.F., Lipton, R.B., Celentano, D.D., Reed M.L. 1992: Prevalence of migraine headache in the United States: relation to age, income, race, and other sociodemographic factors. *JAMA* **267**, 64–49.

Stewart, W.F., Lipton, R.B., Liberman, J. 1996: Variation in migraine prevalence by race. *Neurology* **47**, 52–59.

Thomas, E., Boardman, H.F., Croft, P.R. 2005: Why do older people report fewer headaches? *Gerontology* **51**, 322–328.

Thomas, E., Boardman, H.F., Ogden, H., Millson, D.S., Croft, P.R. 2004: Advice and care for headache: Who seeks it, who gives it? *Cephalalgia* **24**, 740–752.

World Health Organization. 2004: The global burden of disease. http://www.who.int/healthinfo/global_burden_disease/2004_report_update/en/index.html.

Zwart, J-A., Dyb, G., Hagen, K., Ødegård, K.J., Dahl, A.A., Bovim, G., Stovner, L.J. 2003: Depression and anxiety disorders associated with headache frequency. The Nord-Trøndelag Health Study. *Eur J Neurol* **10**, 147–152.

Chapter 14

Pain in children

Gareth T. Jones and Adriana Paola Botello

Introduction

Pain in children is a common phenomenon and, to a large extent, it is a part of the everyday life of the child. Indeed, in the very young, the pain experience may be an important part of life, providing stimuli that help develop pain processing pathways— especially descending inhibitory control from central nervous system sites above the spinal cord, which include an array of neurotransmitters: noradrenaline, serotonin, dopamine, and substance P. There are numerous diseases in childhood with pain as the major presenting symptom. However, these diseases – such as juvenile arthritis and childhood leukaemia – are rare and, from a population perspective, account for only a minor proportion of the overall pain burden in children.

Pain is a symptom, or a syndrome, rather than a disease, without established biomarkers or even gold-standard clinical methods of measurement. Thus, common to all epidemiological pain research, studies examining pain in children can seldom distinguish between the occurrence, and the reporting, of pain. This is particularly important in the very young, who have difficulties expressing pain – or, more correctly, in whom researchers have difficulty accurately measuring pain perception in a way that is demonstrably valid and reliable. There are a number of tools available for the assessment of pain in infants and young children, most of which are used in the clinic or, occasionally, the laboratory setting. Typically, these rely on the observation and categorization of various pain behaviours. However, few of these instruments have been validated for use in population-based research and it is hard, therefore, to determine robust epidemiological estimates of the occurrence of (chronic) pain in the very young. Even in older children, and in adults, an estimate of pain occurrence is a function of many things, including case definition, period of recall, and (particularly pertinent in children) the age group of the population under study. Thus, estimates of pain prevalence in children can vary markedly with the age of study participants, case definition, and study-specific methodological nuances.

Prevalence of pain in children

Perquin et al. (2000), in a large population-based study of children in the Netherlands, found that approximately half of children in the age range of 4–18 years experienced some pain within a 3-month period. Further, nearly half of these children (25% overall) experienced chronic pain – defined as pain that has lasted for longer than 3 months. Consistent with the literature in adults, chronic pain was more common in girls than boys, and increased with age; see Figure 14.1. In Finland, Mikkelsson et al. (1997) demonstrated that around one-third of children reported musculoskeletal pain at least once a week in the past 3 months and a further 40% reported pain once a month over the same period. In terms of the location of these pains: approximately one-third of children reported headache at least once a week; whereas, lower limb pain and neck pain were the most commonly reported musculoskeletal pains, with ~18% and ~15% of children reporting these

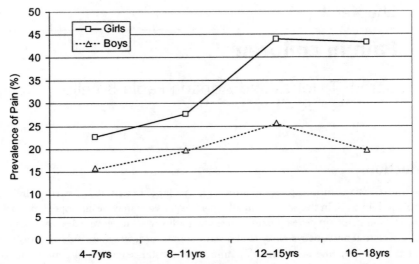

Fig. 14.1 Prevalence of chronic pain in children/adolescents, drawn from data in Perquin et al. (2000).

symptoms at least once a week. In addition, in roughly half of these cases, the leg pain and neck pain coexisted with pain at another site. The relative frequencies of musculoskeletal pain from this study are shown in Figure 14.2. Only 29% of children reported pain 'seldom or never' during the study period.

In this chapter, we discuss the epidemiology of pain in children. It is not our intention to provide a comprehensive review of all epidemiological literature relating to the occurrence of pain in children. Rather, we summarize what we consider to be the key data in the field focusing,

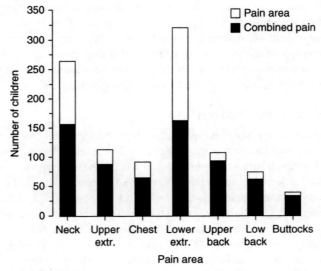

Fig. 14.2 Prevalence of musculoskeletal pain symptoms in children. Reproduced from Mikkelsson et al. (1997). This figure has been reproduced with permission of the International Association for the Study of Pain® (IASP®). The figure may not be reproduced for any other purpose without permission.

in particular, on three of the most common childhood pains: low back pain, abdominal pain, and headache; and focusing where possible on potentially modifiable risk factors.

Low back pain

Descriptive epidemiology

Studies of prevalence of low back pain in children have shown it to be a fairly common condition and, although seldom associated with health service consultation (Watson et al., 2002; Burton et al., 1996; Olsen et al., 1992), there is some evidence that low back pain in childhood is associated with continuing pain in adulthood (Harreby et al., 1995). Salminen et al. (1992a) reported the lifetime cumulative incidence of low back pain to be 30% in Finnish schoolchildren aged 14 years; Olsen et al. (1992), in the United States, reported a lifetime prevalence of 31% in schoolchildren in the age range of 11–17 years; and Troussier et al., (1994) in France, reported cumulative prevalence* of 51% in children in the age range of 6–18 years. Meanwhile Harreby et al. (1999) demonstrated the cumulative life-time prevalence of low back pain in Danish schoolchildren in the age range of 13–16 years to be ~59%. Studies examining low back-pain occurrence over a shorter time interval have also shown high prevalence estimates. In Switzerland, Balagué et al. (1995) demonstrated a 1-year prevalence of back pain of 26% among schoolchildren in the age range of 12–17 years and, in Finland, Taimela et al. (1997) found that the prevalence of 'pain in the low back area that interfered with school work or leisure activities during the previous 12 months' was 18% among children aged 14 and 16 years. Watson et al. (2002) reported a 1-month period prevalence of 24% in English schoolchildren in the age range of 11–14 years, and similar results were found in Denmark: Wedderkopp et al. (2001) found the 1-month prevalence to be 39% in children ranging in age from 8 to 16 years. Further, some studies have shown that as many as 1 child in 20 may be experiencing low back pain at any point in time (Burton et al., 1996; Viry et al., 1999; Troussier et al., 1999).

Consistent with studies in adults (Papageorgiou et al., 1995), low back pain in children increases with age and is more common in girls than boys; see Figure 14.3. Few studies have examined the association between menstruation and low back pain in schoolgirls, although there is some evidence that girls who have passed menarche are no more likely to report low back pain than other girls, after adjusting for age (Jones et al., 2003a). Fairbank et al. (1984) reported an increase in the lifetime cumulative incidence of low back pain from 13% in children aged 12 years, to 41% in those aged 18 years. Similarly, Burton et al. (1996) demonstrated approximately a fourfold increase in lifetime prevalence from 12% in children 11 years old, to 50% in those aged 15 years. Watson et al. (2002) found a doubling in the 1-month prevalence of low back pain between children in England aged 11 (16%) to 14 years (34%), and Balagué et al. (1988) reported a similar increase in the 2-week prevalence in Swiss schoolchildren: from 20% to 32% in children at ages 13 and 17 years, respectively. Masiero et al. (2008) found that, of children in the age range of 13–15 years in Italy, girls were nearly twice as likely to report low back pain as boys (odds ratio (OR): 1.9; 95% confidence interval (95%CI): 1.7–2.2); and Watson et al. (2002) demonstrated

---

* The terms lifetime prevalence, cumulative prevalence, and lifetime cumulative incidence, all essentially mean the same thing – i.e. the ratio of all persons who have ever had an episode of low back pain, to the total number of persons in the population (although, technically, the latter should use population-time as the denominator). Here we have used whichever term was used in the original article, and they can be considered to be interchangeable.

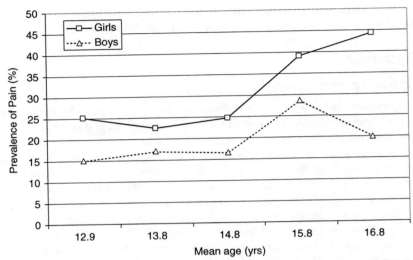

Fig. 14.3 Prevalence of low back pain in children. Data from Grimmer and Williams (2000).

a 50% increase in the odds of low back pain among girls in the age range of 11–14 years, compared to their male counterparts.

Few studies have looked at the onset of low back pain in schoolchildren. In the UK, Jones et al. (2003a) found that ~19% of 933 children in the age range of 12–15 years – known to have been free of low back pain 12 months previously – reported low back pain lasting for 1 day or longer, in the previous month. Further, the occurrence of new-onset low back pain increased with age. Similarly, Brattberg (1994) reported a 2-year incidence of 16%, 22%, and 22% in schoolchildren aged 8, 11, and 13 years, respectively.

Analytical epidemiology

There have been a number of analytical epidemiological studies of the aetiology of low back pain in children of varying quality. However, the majority have been cross-sectional or case-control studies and therefore – irrespective of study quality – are unable to examine the temporal relationship between low back pain and any putative risk factors. In addition, with these study designs, exposure data is collected retrospectively and, as such, is open to a number of potential biases – principally recall bias. Study participants may vary in their ability to accurately report past exposures: this is recall error, but not a bias *per se*. Bias may arise as a result of differential recall between cases and controls, where children with and without low back pain may report exposures with differing degrees of accuracy. In contrast, longitudinal study designs – prospective or retrospective cohort studies – do not suffer from these disadvantages and, therefore, constitute a more robust study design from which to examine aetiology. However, cohort studies are more costly, more time-consuming, and, therefore, less common. Thus, in this section, while we will try and accommodate the best evidence from longitudinal studies where they exist, this will be supplemented with evidence from case-control and cross-sectional studies, as appropriate.

Several studies have examined the relationship between height and weight and childhood low back pain. In terms of height, the evidence is mixed. Some studies have shown an association in boys but not in girls (Nissinen et al., 1994; Salminen et al., 1995; Salminen et al., 1992b), and others have shown, in longitudinal studies, that child stature at baseline does not predict the future onset of symptoms (Kujala et al., 1997). Others have suggested that low back pain is associated with growth, rather than height *per se*, and have demonstrated that children with rapid growth are more likely to report low back pain than other children (Feldman et al., 2001; Poussa et al., 2005). Others, however, have shown no difference in growth between children with and without low back pain (Kujala et al., 1997).

Irrespective of their relationship, from a public health perspective height and growth can, at best, be considered risk markers for low back pain, rather than potentially modifiable risk factors. In terms of modifiable factors, studies can be categorized into four main areas: lifestyle characteristics; mechanical load; psychosocial factors; and general (ill)-health.

Lifestyle characteristics

A number of authors have demonstrated an ~75% increase in the occurrence of low back pain among children engaged in competitive sport (Balagué et al., 1988; Szpalski et al., 2002), and others have shown radiological abnormalities in children who participate in sports involving high mechanical load on the spine (e.g. weightlifting and body building; Duggleby and Kumar, 1997); repeated flexion and extension (e.g. gymnastics and rowing; Duggleby and Kumar, 1997; McMeeken et al., 2001; Harvey and Tanner, 1991); and repeated spinal torsion (e.g. golf and racket sports; Duggleby and Kumar, 1997; Sward et al., 1990). Participation in sports at a competitive level may be associated with over-training, and greater exposure to injury, whereas more modest levels of physical activity may be beneficial. However, while a recent prospective study showed a decrease in the probability of low back pain with increasing physical activity (Wedderkopp et al., 2008), another demonstrated no such effect: compared to children undertaking <100 min of exercise at school per week, those engaging in >3 h experienced a very small, and non-significant, increase in the risk of symptom onset (risk ratio (RR): 1.1; 95%CI: 0.6–1.8; Jones et al., 2003a).

Few studies have examined the role of sedentary activity in the aetiology of low back pain in children. Gunzburg et al. (1999) demonstrated an increase in the occurrence of low back pain in children who play video games for >2 h per day, but failed to demonstrate the same relationship with watching television for >2 h. In contrast, Troussier et al. (1994) demonstrated a dose–risk relationship whereby, compared to watching no television, children who watched <1 h (OR: 1.1; 95%CI: 0.7–1.6), 1–2 h (OR: 1.8; 95%CI: 1.1–2.7), and >2 h (OR: 2.7; 95%CI: 1.4–5.2) experienced an increase in the likelihood of low back pain. Other studies have shown similar results (Balagué et al., 1988).

Prospectively, Jones et al. (2003a) showed no relationship between sedentary activity (using a composite index of time spent watching television, playing video games, and/or using the computer) and risk of low back pain onset, suggesting that, in the case of any relationship observed cross-sectionally, the increase in sedentary activity may occur as a consequence of (or, if not a consequence, at least subsequent to) low back pain, and not as its precursor. Supporting this, a number of authors have examined the relationship between body weight, or body mass index (BMI), and childhood low back pain. While some have found that children reporting low back pain are heavier (Fairbank et al., 1984), others have reported no significant difference in weight and/or BMI between those with or without low back pain (Salminen et al., 1992b; Grimmer and Williams, 2000; Watson et al., 2002). Crucially, of the few prospective studies that have been conducted, the evidence suggests that baseline weight does not predict future low back pain (Nissinen et al., 1994; Salminen et al., 1995).

Mechanical load

Over the last decade there have been many claims in the media and lay-press about heavy schoolbags 'causing' back pain in children. Until recently, however, there was little robust epidemiological evidence in this area. Much of the initial work focused on subjective measures of schoolbag weight and several studies demonstrated an association between low back pain and the perception of schoolbag weight (Szpalski et al., 2002; Gunzburg et al., 1999; Negrini et al., 1998). Watson et al. (2003) gave children a spring balance and a diary to provide an objective measure of mechanical load over a whole school week. These authors found that the 20% of children with the heaviest schoolbags were no more likely to report low back pain than the 20% of children with the lightest loads (OR: 0.9; 95%CI: 0.6–1.4). Further, this study demonstrated a protective effect of high relative bag weight (ratio of bag weight to body weight): compared with children carrying <6.6% of their body weight, those carrying >13.6% experienced a 40% reduction in the occurrence of low back pain (OR: 0.6; 95%CI: 0.4–1.0; Watson et al., 2003). Others, however, have shown conflicting findings: Viry et al. (1999) found that children who carried a relative schoolbag weight of >20% experienced a more than twofold increase in the likelihood of low back pain (OR: 2.2; 95%CI: 0.8–5.8).

Jones et al. (2003a) examined the relationship between schoolbag weight and low back-pain onset prospectively. These authors reported no association between schoolbag weight ($RR_{\text{5th versus 1st quintile}}$: 1.2; 95% CI: 0.7–2.1), or relative bag weight (RR5th versus 1st quintile: 0.8; 95% CI: 0.5–1.3)*, and the risk of low back-pain onset over a 12-month period (Jones et al., 2003). However, there was some evidence of a dose–risk relationship between schoolbag weight and low back-pain onset among children who walk to school, and those who do not use a locker – i.e. among those children who are exposed to their bag weight for the longest periods of time.

Psychosocial factors

A number of studies have examined the role of psychological and psychosocial factors in the epidemiology of low back pain in childhood. Balagué et al. (1995) demonstrated a small but significant decrease in the lifetime prevalence of low back pain associated with a 1-quintile increase in positive affect score, as assessed by the Children's Depression Scale (Tisher et al., 1983); (OR: 0.8; 95%CI: 0.7–0.96), and, similarly, a rise in prevalence associated with increases in negative affect (Balagué et al., 1995). Meanwhile, in Swedish schoolchildren, Brattberg (1994) found strong and significant effects between back pain and a number of adverse psychosocial indicators: fear of schoolmates (OR: 2.4; 95%CI: 1.1–5.3); loneliness (OR: 3.6; 95%CI: 1.2–11.1); difficulty making friends (OR: 2.1; 95%CI: 1.1–4); feeling of being an outsider (OR: 2.1; 95%CI: 1.1–3.8); victim of bullying (OR: 2.1; 95%CI: 1.1–3.6); and passive reaction to bullying (OR: 3.4; 95%CI: 1.6–7.3), although it is unclear how these concepts were measured (Brattberg, 1994). In the UK, using the Strengths and Difficulties Questionnaire (Goodman, 1997), Watson et al. (2002) demonstrated a similar relationship between low back pain 'lasting for one day or longer in the past month' and conduct problems (OR: 3.5; 95%CI: 2.4–4.9); emotional problems (OR: 3.1; 95%CI: 2.3–4.3); hyperactivity (OR: 1.6; 95%CI: 1.2–2.2); and peer problems (OR: 1.5; 95%CI: 1.1–2).

There is little prospective evidence in this area. However, Jones et al. (2003a) followed up the cohort of Watson et al. (2002) and demonstrated that psychosocial difficulties in general (RR: 1.6; 95%CI: 1.1–2.3), and conduct problems in particular (RR: 2.5; 95%CI: 1.7–3.7), significantly predicted, not only the occurrence of low back pain, but the onset of symptoms among children initially free of low back pain.

---

* Risk estimates not given in original article.

General health

One potential mechanism for the relationship between adverse psychosocial factors and low back pain is somatization – i.e. the manifestation of emotional or psychological distress as physical symptoms. As described by Servan-Schreiber et al. (2000), somatization can include the 'stress-related exaggeration of common symptoms, such as headache, light-headedness, or low back pain in the context of, for example, a divorce, new family member or new job' (Servan-Schreiber et al., 2000). In children, somatization may manifest itself in the context of behavioural and peer-relationship difficulties described above. It is plausible, therefore, that children with low back pain may be more likely also to report other 'somatic' symptoms.

Vikat et al. (2000) demonstrated an increase in the likelihood of low back pain in children with increasing number of psychosomatic symptoms. Similarly, Watson et al. (2002) found that children with low back pain were ~3 times more likely to report headache (OR: 3.5; 95%CI: 2.5–5.0); abdominal pain (OR: 3.1; 95%CI: 2.1–4.7); sore throats (OR: 2.7; 95%CI: 1.9–3.7); and day-time tiredness (OR: 3.1; 95%CI: 2.3–4.2) than other children. Prospectively, Jones et al. (2003a) found that these common symptoms – headache, sore throat, and abdominal pain – not only co-occurred with low back pain but, in the absence of low back pain, were associated with between a 50% and 80% increase in the risk of future low back-pain onset.

Abdominal pain

Descriptive epidemiology

Recent data from the US National Longitudinal Study of Adolescent Health suggests that abdominal pain is one of the most commonly occurring symptoms in adolescents, with a prevalence of ~18% (Rhee et al., 2005). This is consistent with data from the UK, which suggests that ~20% of children report abdominal symptoms (Hotopf et al., 1998). Predictably, prevalence is higher in primary care attendees: Huang et al. (2000) demonstrated a prevalence of 44%. Despite this, on physical examination, seldom is a definitive diagnosis made. Devanarayana et al. (2008) found that fewer than one-quarter of children with recurrent abdominal pain had an organic cause – including chronic constipation, urinary tract infection, and gastro-oesophageal reflux disease. Further, in a recent review, Chitkara et al. (2005) demonstrated an absence of evidence relating *Helicobacter pylori* (*H. Pylori*) infection to recurrent abdominal pain. For the most part, childhood abdominal pain is commonly considered to be functional in origin – i.e. with no discernable underlying pathology. This notwithstanding, there is some evidence from national birth cohorts that children with abdominal pain are at increased risk of irritable bowel syndrome, other 'unexplained' symptoms, and psychiatric disorders, as adults (Hotopf et al., 1998; Hotopf et al., 2000; Jones et al., 2007; Howell et al., 2005).

The term recurrent abdominal pain was coined ~50 years ago by Apley and Naish as 'abdominal pain that presents at least three times over a minimum period of three consecutive months and interferes with daily activities (school attendance and performance, participation in sports and extracurricular activities)' (Apley and Naish, 1958). They conducted a survey of 1000 school children and found that 11% reported abdominal pain, with a higher prevalence in girls (12.3%) than boys (9.5%). Prevalence varied with age, and demonstrated a pre-teens peak; see Figure 14.4.

Chitkara et al. (2005) conducted a systematic review of the published literature on the epidemiology of recurrent abdominal pain in Western countries. These authors found that, among studies that ascertained cases by child questionnaire alone, prevalence ranged from 8% to 19%, much of the variation being explained by disease definition and subject age. In contrast, based on

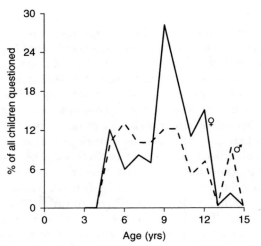

Fig. 14.4 Prevalence of abdominal pain in children. Reproduced from Apley and Naish (1958), with permission from BMJ Publishing Group Ltd.

parental questionnaire or interview, prevalence ranged from 2.4% to 16%. Finally, studies that used a combination of parent and child questionnaires estimated the prevalence to range between 0.3% and 10.8%. In the Far East, Boey et al. (2000) demonstrated that 10.2% of Malaysian schoolchildren in the age range of 11–16 years reported 'abdominal pain occurring at least three times over a period of at least three months, interfering with normal daily activity'; whereas a second study by the same authors, using the same case definition and in a similar setting, found a prevalence of 41.2% in children in the age range of 11–12 years (Boey and Yap, 1999).

In a recent high-quality study in the UK, Ramchandani et al. (2005) demonstrated that, while the 1-year prevalence of any abdominal pain is high: (40% in children aged 3.5 years, rising to 55% in those ~7 years), recurrent abdominal pain – defined as abdominal pain on >5 occasions – was less common: 3.8% and 11.8%, respectively.

Analytical epidemiology

The majority of studies of abdominal pain in children have sought organic causes for symptoms, or have involved patient populations. Because of the selected nature of these populations, the external validity of these findings is uncertain. Instead, it is important to focus on studies of children in the general population, or in school-based samples.

Lifestyle characteristics

A number of studies have examined the role of diet and obesity in the epidemiology of recurrent abdominal pain in children. While some have suggested that lactose intolerance may play a role in the aetiology of the condition (Liebman, 1979; Barr et al., 1979), others have demonstrated a similar prevalence of lactase deficiency in symptomatic and symptom-free children (Lebenthal et al., 1981).

Paulo et al. (2006) found that low fibre intake was associated with the occurrence of recurrent abdominal pain. Similarly, Malaty et al. (2007) found that poor diet – characterized by low levels of fruit and vegetable consumption – was associated with the occurrence of recurrent abdominal pain (OR: 2.6; 95%CI: 1.1–6.2 and 1.5; 0.9–3.2, respectively). These authors also found that children above the 95th percentile of BMI were more likely to report recurrent abdominal pain than other children. Focusing only on anthropometric characteristics, rather than diet, El-Metwally et al. (2007a) recorded body weight and BMI in children free of abdominal pain, and followed them up over 4 years, to determine the onset of chronic symptoms. They found that neither baseline weight nor BMI was associated with an increase in the risk of chronic abdominal pain onset $(OR_{>50th\ percentile}: 1.2; 95\%CI: 0.6–2.5$ and $1.2; 0.6–2.5$, respectively for boys; and $1.0; 0.5–1.1$ and $0.8; 0.5–1.2$ for girls); (El Metwally et al., 2007a).

Psychosocial factors

In a large population-based study of parents and children in the UK – the Avon Longitudinal Study of Parents and Children (ALSPAC) study (Golding et al., 2001) – Ramchandani et al. (2005) examined the epidemiology of recurrent abdominal pain in children in the age range of 2–6 years. These authors found that girls were significantly more likely to report abdominal pain than boys (OR: 1.6; 95%CI: 1.4–1.8), as were those from higher socioeconomic backgrounds $(OR_{social\ class\ I/II}: 1.2; 95\%CI: 1–1.3;$ and $OR_{mother\ educated\ to\ degree\ level}: 1.4; 95\%CI: 1.2–1.7)$; (Ramchandani et al., 2005). A significant association was also found with maternal psychological symptoms including anxiety (OR: 1.8; 95%CI: 1.3–2.4) and depression (OR: 1.9; 95%CI: 1.3–2.3). However, no significant associations were observed between child abdominal pain and paternal psychological symptoms*. The same authors subsequently demonstrated that maternal anxiety was also a strong predictor of adverse outcomes (further abdominal pain, school absence, and anxiety disorder; Ramchandani et al., 2007). Whether parental psychological status is modifiable – especially for the good of the child – is a moot point. A number of studies, however, have examined the role of psychological and psychosocial factors in the child.

Hyams et al. (1996) reported that anxiety was significantly higher in children with abdominal pain or irritable bowel-type symptoms ($P < 0.05$) and that, among those with pain, anxiety was associated with frequency ($P < 0.001$) and duration ($P < 0.001$). Ramchandani et al. (2005) found strong cross-sectional associations between abdominal pain and the various components of the Strengths and Difficulties Questionnaire (Goodman, 1997) among children aged 7 years. Children with a high 'total psychosocial difficulties' score (i.e. top 10% of respondents) experienced more than a doubling in the likelihood of abdominal pain (OR: 2.3; 95%CI: 1.9–2.8) and, in particular, children with emotional problems experienced a similar increase in the odds of symptoms (OR: 2.1; 95%CI: 1.7–2.7). Hyperactivity, conduct problems, and peer problems were also significantly associated, but to a slightly lesser extent. Among younger children (3.5 years), similar effects were observed with sub-scales of the Rutter Parental Scale for Pre-school Children (Elander and Rutter, 1996).

In a longitudinal study, El-Metwally et al. (2007) identified children who were free of abdominal pain and followed them for 4 years. Following a change in taxonomy proposed by the Subcommittee on Chronic Abdominal Pain of the American Academy of Pediatrics (Di Lorenzo et al., 2005), cases (chronic abdominal pain) were identified as those children who reported abdominal pain 1 year after baseline (by definition, new onset abdominal symptoms), and still reported pain at four years; however, recurrent (intermittent) cases and persistent cases were not separated. These authors found that among children in the age range of 11–14 years at baseline,

---

* Data provided in the paper under 'parental psychological symptoms' refers to 'mother' and the 'partner'. No information is actually given on whether this is the child's father. However, for the purposes of the current review it is assumed that, for the majority, this will be the case.

although 43% of children reported new-onset abdominal pain after 1 year, only around half of these children still reported symptoms 3 years subsequently. At baseline, psychosocial factors were assessed using the Strengths and Difficulties Questionnaire. These authors found that, in boys, new-onset chronic abdominal pain was predicted by baseline psychosocial difficulties (OR: $_{>50th\ percentile:\ 2.9}$; 95%CI: 1.5–5.9), conduct problems (OR: 2.4; 95%CI: 1.2–4.9) and a lack of school enjoyment (OR: 2.7; 95%CI: 1.3–5.5). In contrast, in girls, there were no consistent, significant, or sizeable associations between psychosocial factors and the onset of chronic abdominal symptoms (El Metwally et al., 2007).

Boey and Yap et al. (1999) examined the relationship between recurrent abdominal pain and exposure to recent stressful life events – including parental divorce or remarriage; hospitalization of the child, or a close relative; and failure in, or suspension from, school. They found that the parents of children with abdominal pain were ~3 times more likely to report that the child had experienced one or more stressful events, compared with other parents (OR: 2.9; 95%CI: 1.3–6.7; Boey and Yap, 1999). A further study by the same research group examined this in more detail (Boey and Goh, 2001). Death of a close family member was associated with a twofold increase in the likelihood of recurrent abdominal pain (OR: 2.0; 95%CI: 1.4–2.9) with a greater effect being observed with the death of a sibling (OR: 4.5; 95%CI: 1.5–13.5) or parent (OR: 3.6; 95%CI: 1.4–9.5) than a grandparent (OR: 1.8; 95%CI: 1.2–2.6). Similarly, hospitalization of a close relative was also associated with an increase in the occurrence of abdominal pain, although no differential effect was observed between siblings (OR: 2.0; 95%CI: 1.2–3.2), parents (OR: 2.0; 95%CI: 1.3–3.2), or grandparents (OR: 2.1; 95%CI: 1.4–3). Hospitalization of the index child was also associated with an increased likelihood of abdominal symptoms (OR: 2.6; 95%CI: 1.5–4.5), although, from this cross-sectional study, it is not clear whether this hospitalization was prior to, or subsequent to, the onset of symptoms. Boey and Goh (2001) also examined the association between life events related to changes in home circumstances and at school, and the occurrence of recurrent abdominal pain. Children with abdominal pain were more likely to report a recent change of address (OR: 2.0; 95%CI: 1.4–2.9); change in occupation of an immediate family member (OR: 2.4; 95%CI: 1.6–3.7); failure in a major school examination (OR: 2.4; 95%CI: 1.7–3.5), or being bullied at school (OR: 2.5; 95%CI: 1.5–4.2; Boey and Goh, 2001).

From cross-sectional studies, it is impossible to distinguish the temporal relationship between abdominal pain and these risk markers but, while it is possible to argue the case for reverse causality for some of the exposures (e.g. the occurrence of abdominal symptoms may increase the likelihood of exam failure), this is harder for others. However, the observed relationships may also (at least partly) be explained by recall bias. While one would anticipate that recall of some of these events – such as the death of a parent or sibling – would be equally well recalled by all children, it may be that children with abdominal pain better recall some events compared to other children, or perhaps even over-report their occurrence, thus exaggerating the true association of interest. Unfortunately, there is a paucity of prospective data in this field.

Headache/migraine

Descriptive epidemiology

Headache in childhood is very common. Anoniuk et al. (1998) found that, in Brazil, the lifetime prevalence of self-reported headache among children in the age range of 10–14 years was 93.5%, with a 1-year prevalence of 90%. Further, this data was verified by parental report: 93.3% and 89.8%, respectively. In the USA, Rhee et al. (2005) found that headache was the most prevalent complaint (29%) among the adolescent population according to a national survey conducted in

20 000 youngsters, and Brattberg (1994), using a broad definition of headache – pain in the head or in the neck – reported a prevalence of 48% in children aged between 8 years and 17 years in Sweden. Further, these authors found that cumulative incidence over a 2-year period was 37%.

In terms of headache and migraine, disease definition has been applied inconsistently – particularly with respect of the criteria relating to the severity of attack, and the frequency. Disease definition has changed over time and it was not until 1988 that an expert-panel consensus definition was established. With a modification from the definition in adults, migraine in children was defined as the occurrence of at least five episodes of headache, lasting between 2 and 48 h, with at least two of the following criteria: (a) unilateral location; (b) pulsating quality; (c) inhibition of daily activities; or (d) aggravation by physical activity; plus at least one of: (a) nausea/vomiting; or (b) phono-/photophobia (International Headache Society, 1988). Additional visual criteria were stipulated for migraine with aura. Using these criteria, Abu-Arafeh and Russell (1994) determined the prevalence of migraine headache in a large sample of >1750 schoolchildren, representative of the wider schoolchild population, in Aberdeen, UK. They found that the prevalence of migraine in children in the age range of 5–15 years was 10.6%, rising from 3–4% in children in the age range of 5 years to ~14% in those aged 15 years; see Figure 14.5. Using the same disease definition Barea et al. (1996) found the 1-year prevalence of migraine headache to be 9.9% among schoolchildren in the age range of 10–18 years in Brazil, although no increase in prevalence with age was observed. These authors also reported a 1-year prevalence for tension-type headache of 72.8% (Barea et al., 1996).

Few studies have examined the onset of headache or migraine. However, using a slightly different definition of migraine to those used above (Vahlquist, 1955)*, Anttila et al. (2006) reported that the incidence in children aged 7 years, in Finland, was 133.2 per 1000 person-years.

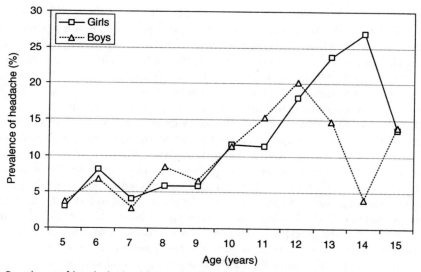

Fig. 14.5 Prevalence of headache in children. Data from Abu-Arafah and Russell (1994).

* Although published recently, this study deliberately replicated the methods and definitions used in a previous study, prior to the introduction of standardized classification criteria.

Incidence was slightly higher in girls (136.8 per 1000 person-years) than boys (129.5 per 1000 person-years) and increased from 19.7 per 1000 person-years in 1974 to 58.6 per 1000 person-years in 1992 (boys and girls combined). Others have reported similar findings: Dooley et al. (2005) found that 26% of children between 12 and 13 years of age reported headaches at least once a week, compared with 31% of those in the age range of 14–15 years. In addition, Carlsson (1996) found that 26% of Swedish schoolchildren reported headache 'once a month or more' with an increase in occurrence with age, and an excess in girls. Others have shown – in younger children (age: 6 years) – no difference in the lifetime prevalence of headache 'disturbing daily activities' between boys and girls (16.6% and 15.3% respectively Aromaa et al., 1998.)

Analytical epidemiology

A number of studies have examined the epidemiology of headache/migraine in children and, like abdominal pain, many come from the clinical setting. The concern with chronic headaches, in children and adults alike, is of serious intra-cranial pathology. However, Abu-Arafeh and Macleod (2005) demonstrated that this is seldom the cause of such symptoms: in a study of 815 children with mean headache duration of >21months, fewer than 0.5% had headaches related to active intra-cranial pathology. This notwithstanding, in a case-series of patients attending clinic with chronic daily headache, Abu-Arafeh found that around one-third had at least one underlying disease that may have contributed to the pathogenesis of the headache (Abu-Arafeh, 2001). However, clinic populations are highly selected and it is difficult for epidemiological studies to disentangle the aetiological risk factors for headache and migraine *per se*, and the risk markers (including factors such as parental behaviour) for consultation. Here, again, we try to focus on population-based epidemiological studies.

Health

In a longitudinal study, Aromaa et al. (1998) found that poor child health was associated with the occurrence of child headache: long-term childhood disease, reported at 5 years, significantly predicted headache occurrence at 6 years (OR: 1.8; 95%CI: 1.1–3). However, maternal assessment of infant poor health at 9 months was even more strongly associated (OR: 2.5; 95%CI: 1.1–5.8); (Aromaa et al., 1998). Gordon et al. (2004) in a large survey of Canadian schoolchildren in the age range of 12–13 years demonstrated that frequent headache occurrence (headaches 'about once a week or more often') was significantly associated with self-rated mental health. While children who reported that they were happy with life or perceived a good future, experienced a protective effect (OR: 0.30; 95%CI: 0.21–0.43 and OR: 0.33; 95%CI: 0.22–0.5, respectively), those who reported negative feelings experienced a significant increase in the likelihood of headaches: ORs ranging from 2.0 (95%CI: 1.5–2.8) for high parental rejection, to 5.8 (95%CI: 4.1–8.2) for 'being relatively depressed'. Dooley et al. (2005) followed up this cohort and examined the risk factors for headache longitudinally among children aged, now, 14–15 years old. They found that happiness with life and perception of a good future remained protective (OR: 0.48; 95%CI: 0.36–0.65 and 0.43; 0.31–0.60, respectively), whereas negative responses at 12–13 years of age were associated with an increase in the likelihood of headache occurrence at 14–15 years: $OR_{feeling\ unhappy,\ sad\ or\ depressed}$: 5.6 (95%CI: 2.1–3.2); $OR_{negative\ self-image}$: 2.6 (95%CI: 2.0–3.5); $OR_{anxiety\ or\ emotional\ disorder}$: 3.8 (95%CI: 2.8–5.1) and $OR_{high\ parental\ rejection}$: 2.5 (95%CI: 1.9–3.4); (Dooley et al., 2005).

Isik et al. (2007) examined the relationship between poor sleep and headache occurrence in 2228 Turkish schoolchildren in the age range of 6–13 years. These authors found strong and significant associations between a number of different sleep characteristics and the occurrence of non-migraine headache, including snoring (OR: 1.4; 95%CI: 1.1–1.7); sleep vocalizations (OR: 1.9; 95%CI: 1.5–2.3); nightmares (OR: 1.9; 95%CI: 1.6–2.4); and night sweating (OR: 2.2; 95%CI: 1.8–2.7); (Isik et al., 2007). Further, even stronger associations were observed with migraine: snoring (OR: 2.0; 95%CI: 1.2–3.2); sleep vocalizations (OR: 3.6; 95%CI: 2.2–5.9); nightmares (OR: 7.1; 95%CI: 4.1–12.4); and night sweating (OR: 4.0; 95%CI: 2.4–6.7). Others have also demonstrated a relationship between sleep problems and headache occurrence longitudinally. Aromaa et al. (1998) found that, at 3 years, difficulties falling asleep either occasionally (OR: 3.2; 95%CI: 0.7–1.7) or every night (OR: 3.2; 95%CI: 1.5–7.2) were associated with a threefold increase in the likelihood of headaches at age 6 years.

Behavioural factors

A number of studies have examined the relationship between childhood behavioural factors and the occurrence of headache. Brattberg (1994) found, cross-sectionally, that children who reported loneliness or a passive reaction to bullying experienced a three- to fourfold increase in head/neck pain (OR: 3.6; 95%CI: 1.4–9.9; and OR: 3.5; 95%CI: 1.8–6.9, respectively). Fear of schoolmates (OR: 2.6; 95%CI: 1.4–5.1), having been bullied (OR: 2.2; 95%CI: 1.4–3.4), and feeling like an outsider (OR: 1.8; 95%CI: 1.1–3.1) were also associated with an increase in the likelihood of symptoms (Brattberg, 1994).

Longitudinally, Aromaa et al. (1998) demonstrated that behavioural problems at age 5 years significantly predicted headache occurrence at 6 years (OR: 2.7; 95%CI: 1.1–6.4), as did concentration difficulties (OR: 2.3; 95%CI: 1.3–4.2), and, conversely, high levels of sociability (OR: 1.5; 95%CI: 1–2.2). In another prospective study, Dooley et al. (2005) focused not on behavioural characteristics *per se*, but on the child's perception of school. These authors found that while positive feelings about school at age 12–13 years (OR: 0.63; 95%CI: 0.51–0.77) and the perception of being fairly treated by teachers (OR: 0.57; 95%CI: 0.45–0.71) were associated with reductions in the likelihood of headache at 14–15 years, lower perception of school achievement and excessive parental academic expectations were associated with increases in the likelihood of future symptoms (OR: 1.7; 95%CI: 1.1–2.6 and OR: 1.5; 95%CI: 1.2–1.8, respectively). Interestingly, a feeling of being left out at school, which these authors had previously shown to be associated with headache symptoms cross-sectionally (OR: 1.5; 95%CI: 1.2–1.8; Gordon et al., 2004), was not significantly associated with future headache symptoms (Dooley et al., 2005).

Adverse events

Juang et al. (2004) examined the relationship between childhood adversity and chronic daily headache. From a population survey of 4645 Taiwanese schoolchildren, 58 children were identified with chronic daily headache (headache for >2 h per day, on >15 days per month) plus 58 controls. These authors found that a poor family environment, characterized by factors such as parental illness, separation, hostility, and neglect was associated with an eightfold increase in the likelihood of headache (OR: 8.3; 95%CI: 2.3–30.). In particular, parental divorce was associated with a nearly sixfold increase in the likelihood of symptoms (OR: 5.8; 95%CI: 1.2–28). Physical abuse was also strongly associated: 10% of cases reported abuse, compared with zero controls (thus, an OR is not calculable).

Other pains (widespread body pain)

We have described each of the most prevalent pains affecting school-aged children: low back pain, recurrent abdominal pain, and headache. However, a number of authors have studied other pain(s) in young populations. El-Metwally et al. (2007b) reported that 21.5% of Finnish children in the age range of 9–13 years (at baseline) reported non-traumatic musculoskeletal pain, all of whom were free of musculoskeletal pain one year previously. Girls were more likely to report new-onset pain than boys (OR: 1.6; 95%CI: 1.2–2.1) and onset was predicted by baseline symptoms, sleep problems, and depressive feelings. With the exception of gender, these factors also predicted the onset of traumatic pain, as did increased frequency of physical exercise (El-Metwally et al., 2007b).

These authors also looked at the onset of widespread body pain. They found that, among children free of widespread pain at baseline, 18% reported new-onset widespread pain at 1-year follow-up (Mikkelsson et al., 2008). Girls were more likely to experience new-onset widespread pain than boys (OR: 1.4; 95%CI: 1.1–1.9). In addition, children who reported depressiveness (OR: 1.5; 95%CI: 1.1-2.1) and those who reported various regional pains at baseline ($OR_{neck pain}$: 1.7; 95%CI: 1.1–2.4; $OR_{upper back pain}$: 2.1; 95%CI: 1.1–4.1; and $OR_{lower back pain}$: 3.0; 95%CI: 1.6–5.7) were also at increased risk. In the UK, Jones et al. (2003b) also looked at the onset of widespread body pain. These authors demonstrated that, among 1081 children in the age group 11–14 years (at baseline) who were free of widespread pain, 8% reported new-onset widespread pain at 1-year follow-up. Female gender was associated with the onset of symptoms, although not significantly so (RR: 1.4; 95%CI: 0.9–2.2). However, behavioural and emotional characteristics – in particular, conduct problems (RR: 2.6; 95%CI: 1.4–4.8) – and the occurrence of baseline somatic symptoms, in particular headaches (RR: 2.5; 95%CI: 1.2–5.4) and abdominal pain (RR: 2.0; 95%CI: 1–4.1), were associated with symptom onset.

Summary

We have focused, deliberately, on the most common non-specific pain(s) affecting children of school age, and the reader is directed elsewhere for information concerning pain of specific and obvious aetiology, such as childhood diseases, or pain following physical trauma. These have their own epidemiology and are beyond the scope of the current chapter.

Many of the pains experienced in childhood share common risk markers: it would appear that children who experience any (painful) symptoms are more likely also to report whatever pain is under investigation. Similarly, adverse behavioural characteristics and poor social behaviour and interaction are associated with childhood pain. Although, hitherto, we have given little consideration to familial factors this is not to say they are not important. To the contrary, there is some evidence that children within families who report headache are more likely themselves to report headache (Aromaa et al., 1998; Laurell et al., 2005). However, the evidence with respect to musculoskeletal pain is less clear (Jones et al., 2004). Further, it is hard to determine what any associations between child pain and family history actually represent. The relationship may reflect shared genetic factors, shared environment, or learned pain behaviour – and, in fact, is probably a function of all three. As such, it is difficult to disentangle the nature of these relationships and, to date, no-one has done so satisfactorily. Similarly, there is increasing evidence that stressful or adverse life events are associated with pain in the child. However, we need to understand more about the mechanisms that underpin these relationships. The challenge for future research is not only to identify and help alleviate the occurrence of pain in children, but also to improve the identification of children at high risk of persistent symptoms. There is now evidence to suggest that the pain experience in childhood is an important predictor of (chronic) pain in adulthood (Harreby et al., 1995; Hotopf et al., 2000; Jones et al., 2007). This is emerging as potentially the most powerful model on which to base public health research into the prevention of chronic pain in populations. It is crucial, therefore, that we understand the aetiology and mechanisms of pain in childhood, so that we are able to design, test, and implement effective interventions that – hopefully – can alter the long-term symptom trajectory.

References

Abu-Arafeh, I. 2001: Chronic tension-type headache in children and adolescents. *Cephalalgia* **21**, 830–6.

Abu-Arafeh, I. and Macleod, S. 2005: Serious neurological disorders in children with chronic headache *Arch.Dis.Child* **90**, 937–40.

Abu-Arafeh, I. and Russell, G. 1994: Prevalence of Headache and Migraine in Schoolchildren. *Br.Med.J* **309**, 765–9.

Anoniuk, S., Kozak, M.F., Michelon, L. and Montemor Netto, M.R. 1998: Prevalence of headache in children of a school from Curitiba, Brazil, comparing data obtained from children and parents. *Arquivos de Neuro-Psiquiatria* **56**, 726–33.

Anttila, P., Metsahonkala, L. and Sillanpaa, M. 2006: Long-term trends in the incidence of headache in Finnish schoolchildren. *Pediatrics* **117**, E1197–E1201.

Apley, J. and Naish, N. 1958: Recurrent abdominal pains: a field study of 1000 school children. *Arch.Dis. Child* **33**, 165–70.

Aromaa, M., Rautava, P. and Helenius, H. 1998: Factors of early life as predictors of headache in children at school entry. *Headache* **38**, 23–30.

Balagué, F., Dutoit, G. and Waldburger, M. 1988: Low back pain in schoolchildren: An epidemiological study. *Scand.J.Rehabil.Med.* **20**, 175–9.

Balagué, F., Skovron, M.L., Nordin, M., Dutoit, G., Pol, L.R. and Waldburger, M. 1995: Low back pain in school children: a study of familial and psychological factors. *Spine* **20**, 1265–70.

Barea, L.M., Tannhauser, M. and Rotta, N.T. 1996: An epidemiologic study of headache among children and adolescents of southern Brazil. *Cephalalgia* **16**, 545–9.

Barr, R.G., Levine, M.D. and Watkins, J.B. 1979: Recurrent Abdominal-Pain of Childhood Due to Lactose-Intolerance – Prospective-Study. *N.Engl.J.Med* **300**, 1449–52.

Boey, C.C.M. and Goh, K.L. 2001: The significance of life-events as contributing factors in childhood recurrent abdominal pain in an urban community in Malaysia. *J.Psychosom.Res* **51**, 559–62.

Boey, C.C.M. and Yap, S.B. 1999: An epidemiological survey of recurrent abdominal pain in a rural Malay school. *J.Paediatrics.Child.Health* **35**, 303–5.

Boey, C.C.M., Yap, S.B. and Goh, K.L. 2000: The prevalence of recurrent abdominal pain in 11-to 16-year-old Malaysian schoolchildren. *J.Paediatrics.Child.Health* **36**, 114–16.

Brattberg, G. 1994: The incidence of back pain and headaches among Swedish school children. *Qual.Life Res* **3**, S27–S31.

Burton, A.K., Clarke, R.D., McClune, T.D. and Tillotson, K.M. 1996: The natural history of low back pain in adolescents. *Spine* **21**, 2323–8.

Carlsson, J. 1996: Prevalence of headache in schoolchildren: relation to family and school factors. *Acta Paediatr* **85**, 692–6.

Chitkara, D.K., Rawat, D.J. and Talley, N.J. 2005: The epidemiology of childhood recurrent abdominal pain in Western countries: A systematic review. *Am.J.Gastroenterol* **100**, 1868–75.

Devanarayana, N.M., de Silva, D.G., de Silva, H.J. 2008: Aetiology of recurrent abdominal pain in a cohort of Sri Lankan children. *J.Paediatrics.Child.Health* **44**(4), 195–200.

Di Lorenzo, C., Colletti, R.B., Lehmann, H.P., Boyle, J.T., Gerson, W.T., Hyams, J.S. et al. 2005: Chronic abdominal pain in children: A clinical report of the American Academy of Pediatrics and the North American Society for Pediatric Gastroenterology, Hepatology and Nutrition. *J.Pediatr.Gastroenterol. Nutr* **40**, 245–8.

Dooley, J.M., Gordon, K.E. and Wood, E.P. 2005: Self-reported headache frequency in Canadian adolescents: validation and follow-up. *Headache* **45**, 127–31.

Duggleby, T. and Kumar, S. 1997: Epidemiology of juvenile low back pain: a review. *Disabil.Rehabil* **19**, 505–12.

Elander, J. and Rutter, M. 1996: Use and development of the Rutter parents' and teachers' scales. *Intl.J.Methods.Psych.Res* **6**, 63–78.

El Metwally, A., Halder, S., Thompson, D., Macfarlane, G.J. and Jones, G.T. 2007a: Predictors of abdominal pain in schoolchildren: a 4-year population-based prospective study. *Arch.Dis.Child* **92**, 1094–8.

El-Metwally, A., Salminen, J.J., Auvinen, A., Macfarlane, G. and Mikkelsson, M. 2007b: Risk factors for development of non-specific musculoskeletal pain in preteens and early adolescents: a prospective 1-year follow-up study. *BMC Musculoskeletal Disorders* **8**, 46.

Fairbank, J.C.T., Pynsent, P.B., van Poortvliet, J.A. and Phillips, H. 1984: Influence of anthropometric factors and joint laxity in the incidence of adolescent back pain. *Spine* **9**, 461–3.

Feldman, D.E., Shrier, I., Rossignol, M. and Abenhaim, L. 2001: Risk factors for the development of low back pain in adolescence. *Am.J.Epidemiol* **154**, 30–6.

Grimmer, K. and Williams M. 2000: Gender-age environmental associates of adolescent low back pain. *Appl.Ergon* **31**, 343–60.

Golding, J., Pembrey, M. and Jones, R. 2001: ALSPAC-The Avon Longitudinal Study of Parents and Children - I. Study methodology. *Paediatric and Perinatal Epidemiology* **15**, 74–87.

Goodman, R. 1997: The Strengths and Difficulties Questionnaire: a research note. *J.Child Psychol.Psychiatry* **38**, 581–6.

Gordon, K.E., Dooley, J.M. and Wood, E.P. 2004: Self-reported headache frequency and features associated with frequent headaches in Canadian young adolescents. *Headache* **44**, 555–61.

Gunzburg, R., Balagué, F., Nordin, M., Szpalski, M., Duyck, D., Bull, D., et al. 1999: Low back pain in a population of school children. *Eur.Spine J* **8**, 439–43.

Harreby, M., Neergaard, K., Hesselsoe, G. and Kjer, J. 1995: Are radiologic changes in the thoracic and lumbar spine of adolescents risk factors for low back pain in adults? A 25-year prospective cohort study of 640 school children. *Spine* **20**, 2298–302.

Harreby, M., Nygaard, B., Jessen, T., Larsen, E., Storr-Paulsen, A., Lindahl, A. et al. 1999: Risk factors for low back pain in a cohort of 1389 Danish school children: an epidemiologic study. *Eur.Spine J* **8**, 444–50.

Harvey, J. and Tanner, S. 1991: Low back pain in young athletes. A practical approach. *Sports Med* **12**, 394–406.

Hotopf, M., Carr, S., Mayou, R., Wadsworth, M. and Wessely, S. 1998: Why do children have chronic abdominal pain, and what happens to them when they grow up? Population based cohort study. *Br. Med.J* **316**, 1196–200.

Hotopf, M., Wilson-Jones, C., Mayou, R., Wadsworth, M. and Wessely, S. 2000: Childhood predictors of adult medically unexplained hospitalisations. Results from a national birth cohort study. *Br.J.Psychiatry* **176**, 273–80.

Howell, S., Poulton, R. and Talley, N.J. 2005: The natural history of childhood abdominal pain and its association with adult irritable bowel syndrome: Birth-cohort study. *Am.J.Gastroenterol* **100**, 2071–8.

Huang, R.C., Palmer, L.J. and Forbes, D.A. 2000: Prevalence and pattern of childhood abdominal pain in an Australian general practice. *J.Paediatrics.Child.Health* **36**, 349–53.

Hyams, J.S., Burke, G., Davis, P.M., Rzepski, B. and Andrulonis, P.A. 1996: Abdominal pain and irritable bowel syndrome in adolescents: a community-based study. *J.Pediatrics* **129**, 220–6.

International Headache Society. 1988: Classification and diagnostic criteria for headache disorders, cranial neuralgias and facial pain. Headache Classification Committee of the International Headache Society. *Cephalalgia* **8**, 1–96.

Isik, U., Ersu, R.H., Ay, P., Save, D., Arman, A.R., Karakoc, F., et al. 2007: Prevalence of headache and its association with sleep disorders in children. *Pediatric Neurology* **36**, 146–51.

Jones, G.T., Silman, A.J. and Macfarlane, G.J. 2003b: Predicting the onset of widespread body pain among children. *Arthritis & Rheumatism* **48**, 2615–21.

Jones, G.T., Silman, A.J. and Macfarlane, G.J. 2004: Parental pain is not associated with pain in the child: a population based study. *Ann.Rheum.Dis* **63**, 1152–4.

Jones, G.T., Silman, A.J., Power, C. and Macfarlane, G.J. 2007: Are common symptoms in childhood associated with chronic widespread body pain in adulthood? Results from the 1958 British Birth Cohort Study. *Arthritis & Rheumatism* **56**, 1669–75.

Jones, G.T., Watson, K.D., Silman, A.J., Symmons, D.P. and Macfarlane, G.J. 2003a: Predictors of low back pain in British schoolchildren: a population-based prospective cohort study. *Pediatrics* **111**, 822–8.

Juang, K.D., Wang, S.J., Fuh, J.L., Lu, S.R. and Chen, Y.S. 2004: Association between adolescent chronic daily headache and childhood adversity: a community-based study. *Cephalalgia* **24**, 54–9.

Kujala, U.M., Taimela, S., Oksanen, A. and Salminen, J.J. 1997: Lumbar mobility and low back pain during adolescence. A longitudinal three-year follow-up study in athletes and controls. *Am.J.Sports Med* **25**, 363–8.

Laurell, K., Larsson, B. and Eeg-Olofsson, O. 2005: Headache in schoolchildren: Association with other pain, family history and psychosocial factors. *Pain* **119**, 150–8.

Lebenthal, E., Rossi, T.M., Nord, K.S. and Branski, D. 1981: Recurrent Abdominal-Pain and Lactose Absorption in Children. *Pediatrics* **67**, 828–32.

Liebman, W.M. 1979: Recurrent Abdominal-Pain in Children - Lactose and Sucrose Intolerance - Prospective-Study. *Pediatrics* **64**, 43–5.

Malaty, H.M., Abudayyeh, S., Fraley, K., Graham, D.Y., Gilger, M.A. and Hollier, D.R. 2007: Recurrent abdominal pain in school children: effect of obesity and diet. *Acta Paediatr* **96**, 572–6.

Masiero, S., Carraro, E., Celia, A., Sarto, D. and Ermani, M. 2008: Prevalence of nonspecific low back pain in schoolchildren aged between 13 and 15 years. *Acta Paediatr* **97**, 212–16.

McMeeken, J., Tully, E., Stillman, B., Nattrass, C., Bygott, I.L. and Story, I. 2001: The experience of back pain in young Australians. *Man.Ther* **6**, 213–20.

Mikkelsson, M., El-Metwally, A., Kautiainen, H., Auvinen, A., Macfarlane, G.J. and Salminen, J.J. 2008: Onset, prognosis and risk factors for widespread pain in schoolchildren: A prospective 4-year follow-up study. *Pain* **138**, 681–7.

Mikkelsson, M., Salminen, J.J. and Kautiainen, H. 1997: Non-specific musculoskeletal pain in preadolescents. Prevalence and 1-year persistence. *Pain* **73**, 29–35.

Negrini, S., Carabalona, R., Pinochi, G., Malengo, R. and Sibilla, P. 1998: Backpack and back pain in schoolchildren: is there a direct relationship? *J.Bone & Joint Surgery - British Volume* **80B**, 247.

Nissinen, M., Heliövaara, M., Seitsamo, J., Alaranta, H. and Poussa, M. 1994: Anthropometric measurements and the incidence of low back pain in a cohort of pubertal children. *Spine* **19**, 1367–70.

Olsen, T.L., Anderson, R.L., Dearwater, S.R., Kriska, A.M., Cauley, J.A., Aaron, D.J., et al. 1992: The epidemiology of low back pain in an adolescent population. *Am.J.Public Health* **82**, 606–8.

Papageorgiou, A.C., Croft, P.R., Ferry, S., Jayson, M.I.V. and Silman, A.J. 1995: Estimating the prevalence of low back pain in the general population. Evidence from the South Manchester Back Pain Survey. *Spine*; **20**, 1889–94.

Paulo, A.Z., Amancio, O.M.S., de Morais, M.B. and Tabacow, K.M.M.D. 2006: Low-dietary fiber intake as a risk factor for recurrent abdominal pain in children. *European Journal of Clinical Nutrition* **60**, 823–7.

Perquin, C.W., Hazebroek-Kampschreur, A.A.J.M., Hunfield, J.A.M., Bohnen, A.M., Suijlekom-Smit, L.W.A., Passchier, J., et al. 2000: Pain in children and adolescents: a common experience. *Pain* **87**, 51–8.

Poussa, M.S., Heliovaara, M.M., Seitsamo, J.T., Kononen, M.H., Hurmerinta, K.A. and Nissinen, M.J. 2005: Anthropometric measurements and growth as predictors of low-back pain: a cohort study of children followed up from the age of 11 to 22 years. *Eur.Spine J* **14**, 595–8.

Ramchandani, P.G., Fazel, M., Stein, A., Wiles, N. and Hotopf, M. 2007: The impact of recurrent abdominal pain: predictors of outcome in a large population cohort. *Acta Paediatr* **96**, 697–701.

Ramchandani, P.G., Hotopf, M., Sandhu, B. and Stein, A. 2005: The epidemiology of recurrent abdominal pain from 2 to 6 years of age: Results of a large, population-based study. *Pediatrics* **116**, 46–50.

Rhee, H., Miles, M.S., Halpern, C.T. and Holditch-Davis, D. 2005: Prevalence of recurrent physical symptoms in U.S. adolescents. *Pediatric Nursing* **31**, 314–19.

Salminen, J.J., Erkintalo, M., Laine, M. and Pentti, J. 1995: Low back pain in the young. A prospective three-year follow-up study of subjects with and without low back pain. *Spine* **20**, 2101–7.

Salminen, J.J., Maki, P., Oksanen, A. and Pentti, J. 1992b: Spinal mobility and trunk muscle strength in 15-year-old schoolchildren with and without low-back pain. *Spine* **17**, 405–11.

Salminen, J.J., Pentti, J. and Terho, P. 1992a: Low back pain and disability in 14-year-old schoolchildren. *Acta Paediatr* **81**, 1035–9.

Servan-Schreiber, D., Kolb, N.R. and Tabas, G. 2000: Somatizing patients: Part I. Practical diagnosis. *Am.Fam.Physician* **61**, 1073–8.

Sward, L., Eriksson, B. and Peterson, L. 1990: Anthropometric characteristics, passive hip flexion, and spinal mobility in relation to back pain in athletes. *Spine* **15**, 376–82.

Szpalski, M., Gunzburg, R., Balagué, F., Nordin, M. and Melot, C. 2002: A 2-year prospective longitudinal study on low back pain in primary school children. *Eur.Spine J* **11**, 459–64.

Taimela, S., Kujala, U.M., Salminen, J.J. and Viljanen, T. 1997: The prevalence of low back pain among children and adolescents: a nationwide, cohort-based questionnaire survey in Finland. *Spine* **22**, 1132–6.

Tisher, M. and Lang, M. 1983: The Children's Depression Scale: Review and Further Developments. In Cantwell DP, Carlson GA, eds. *Affective Disorders in Childhood and Adolescence – An Update*, Lancaster: MTP.

Troussier, B., Davoine, P., de Gaudemaris, R., Fauconnier, J. and Phelip, X. 1994: Back pain in school children. A study among 1178 pupils. *Scand.J.Rehabil.Med* **26**, 143–6.

Troussier, B., Marchou-Lopez, S., Pironneau, S., Alais, E., Grison, J., Prel, G., et al. 1999: Back pain and spinal alignment abnormalities in schoolchildren. *Rev.Rhum.Engl.Ed* **66**, 370–80.

Vahlquist, B. 1955: Migraine in children. *Int Arch Allergy* **7**, 348–55.

Vikat, A., Rimpela, M., Salminen, J.J., Rimpela, A., Savolainen, A. and Virtanen, S.M. 2000: Neck or shoulder pain and low back pain in Finnish adolescents. *Scand.J.Pub.Health* **28**, 164–73.

Viry, P., Creveuil, C. and Marcelli, C. 1999: Nonspecific back pain in children. A search for associated factors in 14-year-old schoolchildren. *Rev.Rhum.Engl.Ed* **66**, 381–8.

Watson, K.D., Papageorgiou, A.C., Jones, G.T., Taylor, S., Symmons, D.P., Silman, A.J. et al., 2002: Low back pain in schoolchildren: occurrence and characteristics. *Pain* **97**, 87–92.

Watson, K.D., Papageorgiou, A.C., Jones, G.T., Taylor, S., Symmons, D.P., Silman, A.J. et al., 2003: Low back pain in schoolchildren: the role of mechanical and psychosocial factors. *Arch.Dis.Child* **88**, 12–17.

Wedderkopp, N., Leboeuf-Yde, C., Andersen, L.B., Froberg, K. and Hansen, H.S. 2001: Back pain reporting pattern in a Danish population-based sample of children and adolescents. *Spine* **26**, 1879–83.

Wedderkopp, N., Kjaer, P., Hestbeck, L., Korsholm, L. and Leboeuf-Yde, C. 2008: High-level physical activity in childhood seems to protect against low back pain in early adolescence. *The Spine Journal* doi:10.1016/j.spinee.2008.02.003.

Chapter 15

Life-course influences on chronic pain in adults

Gary J. Macfarlane

Introduction

Early studies on the epidemiology of chronic pain focused on adults and principally were concerned with the evaluation of short- and medium-term risk factors for the onset of such pain. Given that potential risk factors for the onset of an episode of pain may be modified by the previous experience of pain, early cohort studies sought to investigate first onset of regional pain (e.g. back pain). Such studies faced the difficulty that few people in adult life were experiencing the onset of such regional pain for the first time. Those doing so were very much a minority of all persons experiencing episodes of back pain. Secondly, when asked, many people who did have an episode of, e.g. back pain in adult life, reported that the first onset had been many years previously and indeed many reported a first onset in the teenage years. Subsequent studies of back pain, and other pain, in children confirmed that the experience of previous earlier pain was common (Watson et al., 2003).

Researchers began to appreciate the importance of studying the epidemiology of pain across the life-course. The productivity of such an approach had been appreciated previously in other areas of medicine. The developmental model of disease has provided strong evidence in relation to cardiovascular disease (Barker, 2004), while the life-course approach has demonstrated early-life or 'critical period' influences across a variety of health outcomes (Strachan et al., 2007), mortality (Hart et al., 1998), and lifestyle factors which are strongly related to ill-health (Graham et al., 2006; Caldwell et al., 2008).

In comparison, the study of life-course influences on the report of chronic pain in adulthood is in its infancy. The earliest consideration of these factors was in two studies published in an issue of *Arthritis and Rheumatism* in 1995. Both studies concerned fibromyalgia: a syndrome of chronic widespread pain (CWP) in the absence of an attributable pathology, accompanied by a high count of tender points at various specified locations in the body. In the first case-control study of 40 fibromyalgia female patients and 42 controls, reported sexual abuse was high both in cases (65%) and controls (52%) and was not statistically significantly different between the two groups. However, amongst the patients with fibromyalgia, the report of sexual abuse was associated with the number and severity of symptoms, including pain (Taylor et al., 1995). Although this study did collect information on when any reported abuse occurred (i.e. childhood, adolescence or adulthood), it was not reported separately in the manuscript.

The second case-control study, of 83 female patients with fibromyalgia and 161 consecutively sampled non-fibromyalgia female controls, also found a high level of physical and sexual abuse amongst cases (53%) and controls (42%) which was not significantly different between the groups. However, frequent and severe abuse was associated with fibromyalgia, and when data was analysed by when the reported abuse occurred, cases reported a significant excess of sexual abuse in childhood (37% vs. 22%; $P = 0.01$), sexual abuse in childhood and adulthood (17% vs. 6%; $P = 0.004$), and physical abuse in childhood (13% vs. 4%; $P < 0.001$; Boisset-Pioro et al., 1995).

A subsequent study found that, amongst patients with fibromyalgia, those who reported abuse were more likely to have high health care usage as well as greater levels of pain, fatigue, disability, and stress (Alexander et al., 1998). McBeth et al. (1999) in a population study demonstrated that the report of traumatic events in childhood was associated with a higher tender point count in adulthood. Such results led to consideration of how such traumatic events may be associated with chronic pain symptoms and, in particular, how they may have long-term influences. However, such studies also have methodological shortcomings, which hamper their interpretation. Therefore, replication and, importantly, more rigorous studies were required before the role of such early-life factors could be assessed.

This chapter reviews the evidence to date on whether events early in life can exert influences on the reporting of chronic pain in adulthood.

Epidemiology of pain in childhood

The topic of pain in children is covered in detail in Chapter 14, but there are several pertinent conclusions that are important to mention in the context of considering life-course influences on pain. Firstly, although pain is an uncommon reason for children to seek medical care, reported pain in children is common. The most common types of pain amongst children aged 14 years are headache, abdominal pain, and back pain, and they are frequently reported as causing functional limitation (Salminen et al., 1992). Secondly, there is a continuity of symptom patterns over time. In the Avon Longitudinal Study of Parents and Children (ALSPAC), children whose parents reported they had recurrent abdominal pain at 2 years, were 9 times more likely to have the same report at the age of four years (in comparison to those children whose parents did not report they had recurrent abdominal pain at the age of 2 years; Ramchandani et al., 2005). Thirdly, risk factors (or at least risk markers) have been identified for pain in children and there are common features across different types of pain. As an example from the ALSPAC study above, recurrent abdominal pain at the age of 6 years was strongly associated with emotional problems, conduct problems, hyperactivity, and peer problems, in the child. They were also predicted by factors in the first year of life: maternal anxiety, paternal anxiety, and parental reports of child temperament problems such as irregular feeding and sleeping (Ramchandani et al., 2006). Similar results have been found for behavioural and emotional factors predicting, amongst children in the age range of 11–14 years free of low back pain, those who would report back pain 12 months subsequently (Jones et al., 2003). In contrast, studies in children have failed to show an important role, except at the extremes of exposure, for mechanical injury in the development of musculoskeletal disorders (Jones and Macfarlane, 2005). Fourthly, children who report one type of pain symptom are more likely to report other pain symptoms and other common non-pain symptoms (Watson et al., 2003).

Do children who report pain become adults who report chronic pain?

In an early study, Harreby et al. (1995) reported on 481 subjects evaluated at 13 and 38 years of age in Denmark. Information collected at recruitment was used to try to predict low back pain in adults. Those children who reported back pain had a twofold increased odds of reporting back pain as an adult. This study had little other information to allow the nature and possible mechanisms of such a relationship to be evaluated. Birth-cohort studies are particularly useful in evaluating the continuity of symptoms and, using the British 1958 Birth Cohort Study, which recruited ~17 000 babies born during 1 week of that year and their parents (Power et al., 1992), Fearon and Hotopf (2001) demonstrated that children whose parents reported that they had headache during child-hood were approximately twice as likely to themselves report headache at age 33. In addition, they were also significantly more likely as adults to report multiple physical symptoms and psychiatric morbidity. A second British Birth Cohort Study (commenced in 1946) has partly confirmed these findings. Although children with abdominal pain were not significantly more likely to report abdominal pain or headache as adults, they were significantly more likely to report common somatic symptoms generally, and to have had a mental disorder diagnosed (Hotopf et al., 1998), and children with persistent abdominal pain were significantly more likely by age 45 to have been admitted to hospital with medically unexplained symptoms (2.95 per 1000 person-years at risk) in comparison to those children who did not have persistent childhood abdominal pain (0.76 per 1000 person-years; Hotopf et al., 2000). Supporting this link across the life-course, Jones et al. (2007a) reported that children who were reported at age 7 by their mothers to complain of multiple common childhood symptoms were themselves, at age 45, 1.5 times (95% confidence interval (CI): 1.03–2.3) more likely to report chronic widespread body pain.

Is chronic pain in adulthood linked to the reporting of specific events in childhood?

Evidence from case-control studies

A case-control study in Germany recruited, from a university hospital outpatient department, a group of 38 patients with fibromyalgia, 71 with somatoform pain disorders (mainly back pain) and 44 with 'medically explained' chronic pain (mainly neuropathic pain). All subjects were administered the Structured Biographical Interview for Pain Patients, which demonstrated that fibromyalgia patients reported poor relationships with their mother, poorer relationships with their father, and generally felt less secure (Imbierowicz and Egle., 2003). Further, the authors constructed a scale of childhood adversities, giving greater weight to those thought to have a greater impact (e.g. death of father or mother compared with poor financial situation). This dem-onstrated that fibromyalgia patients reported the greatest level of childhood adversity, followed by the somatoform pain-disorder patients, while the patients with 'medically explained' pain had the lowest levels.

A case-control study of adults in the age range of 18–65 years with CWP, the cardinal symptom of the fibromyalgia syndrome, in the northwest region of England attempted to address the issue of whether associations based on subject reports could be explained by recall bias. The study asked about the occurrence of a series of events prior to age 16: serious illness of parents, separation from or death of parents, hospitalizations, operations, and abuse. Without exception, all these events were reported significantly more frequently amongst cases with CWP compared to controls without CWP. The events of hospitalizations and operations afforded the opportunity, however, also to collect this information from medical records. Therefore, this information was extracted by study personnel blind to the reports from individual subjects. When the association was evaluated using data from medical records, there was no longer any association between case/control status and childhood operations, and the association with hospitalizations was attenuated and no longer statistically significant. The reason for this was that subjects with CWP who had an operation noted in their records always reported it at interview, whereas approximately half the controls with documented operations did not report them at interview. This study therefore provided strong evidence of differential recall depending on current health status (McBeth et al., 2001).

A retrospective cohort study which also addressed this issue was a study in the US Mid-West which identified a cohort of children ('exposed') whose parents had been prosecuted because of some aspect of lack of care (such as neglect or abuse), and a cohort of children ('non-exposed') whose parents had not. When followed up in adult life, Raphael et al. (2001) enquired about pain problems: there was no difference between the exposed and non-exposed cohorts. However, using the same subjects, she asked them to retrospectively rate the quality of care from their parents. When they relied on this information (rather than the documented evidence), adults who rated their care in childhood as poor reported significantly more pain problems than those who did not. Taking the results of these last two studies together, one could conclude that the association between pain problems in adulthood may be with recall of childhood events rather than with the actual events themselves.

Evidence from cohort studies

A more epidemiologically rigorous approach to evaluating possible relationships is through cohort studies which can eliminate the issue of recall bias. However, there are few cohort studies available which allow the detailed evaluation of both the relevant early-life events, such as psychological, psychosocial, and physically traumatic events, as well as an evaluation of chronic pain in adult life. One such study is the, previously mentioned, 1958 Birth Cohort Study. This is a study of all persons born in the UK during 1 week in 1958. The participants have been followed up periodically through life, most recently when participants were aged 45. Information available prior to age 7, from the child's mother, includes psychosocial factors (e.g. separation from mother, institutional care), health-related factors (e.g. common childhood symptoms, poor health, operations, and hospitalizations), and physically traumatic events (such as motor vehicle accidents). This study has demonstrated several important findings in relation to the development of CWP in adulthood. There was no relationship between CWP at age 42 and previous operations, hospitalizations, and/or poor child health reported by the mother when the child was 7 years old. However, if the child had been hospitalized following a motor vehicle accident, they were ~50% more likely to report CWP themselves at age 45. The adult self-report of CWP was also related to being in institutional care and having been separated from their mother prior to age 7: indeed, the longer the period of separation from the mother, the higher the risk of adult CWP (Jones et al., 2007b).

Biological pathways linking early life events with chronic pain in adulthood

If some events in childhood are linked to chronic pain in adulthood what are the biological mechanisms that might link them?

Firstly, some studies have demonstrated differences in pain thresholds between subjects with and without the report of specific events in childhood. Buskila et al. (2003) in Israel performed a retrospective cohort study of 120 children in the age range of 12–18 years who either had been born prematurely or were full-term deliveries. The group who were born prematurely demonstrated a higher tender point count and a decreased pain threshold. However, it was of note that most of the group born prematurely did not, at follow-up, report pain or related symptoms. A further retrospective cohort study of 69 children in Germany examined three groups: a) preterm children admitted to intensive care, b) full-term children admitted to intensive care, and c) full-term children not admitted to intensive care. At the age of 9–14 years the groups admitted to intensive care (both pre- or full term) exhibited increased perceptual heat sensitization but also an increased heat pain threshold (Hermann et al., 2006).

Secondly, there has been interest in the hypothalamic–pituitary–adrenal (HPA) axis in mediating the effects of stressful life events. Altered function of the HPA axis has been linked to the report of both regional and widespread pain in adults (Griep et al., 1998). Grunau et al. (2007) followed three groups of children from birth. Included in the study were extremely low gestational age (23–28 weeks), very low gestational age (29–32 weeks), and full-term babies. At 3 months after birth, the full-term babies had significantly higher basal cortisol levels. This difference had disappeared by 6 months. By 9 months (and persisting at 18 months), there were higher levels amongst those babies who were of extremely low gestational age. Emphasizing the potential importance of such changes in HPA-axis function, McBeth et al. (2007) identified adults free of CWP) but who were considered at high risk of its development because of a high number of somatic symptoms and aspects of illness behaviour. They assessed the HPA-axis function of these 'high-risk' subjects and then re-assessed their pain status 12 months later. Amongst this high-risk group, those who did develop CWP were more likely (at the time of recruitment) to fail to suppress their HPA axis after low-dose dexamethasone and were more likely to have a flattened diurnal rhythm of salivary cortisol, i.e. to have higher evening and lower morning levels.

The relevance of early life events to managing chronic pain

So what relevance does this have to management? Patients often attribute the onset of their symptoms to an adverse life event and often to such an event in childhood. It can be useful to acknowledge to patients, therefore, that scientific studies have shown that persons with chronic pain are more likely to recall early-life adverse events and that some of those adverse events are associated with long-term effects on health. Acknowledging this possible link can then allow one to move on to the management of such symptoms including the use of behavioural therapies. It has further been shown that the response to treatment may be influenced by the report of early-life events such as sexual abuse. Creed et al. (2005) conducted an intervention study for patients with severe irritable bowel syndrome. Patients were randomly assigned to eight sessions of individual psychotherapy, 3 months of treatment with paroxetine (an antidepressant medication), or usual care by the primary care physician and gastroenterologist. Patients who reported sexual abuse had more severe symptoms and poorer functioning. Moreover, amongst those who received the individual psychotherapy sessions, patients who reported childhood sexual abuse demonstrated improvements in outcome (using the Symptom Checklist 90 somatization score) while those who did not report such abuse symptoms did not improve.

Conclusion

The study of the role of early-life events, with respect to pain in adulthood, is relatively new. The early studies had important methodological limitations. They were retrospective and, therefore, were studying the relationship between chronic pain (mainly fibromyalgia) and recall of childhood events. Subsequent studies using alternative methodologies have demonstrated differential recall of past events between persons with and without current chronic pain. Nevertheless, prospective studies have demonstrated an association between some events early in life and the report of chronic pain in adulthood. These events include hospitalization for a motor vehicle accident and separation from one's mother. The report (by the mother) of childhood common symptoms is also a marker for persons who are more likely to report chronic pain as an adult. Thus, having established that there is a link between experiences and the experience of pain across the life-course, the usefulness of these observations needs to be determined in terms of understanding the biological mechanisms linking these. Only by understanding these can we then consider how interventions can potentially interrupt this life trajectory and contribute to prevention of chronic pain in adulthood.

References

Alexander RW, Bradley LA, Alarcón GS, Triana-Alexander M, Aaron LA, Alberts KR, et al. 1998: Sexual and physical abuse in women with fibromyalgia: association with outpatient health care utilization and pain medication usage. *Arthritis Care Res* **11**(2), 102–115.

Barker DJ. 2004: The developmental origins of chronic adult disease. *Acta Paediatr Suppl* **93**(446):26–33.

Boisset-Pioro MH, Esdaile JM, Fitzcharles MA. 1995: Sexual and physical abuse in women with fibromyalgia syndrome. *Arthritis Rheum* **38**(2), 235–241.

Buskila D, Neumann L, Zmora E, Feldman M, Bolotin A, Press J. 2003: Pain sensitivity in prematurely born adolescents. *Arch Pediatr Adolesc Med* **157**(11), 1079–1082.

Caldwell TM, Rodgers B, Clark C, Jefferis BJ, Stansfeld SA, Power C. 2008: Lifecourse socioeconomic predictors of midlife drinking patterns, problems and abstention: findings from the 1958 British Birth Cohort Study. *Drug Alcohol Depend* **1**;**95**(3), 269–278. Epub 2008 Mar 12.

Creed F, Guthrie E, Ratcliffe J, Fernandes L, Rigby C, Tomenson B,et al. 2005: Reported sexual abuse predicts impaired functioning but a good response to psychological treatments in patients with severe irritable bowel syndrome. *Psychosom Med* **67**(3), 490–499.

Fearon P and Hotopf M. 2001: Relation between headache in childhood and physical and psychiatric symptoms in adulthood: national birth cohort study. *BMJ* **12**;**322**(7295), 1145.

Graham H, Francis B, Inskip HM, Harman J; SWS Study Team. 2006: Socioeconomic lifecourse influences on women's smoking status in early adulthood. *J Epidemiol Community Health* **60**(3), 228–233.

Griep EN, Boersma JW, Lentjes EG, Prins AP, Van der Korst JK, de Kloet ER. 1998: Function of the hypothalamic-pituitary-adrenal axis in patients with fibromyalgia and low back pain. *J Rheumatol* **25**,1374–1381.

Grunau RE, Haley DW, Whitfield MF, Weinberg J, Yu W, Thiessen P. 2007: Altered basal cortisol levels at 3, 6, 8 and 18 months in infants born at extremely low gestational age. *J Pediatr.* **150**(2), 151–156.

Harreby M, Neergaard K, Hesselsøe G, Kjer J. 1995: Are radiologic changes in the thoracic and lumbar spine of adolescents risk factors for low back pain in adults? A 25-year prospective cohort study of 640 school children. *Spine* **1**;**20**(21), 2298–2302.

Hart CL, Smith GD, Blane D. 1998: Inequalities in mortality by social class measured at 3 stages of the lifecourse. *Am J Public Health* **88**(3), 471–474.

Hermann C, Hohmeister J, Demirak S, Zohsel K, Flor H. 2006: Long-term alteration of pain sensitivity in school-aged children with early pain experiences. *Pain.* **125**, 278–85.

Hotopf M, Carr S, Mayou R, Wadsworth M, Wessely S. 1998: Why do children have chronic abdominal pain, and what happens to them when they grow up? A population-based cohort study. *BMJ* **316**, 1196–1200.

Hotopf M, Wilson-Jones C, Mayou R, Wadsworth M, Wessely S. 2000: Childhood predictors of adult medically unexplained hospitalisations. Results from a national birth cohort study. *Brit J Psychiatry* **176**, 273–1280

Imbierowicz K and Egle UT. 2003:Childhood adversities in patients with fibromyalgia and somatoform pain disorder. *Eur J Pain* **7**(2), 113–119.

Jones GT and Macfarlane GJ. 2005: Epidemiology of low back pain in children and adolescents. *Arch Dis Child* **90**(3), 312–316.

Jones GT, Power C, Macfarlane GJ. 2007b: Physical adversity and poor social environment in childhood increase the risk of chronic widespread pain in adulthood – results from the 1958 British Birth Cohort Study. *Arthritis Rheum* **56**, S305.

Jones GT, Watson KD, Silman AJ, Symmons DP, Macfarlane GJ. 2003: Predictors of low back pain in British schoolchildren: a population-based prospective cohort study. *Pediatrics* **111**(4 Pt 1), 822–828.

Jones GT, Silman AJ, Power C, Macfarlane GJ. 2007a: Are common symptoms in childhood associated with chronic widespread body pain in adulthood? Results from the 1958 British Birth Cohort Study. *Arthritis Rheum* **56**(5), 1669–1675.

McBeth J, Silman AJ, Gupta A, Chiu YH, Ray D, Morriss R, et al. 2007: Moderation of psychosocial risk factors through dysfunction of the hypothalamic-pituitary-adrenal stress axis in the onset of chronic widespread musculoskeletal pain: findings of a population-based prospective cohort study. *Arthritis Rheum* **56**(1), 360–371.

McBeth J, Morris S, Benjamin S, Silman AJ, Macfarlane GJ. 2001: Associations between adverse evesnts in childhood and chronic widespread pain in adulthood: are they explained by differential recall? *J Rheumatol* **28**(10), 2305–2309.

McBeth J, Macfarlane GJ, Benjamin S, Morris S, Silman AJ. 1999: The association between tender points, psychological distress, and adverse childhood experiences: a community-based study. *Arthritis Rheum* **42**(7), 1397–1404.

Power C. 1992: A review of child health in the 1958 birth cohort: National Child Development Study. *Paediatr Perinat Epidemiol* **6**(1), 81–110. Review.

Ramchandani PG, Hotopf M, Sandhu B, Stein A; ALSPAC Study Team. 2005: The epidemiology of recurrent abdominal pain from 2 to 6 years of age: results of a large, population-based study. *Pediatrics* **116**(1), 46–50.

Ramchandani PG, Stein A, Hotopf M, Wiles NJ; ALSPAC STUDY TEAM. 2006: Early parental and child predictors of recurrent abdominal pain at school age: results of a large population-based study. *J Am Acad Child Adolesc Psychiatry* **45**(6), 729–736.

Raphael KG, Widom CS, Lange G. 2001: Childhood victimization and pain in adulthood: a prospective investigation. *Pain* **92**(1-2), 283–293.

Salminen JJ, Pentti J, Terho P. 1992: Low back pain and disability in 14-year-old schoolchildren. *Acta Paediatr* **81**(12), 1035–1039.

Strachan DP, Rudnicka AR, Power C, Shepherd P, Fuller E, Davis A, et al. 2007:Lifecourse influences on health among British adults: effects of region of residence in childhood and adulthood. *Int J Epidemiol* **36**(3), 522–531. Epub 2007 Jan 25.

Taylor ML, Trotter DR, Csuka ME. 1995: The prevalence of sexual abuse in women with fibromyalgia. *Arthritis Rheum* **38**(2), 229–234.

Watson KD, Papageorgiou AC, Jones GT, Taylor S, Symmons DP, Silman AJ, et al. 2003: Low back pain in schoolchildren: the role of mechanical and psychosocial factors. *Arch Dis Child* **88**(1), 12–17.

Chapter 16

Pain in older people

Elaine Thomas[1]

Introduction

The assessment of pain in older adults is a challenging process (Hadjistavropoulus et al., 2007). With the continued and projected growth of the older population, pain and its effect on functioning and health care-seeking behaviour in older adults will become an increasing concern (Badley and Crotty, 1995). The specific topic of pain in older adults is under-investigated, with few studies exclusively concerned with older adults or including sufficient numbers of older adults to allow robust estimates of prevalence, characteristics, or associations of pain in the oldest age-groups. A systematic review reported that <1% of 4000 research papers published on pain each year focus on older adults (Melding, 1991; American Geriatric Society, 2002). In addition, comparative estimates of the frequency of pain problems are sparse due to the lack of clear and consistent definitions of pain location, duration, and severity, especially in this age-group where issues of cognition and recall might intrude more frequently than in younger age-groups.

This chapter reviews the current literature associated with chronic pain in older adults and focuses specifically on the size, impact, and commonest causes of the problem in the community and primary care, possible explanations for the difference in the pain experience in older adults, projections of the future size of the problem and suggestions for where best to focus efforts to reduce the problem.

The size of the problem

Although much work in the field of pain research in older adults has been carried out in specialist pain clinics, the selectivity of the participants in this setting leads to questions about the wider applicability of the findings to public health and aetiological aspects of the problem in this age-group (Crombie and Davies, 1998). To get a fuller picture of the burden of pain, researchers need to turn to the community and primary care (Crombie et al., 1994).

Most of our current understanding of the epidemiology of chronic pain in older adults comes from cross-sectional studies. Whilst these studies do provide useful data, they are limited in that they tell us about a single point in time. Information about the course of pain over time is needed to help determine the degree of persistence, the rate of onset of new symptoms, and factors that can predict these patterns. Therefore, prospective studies have an important role to play and there are a growing number of such studies appearing in the literature.

[1] Some parts of this chapter reflect the content of a chapter entitled "The epidemiology of pain" in *Pain in older people* edited by P. Crome, F. Lally, and C.J. Main (Oxford University Press, 2007), and I am grateful to my co-authors on that chapter (Kate Dunn and Clare Jinks) for allowing me to use some of that content in shaping the current chapter.

Community studies

Chronic pain is common in community-dwelling older adults, with estimates of 18–57% prevalence based on self-report in population surveys. Table 16.1 summarizes the results of a systematic survey which illustrates this range (Harris, 2004). These figures represent a wide range of estimates of the size of the problem, the main reason for such variation being the different definitions used for chronic pain. The majority of the studies using a definition similar to 'persistent or recurrent pain for at least 3–6 months' resulted in estimates of ~50% (Andersson et al., 1993; Birse and Lander, 1998; Elliott et al., 1999; Gerdle et al., 2004; Mäntyselkä et al., 2003). One exception was the noticeably lower estimate reported by Bowsher et al. (1991), which may be a consequence of the method of data collection; responders to the telephone survey were asked whether 'they or anyone else in their household suffered from chronic pain'. Clearly, lower estimates were derived from those studies with more conservative definitions of chronic pain; e.g. in Breivik et al. (2005), individuals needed to have suffered from pain occurring at least twice a week for at least 6 months with severity recorded as at least a score of 5 on a 0–10 numerical rating scale.

The current evidence regarding the influence of gender is almost unequivocal in finding higher levels of chronic pain in females. The evidence for a relationship with age is less clear, with some studies suggesting no relationship with age (Andersson et al., 1993; Blyth et al., 2001; Gerdle et al., 2004) and others suggesting an increase in the reporting of symptoms with increasing age (Birse and Lander, 1998; Bowsher et al., 1991; Brochet et al., 1998; Elliott et al., 1999; Mäntyselka et al., 2003). Only one of these studies reported a clear reduction in symptoms with age (Breivik et al., 2005). Studies examining other measures of pain in older adults such as pain at moderate or severe levels (Brattberg et al., 1996; Scudds and Østby, 2001) or pain that interferes with daily activities (Thomas et al., 2004) suggest that these pain symptoms do increase with age. Interestingly, in all three of these latter studies, the prevalence of 'any pain' was constant with increasing age; it was the more severe disabling subgroups which increased in frequency with age.

In contrast with the number of cross-sectional studies examining chronic pain in older adults, few have gathered data prospectively in this age group to determine the frequency of onset of new chronic pain or the persistence of (or indeed recovery from) existing symptoms. At 4-year follow-up, Elliott et al. (2002) reported, in an adult population, persistence of chronic pain in almost 4 out of 5 persons reporting chronic pain symptoms at recruitment, but no results were given by age-group. A similarly high level of persistence of pain symptoms – here defined as pain that interferes with daily activities – was reported in a 3-year follow-up study of adults aged ≥50 years (Thomas et al., 2007). In a small interview study of 169 independent living adults aged ≥60 years, 90% of responders were in the same pain group (i.e. no pain, pain with no interference, and pain with interference) at three assessments out of a total of five performed over a 2-year period, and 37% reported chronic pain with interference in at least three assessments (Mossey and Gallagher, 2004). Data is also beginning to emerge that the onset of pain following periods free from pain remains substantial in this age-group. Elliott et al. (2002) reported that one in three adults free from chronic pain at recruitment reported painful symptoms 4 years later. In a prospective cohort study of an older adult population, Thomas et al. (2007) reported a 20% incidence of onset of pain that interfered with everyday life at 3-year follow-up among people aged >50 years who had been free of disabling pain in the original baseline survey.

Primary care

Although the population prevalence of chronic pain in older adults is high, only a minority of those with symptoms will seek professional help [e.g. 22% in a 12-month period for hand pain

Table 16.1 Prevalence of chronic pain in population-based studies: data for adults aged ≥45 years

Study	Age (years)	Number in study (45+)	Chronic pain definition	Prevalence(45+)	Prevalence with age (%)									
					45-	50-	55-	60-	65-	70-	75-	80-	85-	90-
Andersson et al., 1993	25–74	924	Persistent or recurrent pain for more than 3/12	*	59	68	62	60	55	52				
Birse & Lander, 1998	18+	129	Recurrent or persistent pain for at least 6/12	56%		37			58				53	
Blyth et al., 2001	15–84	8943	Daily pain for 3/12 in last 6/12	25%	22	24	28	26	28	24	24	26		
Bowsher et al., 1991	15+	477	Pain, on or off, for more than last 3/12	18%	10		19				22			
Breivik et al., 2005	18+	*	Pain for more than 6/12, 2+ times per week and 5+ (on 0-10 scale) in last episode	*		18			14	9			4	
Brochet et al., 1998	68+	741	Daily pain for more than 6/12	32%						27	35			45
Elliott et al., 1999	25+	2482	Pain that had started more than 3/12 ago	57%	52		57		57			62		
Gerdle et al., 2004	18–74	*	Pain for more than 3/12	*			61		56					
Mäntyselka et al., 2003	15–74	2477	Pain for at least 3/12	44%	39	42	44	45	45	46				
			Daily or continuous for at least 3/12	23%	15	19	24	25	26	27				

*Information not available from the manuscript

(Dziedzic et al., 2007), 28% in an 18-month period for knee pain (Bedson et al., 2007)]. Despite this, pain conditions are one of the most frequent reasons for older adults to seek primary health care (Mäntyselkä et al., 2001; Hasselström et al., 2002) and hence represent a significant burden on health services (Roberts et al., 2002; Woolf and Akesson, 2001). In a study based in 25 primary health care centres in Finland, adults aged ≥50 years were responsible for 44% of all consultations in a 4-week period and 48% of these consultations had pain as either a primary or secondary reason for the visit (Mäntyselkä et al., 2001). Similar findings were reported from a 1-year Swedish study based in a single health centre in which adults aged ≥50 years were responsible for more than half of all pain-related consultations, despite making up less than one-third of the registered population (Hasselström et al., 2002).

Impact

The presence of pain at some point during life seems almost inevitable, and a large proportion of people with pain will have periods of their life in which the pain is persistent. Although much of this may be regarded as a normal part of life, the impact of symptoms on everyday life can be substantial and multi-faceted, and can manifest as poor general health, limitations in the activities of daily living, and depression. Moreover, the effects of pain also have an impact at the societal level, in terms of the economy, and health and social services.

Health-related impact

Older adults have been shown to rate 'milder' states of ill health, such as the disability associated with moderate pain, less adversely than younger adults, but, in the context often of multiple morbidities, older people's rating of specific disabilities often reflects their wider health status. When comparing these ratings in older people by disability status, persons with a disability tended to give a worse rating to all the ill health states studied compared to their non-disabled peers (Ebrahim et al., 1991). This latter finding was supported in a study of community dwelling-older adults where the presence of persistent pain was strongly related to reporting poorer general health, despite adjusting for differences in socio-demographic factors and access to medical care (Reyes-Gibby et al., 2002).

In a study of independent-living older age community residents, pain was shown to be strongly related to physical performance. Moreover, the combination of activity-limiting pain and depressive symptoms led to an even greater likelihood of being in the lowest quartile of self-reported physical performance (Mossey et al., 2000). When these individuals were followed-up 2 years later, those with chronic activity-limiting pain were significantly more likely to have persistent problems with physical function (Mossey and Gallagher, 2004).

Depression has been consistently shown to be associated with pain. In a large study of elderly adults in the community, the presence of depressive symptoms showed a strong dose–response relationship with pain, i.e. depression scores were lowest in those with no pain, higher in those with less than daily pain, and highest in those with daily pain (Landi et al., 2005). Similar findings were reported from the Women's Health and Ageing Study (Leveille et al., 2007) where moderate-to-high levels of depressive symptomatology were seen in 5% of those with none or mild pain compared to 18% of those with widespread pain. In a 2-year follow-up study of community-dwelling adults aged ≥65 years, the onset of depression was strongly linked with having moderate-to-severe pain either in the month before baseline or before re-survey, and worsening pain over the study period (Harris et al., 2006). In primary care, moderate-to-severe depressive symptoms have been recorded in 13% of older adults consulting for musculoskeletal pain (Mallen and Peat, 2008) and 19% of patients with osteoarthritis (Rosemann et al., 2007).

Economic impact

There is clearly a substantial demand on the health and social care services as a consequence of the management of older adults with chronic pain conditions. Although total costs related to pain in this age-group are difficult to estimate, data are available for individual conditions, such as the commonest pain syndrome in older people in the UK, namely osteoarthritis (see following paragraphs for more detailed discussion of this condition).

In the UK, the estimated total costs for community and social services in 2001 for osteoarthritis were £248 million, and 36 million working days were lost as a result of this condition in 1999–2000 at a cost of over £3 billion in lost production (Arthritis Research Campaign, 2002). In addition to the costs to the state, there are substantial 'monetary' costs to the individual and their families including treatments not covered by the state, unpaid informal caregivers, and loss of earnings. In a UK general practice study of knee osteoarthritis, median monthly costs of £5 (range: 66p to £150) for complementary medicines and £13.50 (range: £1 to £150) for complementary therapists were reported (Jordan et al., 2004). In a Canadian study of direct and indirect costs to the individual in older adults with disabling hip and knee osteoarthritis, 60% of individuals reported osteoarthritis-related costs with an annual mean of $12 200 CDN (range: $30–$152 660). Indirect costs were reported by almost 90% of individuals with a mean of $12 990 CDN ($110–$149 470), 50% of the indirect costs being attributable to caregiver costs (Gupta et al., 2005).

Validity of measurement tools

A series of studies by Gagliese and co-workers (2003; 2005) suggests that some of the differences in pain reporting in younger and older patients are related to the validity of the tools used to measure pain. Despite no difference in pain intensity (highest, usual, or lowest) and similar clinimetric properties of the McGill Pain Questionnaire (MPQ) in the younger and older patients, older chronic pain patients had a lower overall and sensory component score on the MPQ and also reported fewer descriptors of their pain (Gagliese and Melzick, 2003). These findings were replicated in a second study of surgical patients (Gagliese and Katz, 2003) in which the authors suggested that there are age-related differences in pain qualities, as captured by verbal descriptions of pain, but not in measures of pain intensity. A later study (Gagliese et al., 2005) confirmed these findings and added a suggestion that for measures of pain intensity, the Numerical Rating Scale (NRS) was preferred to the Visual Analogue Scale (VAS) as a measure of pain intensity, since the NRS had superior measurement properties (lower missing data levels and greater face validity), and, importantly, these properties were not age related.

Further evidence regarding the potential effect of age on responses to pain-measurement tools comes from a cohort of older residents (age: ≥60 years) in nursing homes reported by Kamel et al. (2001). Whilst age was strongly related to positive responses to a simple enquiry regarding the presence of pain 'Do you have pain?' (6% in those aged >85 years compared with 15% in those in the age range of 60–85 years), responses to more complex measures of pain presence, such as a VAS or a pain-descriptors scale, were not affected by age.

Causes of chronic pain in older people

The following section discusses the main causes of chronic pain in older people. In terms of the population effect, musculoskeletal pain is the main problem in older adults because of its high prevalence. Comparisons of prevalence estimates of 'any' pain and musculoskeletal pain suggest that the majority of all pain experienced is due to pain in the musculoskeletal system;

Bergman et al. (2001) reported a prevalence estimate of 45% for chronic musculoskeletal pain in participants aged ≥50 years.

The commonest group of chronic musculoskeletal pain conditions in older people is joint pain, notably pain in the knee, hip, hand, and foot. Most of this is classed clinically as 'osteoarthritis', a syndrome of pain and restricted movement in the joints occurring particularly in older people, although only a proportion of pain in these joints is accompanied by definite radiographic changes of osteoarthritis. The distinction between disease and symptom is further evidenced by population studies showing a substantial prevalence of radiographic changes of osteoarthritis occurring without symptoms (McAlindon et al., 1992). Recent evidence, however, has suggested that, among older people with knee pain, the majority will have some evidence of radiographic disease if X-ray views are obtained of the whole joint (Duncan et al., 2007).

Osteoarthritis is the commonest pain-related chronic condition (Ferrell et al., 1990). In the UK, osteoarthritis is responsible for >3 million consultations per year (Arthritis Research Campaign, 2002; ARMA, 2004). The proportion of disability and productivity losses attributable to osteoarthritis has been shown to outweigh most other causes (Hootman and Helmick, 2006). Overall, joint pain is consistently shown to be the most important influence on health-related quality of life in the older population (Alonso et al., 2004).

Osteoarthritis provides a good model of where a combined model for approaches to prevention of chronic pain is plausible (i.e. looking at disease factors and at factors that influence the likelihood of chronic pain developing).

First, tackling factors [such as obesity, injury, occupational over-use of the joint, childhood skeletal abnormalities (Cimmino and Parodi, 2005)] that predispose to the process of cartilage degeneration and bony thickening (the pathology of osteoarthritic change in the joint) will prevent chronic pain at older ages by preventing the underlying disease. However, just how much can be achieved by attempting to prevent cartilage changes is a topic of debate (Felson, 2009). There is good evidence, however, that joint replacement in advanced osteoarthritis is a good means of tertiary prevention of chronic pain, particularly at the knee and hip, by reducing pain and its consequences long-term.

Second, there is the evidence that most chronic joint pain in older people (the clinical syndrome of osteoarthritis), regardless of the extent to which it is associated with radiographic changes in the joint, behaves much like any other chronic pain syndrome – the pain and restricted activity related to any one joint is more severe in the presence of other pains (Croft et al., 2005), and the restricted activity is more related to pain severity, concomitant anxiety and depression, low levels of physical fitness and activity, and attitudes and beliefs about pain, than it is to the degree of radiographic change (O'Reilly et al., 1998).

Primary prevention geared towards improving physical activity, avoiding injury, and improving muscle strength and physical activity levels has specific potential because such changes, especially during the middle adult years, may work both by preventing the joint changes that constitute the disease of osteoarthritis and by reducing the propensity to develop chronic joint pain.

In addition to osteoarthritis and joint pain, some other pathological conditions in older people are assumed to give rise to pain by neuropathic (nerve-damage) mechanisms. However, these conditions, such as shingles and cancer, have a smaller population effect due to their lower prevalence, although the impact on the individual sufferer may be higher.

Musculoskeletal pain: joints

This section concentrates on three specific regional pain syndromes (knee, hip, and hand).

Estimates of the 12-month prevalence of chronic knee pain from large population-based studies of older adults range from 25% to 33%, tend to be higher in females, and show a slight increase with advancing age (McAlindon et al., 1992; O'Reilly et al., 1998; Dawson et al., 2004; Jinks et al., 2004). In the study of Jinks et al. (2004), chronic pain accounted for just over half of all knee pain reported in this population, and almost half of those with chronic knee pain reported at least one consultation with their GP during the 12-month time frame. Despite the age and gender associations with the prevalence estimates, consultation rates for chronic knee pain were not related to either gender or age (Jinks et al., 2004). In a follow-up of those with chronic knee pain previously reported in Dawson et al. (2004), 72% of responders reported chronic knee pain at 1-year (Dawson et al., 2005).

Using a similar definition to that used for knee pain, Dawson et al. (2004) reported lower prevalence estimates for chronic hip pain at 19% in community-dwelling adults aged ≥65 years. Despite this lower prevalence, the persistence of hip pain over a 1-year period was similar to that seen for knee pain (Dawson et al., 2005).

Less research attention has been given to the hand despite it being one of the most common sites of pain in this age-group. Population-based studies have reported that up to 30% of older adults will have hand symptoms in a 1-month period and that more than half the hand pain will be chronic, i.e. symptoms have lasted for >3 months (Dziedzic et al., 2007). Moreover, the prevalence of chronic hand pain is greater in females and increases with increasing age (Dziedzic et al., 2007).

Musculoskeletal pain: chronic widespread pain (CWP)

This is regarded either as a syndrome in its own right, or as representing the concomitant presentation of multiple regional pain syndromes, or in many cases among older people, a generalized form of osteoarthritis.

Pain symptoms often coexist in the same patients, and it is difficult to disentangle whether they are separate conditions with different aetiology and prognosis, or whether they are part of a widespread pain syndrome. One of the most frequently applied definitions for chronic widespread pain is that proposed by the American College of Rheumatology as part of their criteria for fibromyalgia (Wolfe et al., 1990) where pain must be present in two contralateral quadrants of the body and in the axial skeleton. Cross-sectional studies show that CWP symptoms are common-place in older adults, with estimates in the region of 9% (Hunt et al., 1999) to 16% (Croft et al., 1993). Prospective studies provide evidence that CWP symptoms in this age group are persistent: 60% at 1-year follow-up (McBeth et al., 2001) and 43% at 7-year follow-up (Papageorgiou et al., 2002).

Two examples of disease-based chronic pain in older people

Cancer becomes increasingly common with increasing age. Cancer Research UK has collated official statistics from England, Wales, Scotland, and Northern Ireland to determine that 74% of all cancer cases are diagnosed in adults aged ≥60 years, and >30% of cases are in people aged ≥75 years (Cancer Research United Kingdom, 2008). Pain, due to either cancer or its treatment, is reported in up to 70% of all cancer patients and increases to 80–100% in patients with advanced disease (Coyle et al., 1990; Cleeland et al., 1994; Rao and Cohen, 2004). Blyth, in Chapter 21, reviews cancer pain as a chronic pain syndrome.

Data from the USA estimates that there are 1 million cases of herpes zoster, or shingles, each year and that 10–20% of adults will develop such symptoms in their life. The lifetime incidence of shingles in those reaching the age of 85 is ~50%. Moreover, the incidence of symptoms increases almost 10-fold from 1.1 per 1000 person-years in those aged <50 to 10.9 per 1000 person-years in those aged ≥80 (Weinberg, 2007). Herpes zoster, or shingles, can precipitate a chronic pain syndrome, post-herpetic neuralgia, which can cause long-term impaired quality of life (Schmader, 2002).

Why might pain be different in older people?

The following section explores theories from the pain literature as to why older adults may experience or report pain differently to their younger counterparts. These theories will be split into three main headings: potential specific biological factors, pain management, and the validity of tools used to measure pain in older age-groups.

Potential specific biological factors

Any potential biological explanations for differential pain experience with age will depend on the type of pain being described. Here, the interest lies in chronic pain that is 'pain that persists beyond the normal time of healing' (International Association for the Study of Pain, 1986), a definition that acknowledges the potential for maladaptive responses (Sufka, 2000). In acute pain there is a closer link between the neural encoding and processing of the noxious stimulus, i.e. nociception (Loeser and Treede, 2008), and the pain perceived. The situation is more complex in pain of a chronic nature as factors other than nociception, such as cognitions, are thought to play important roles in the pain experience.

Nociception

Gibson and Helme (2001) present a comprehensive review of experimental data examining the effect of ageing on such aspects as pain sensitivity and tolerance. Although they report that the results of individual studies in their review are somewhat contradictory, perhaps due to differences in the populations studied, type of experiments applied, and outcome measures used, it is thought that the weight of evidence does support an age-related decline in pain sensitivity. In summary, older, compared with younger, adults require a higher level of stimulation in order for them to report the presence of pain (Washington et al., 2000; Zheng et al., 2000). Interestingly, the age differences in pain sensitivity generally hold for two of the three main forms of experimental pain stimulation, i.e. thermal and mechanical pressure, whereas there is little evidence regarding the influence of age in electrical pain stimulation. One suggestion given by Gibson and Helme (2001) for these differences relates to the different mechanisms by which these methods 'cause' the noxious stimulation. Thermal and mechanical pressure stimulation methods work through receptor activation and energy transduction to stimulate the sensory fibres, whereas electrical stimulation does this directly. They also suggest that the decline in pain perception could potentially align with the changes in other sensory receptor systems that occur with increasing age, such as touch and vision (Gibson and Helme, 2001).

Clearly, the usefulness of the results of experimental pain studies is strongly related to the degree to which they can represent the complexity of the situation in people experiencing long-term pain conditions. The majority of experimental studies are carried out on healthy controls, i.e. a selective group of older adult 'avoiders' of chronic pain, and tend to generate pain of a controlled and acute nature, which has little, if any, psychological component. One alternative source of 'experimental' data regarding the age-related effects of pain is from surgical studies in which younger and older adults undergoing the same surgery are compared for their pre- and post-operative pain experiences. The evidence with regard to post-operative pain in younger and older adults is conflicting, with some suggesting lower levels of post-operative pain intensity in older adults (Thomas et al., 1998; see also Chapter 19), whilst others suggest no age effect (Gagliese et al., 2000; 2008). Further work from Gagliese et al. (2000) suggests that, in patients undergoing similar operations, older patients expect less post-operative pain intensity and use lower levels of post-operative patient-controlled levels of morphine but use it for longer.

Cognitions

There is a substantial evidence-base to suggest that older people with cognitive problems are less likely to report pain compared to their non-cognitively impaired peers (Huffman and Kunik, 2000), most of the evidence coming from studies based in residential homes. Reynolds et al. (2008) reported a decrease in the prevalence of self-reported pain with increasing levels of cognitive impairment, from 34% in those with no cognitive impairment, to 10% in those with severe cognitive impairment. This study also showed that the presence of diagnoses likely to cause pain did not vary in relation to cognitive impairment status (Reynolds et al., 2008). Similar findings have been found for physician-identified pain; pain was found to be less common in non-communicative residents compared with those who were communicative (Sengstaken and King, 1993). Mäntyselkä et al. (2004) reported the first study to confirm lower pain reporting in those with dementia in a community-dwelling sample; despite similar demographics, participants with dementia were half as likely to report daily pain (23% vs. 40%) and daily pain that interfered with routine activities (19% vs. 36%). In addition to the evidence showing lower rates of pain presenting in older adults with cognitive problems, there is data from both nursing home (Horgas and Tsai, 1998; Reynolds et al., 2008) and community (Mäntyselka et al., 2004) studies to suggest that analgesic medication is prescribed and administered at lower levels in pain patients with cognitive impairment compared to their cognitively intact peers.

The concern from this type of evidence is that pain is being experienced but not expressed or communicated by cognitively impaired older adults, rather than such persons actually experiencing less pain because of their cognitive status (Frampton, 2003). In an experimental study to measure responses to a mildly painful stimulus (venepuncture) in patients with different severity of dementia compared to healthy controls, greater severity of dementia was associated with a blunting of the physiological response, more interference in responding to direct questions regarding pain and anxiety, and an increase in general, rather than pain-specific, facial expressions, independent of age (Porter et al., 1996). In studies of lumbar puncture, results suggest a lower rate of headache after the procedure in elderly persons with dementia (Blennow et al., 1993; Hindley et al., 1995). Frampton (2003) discusses that these changes in the bio-behavioural system are similar to those that occur in the autonomic nervous system in Alzheimer's disease, which produces an inability to 'perceive' and therefore 'prepare psychologically' for an impending event (Schwartz et al., 1991). However, against these results must be contrasted epidemiological findings which compared persons from a general population sample, with and without mild degrees of cognitive complaints (i.e. self-reported difficulties with some items of cognitive function). Self-reported pain was 2.5 times more likely in those with cognitive complaints, independent of concurrent anxiety and depression (Westoby et al., 2009).

Pain management

The management of chronic pain, in general, needs to consider a wide range of options including pharmacological and non-pharmacological treatment (American Geriatric Society, 2002). This review reported that a number of non-pharmacological treatment interventions had been shown to be effective for the treatment of chronic pain, including both physical and psychological modalities. Pharmacotherapy, however, was the most common pain management approach used in older adults.

The distribution, metabolism, and excretion of several drugs alter with advancing age (Milton et al., 2008), and older adults are generally more susceptible to adverse events (American Geriatric Society, 2002). Summarizing the general lack of an evidence-base for pain medication in older adults, Weiner (2002) stated in an editorial that 'a lack of knowledge regarding how to prescribe opioid and non-opioid analgesics certainly contributes to inadequate and potentially toxic pain management regimens for older adults'.

In older adults particularly, the decision to use pharmacological treatments needs to consider the existence of co-morbidities. Co-morbidity is common in older people and hence polypharmacy is common in this age-group, with chronic pain in particular being managed alongside other conditions. In England, ~20% of the population are aged ≥60 (Office for National Statistics, 2006), but this age-group accounted for 57% of prescription items dispensed by community pharmacists in 2003, a figure which equates to an average of 35 items per head (Department of Health, 2004). It has been estimated that one in five adults aged >70 are prescribed at least five different drugs (Rollason and Vogt, 2003). Although polypharmacy has been associated with an increase in a range of adverse events, it is not fully understood whether this is a direct consequence of the interactions of the medications or simply that the receipt of multiple medications is an indicator of greater frailty (Milton et al., 2008).

What is the future for chronic pain in older adults?

It has been estimated that the proportion of the world's population aged >65 will more than double in the next 40 years (from 7.7% in 2008 to 16.5% in 2050) and the over-80-year age-group will more than triple, from 1.5% to 4.9%, in the same time period (US Census Bureau, 2008). Clearly, such large projected increases in groups of society that currently require high resources from the medical and social services has major implications for the provision of such services in the future.

Work from the UK has derived models, using data on the projected ageing of the population together with trends in the health of populations, including rates of obesity and smoking, to examine the effect on disability due to arthritis from 2006 to 2026 (Jagger et al., 2009). In the simplest model, which examined the effect of ageing alone, the percentage of older adults with arthritis would increase by close to 50% by 2026. Under the 'best-case' scenario, of improvements in general health behaviour and treatment, the numbers with arthritis do reduce but due to the larger effect of the increasing population, the size of the reduction is small. However, under the scenario of a general decline in the health of the population, there would be a further 300 000 older people with arthritis (Jagger et al., 2009).

Where best to focus future research resources?

The data presented in this chapter show that there are several areas on which to focus future research into chronic pain in older people. Although this chapter has focused on older adults, the main targets for prevention of chronic pain in this age-group lie at younger ages. This means there is a need to determine the patterns and prognosis of chronic pain over time, both in the general population and primary care, to enable more efficient planning of medical and social care resources and to be able to identify potentially modifiable risk factors for the onset and persistence of such symptoms.

The impact of co-morbidities on both the presentation and treatment of pain is an important issue in older adults. With particular emphasis on cognitive decline, further research on pain presentation in the presence of other co-morbidities will provide a clearer picture of chronic pain and the potential for prevention in 'real life'. In addition, establishing the potential treatment interactions that may occur as a consequence of polypharmacy will aid medical professionals to effectively treat pain in older patients with multiple chronic conditions.

References

Alonso J, Ferrer M, Gandek B, Ware JE Jr, Aaronson NK, Mosconi P,et al; IQOLA Project Group 2004: Health-related quality of life associated with chronic conditions in eight countries: results from the International Quality of Life Assessment (IQOLA) Project. *Qual Life Res* **13**, 283–298.

American Geriatric Society – Panel on Persistent Pain in Older Persons 2002: The management of persistent pain in older persons. *J Am Geriatr Soc* **6**, S205–S224.

Andersson HI, Ejlertsson G, Leden I, Rosenberg C 1993: Chronic pain in a geographically defined general population: studies of difference in age, gender, social class, and pain localization. *Clin J Pain* **9**, 174–182.

ARMA 2004: Standards of Care for people with osteoarthritis. www.arma.uk.net/pdfs/oa06.pdf. [accessed 21 November 2009]

Arthritis Research Campaign 2002: Arthritis: the Big Picture. http://www.arc.org.uk/arthinfo/documents/BigPic.pdf. [accessed 24 August 2009]

Badley EM and Crotty M 1995: An international comparison of the estimated effect of the aging of the population on the major cause of disablement, musculoskeletal disorders. *J Rheumatol* **22**, 1934–1940.

Bedson J, Mottram S, Thomas E, Peat G 2007: Knee pain and osteoarthritis in the general population: what influences patients to consult? *Fam Pract* **24**, 443–453.

Bergman S, Herrström P, Högström K, Petersson I, Svensson B, Jacobsson LTH 2001: Chronic musculoskeletal pain, prevalence rates, and sociodemographic associations in a Swedish population study. *J Rheumatol* **28**, 1369–1377.

Birse T and Lander J 1998: Prevalence of chronic pain. *Can J Pub Health* **89**, 129–131.

Blennow K, Wallin A, Hager O 1993: Low frequency of postlumbar puncture headache in demented patients. *Acta Neurol Scand* **88**, 221–223.

Blyth FM, March LM, Branic AJM, Jorm LR, Williamson M, Cousins MJ 2001: Chronic pain in Australia: a prevalence study. *Pain* **89**, 127–134.

Bowsher D, Rigge M, Sopp L 1991: Prevalence of chronic pain in the British population: A telephone survey of 1037 households. *Pain Clinic* **4**, 223–230.

Brattberg G, Parker MG, Thorsland M 1996: The prevalence of pain among the oldest old in Sweden. *Pain* **67**, 29–34.

Breivik H, Collett B, Ventafridda V, Cohen R, Gallacher D 2006: Survey of chronic pain in Europe: prevalence, impact on daily life, and treatment. *Eur J Pain* **10**, 287–233.

Brochet B, Michel P, Barberger-Gateau P, Dartigues J-F 1998: Population-based study of pain in elderly people: a descriptive survey. *Age Ageing* **27**, 279–284.

Cancer Research United Kingdom 2008: UK cancer incidence statistics by age. http://info.cancerresearchuk.org/cancerstats/incidence/age/?a=5441 [accessed 24 August 2009].

Cimmino and Parodi M 2005: Risk factors for osteoarthritis. *Semin Arthritis Rheum* **34**, 29–34.

Cleeland CS, Gonin R, Hatfield AK 1994: Pain and its treatment in outpatients with metastatic cancer. *N Engl J Med* **330**, 592–596.

Coyle N, Adelhardt J, Foley KM, Portenoy RK 1990: Character of terminal illness in the advanced cancer patient: Pain and other symptoms during the last four weeks of life. *J Pain Symptom Manage* **5**, 83–93.

Croft P, Rigby AS, Boswell R, Schollum J, Silman A 1993: The prevalence of chronic widespread pain in the general population. *J Rheumatol* **20**, 710–713.

Croft P, Jordan K, Jinks C 2005: "Pain elsewhere" and the impact of knee pain in older people. *Arthritis Rheum* **52**, 2350–2354.

Crombie IK and Davies HT 1998: Selection bias in pain research. *Pain* **74**, 1–3.

Crombie I, Davis HTO, Macrae WA 1994: The epidemiology of chronic pain: time for new directions. *Pain* **57**, 1–3.

Dawson J, Linsell L, Zondervan K, Rose P, Carr A, Randall T, et al 2005: Impact of persistent hip or knee pain on overall health status in elderly people: a longitudinal population study. *Arthritis Rheum* **15**, 368–374.

Dawson J, Linsell L, Zondervan K, Rose P, Randall T, Carr A, et al 2004: Epidemiology of hip and knee pain and its impact on overall health status in older adults. *Rheumatology* **43**, 497–504.

Department of Health 2004: Prescriptions dispensed in the community: Statistics for 1993 to 2003, England. [accessed 24 August 2009].

Duncan R, Peat G, Thomas E, Hay E, McCall I, Croft P 2007: Symptoms and radiographic osteoarthritis: not as discordant as they are made out to be? *Ann Rheum Dis* **66**, 86–91.

Dziedzic K, Thomas E, Hill S, Wilkie R, Peat G, Croft PR 2007: The impact of musculoskeletal hand problems in older adults: findings from the North Staffordshire Osteoarthritis Project (NorStOP). *Rheumatology* **46**, 963–967.

Ebrahim S, Brittis SJ, Wu A 1991: The valuation of states of ill-health: the impact of age and disability. *Age Ageing* **20**, 37–40.

Elliott AM, Smith BH, Penny KI, Smith WC, Chambers WA 1999: The epidemiology of chronic pain in the community. *Lancet* **354**, 1248–1252.

Elliott AM, Smith BH, Hannaford PC, Smith WC, Chambers WA 2002: The course of chronic pain in the community: results of a 4-year follow-up study. *Pain* **99**, 299–307.

Felson DT 2009: Developments in the clinical understanding of osteoarthritis. *Arthritis Res Ther* **11**, 203.

Ferrell BA, Ferrell BR, Osterweil D 1990: Pain in the nursing home. *J Am Geriatr Soc* **38**, 409–414.

Frampton M 2003: Experience assessment and management of pain in people with dementia. *Age Ageing* **32**, 248–251

Gagliese L, Gauthier LR, Macpherson AK, Jovellanos M, Chan VW 2008: Correlates of postoperative pain and intravenous patient-controlled analgesia use in younger and older surgical patients. *Pain Med* **9**, 299–314.

Gagliese L, Jackson M, Ritvo P, Wowk A, Katz J 2000: Age is not an impediment to effective use of patient-controlled analgesia by surgical patients. *Anesthesiology* **93**, 601–610.

Gagliese L and Katz J 2003: Age differences in postoperative pain are scale dependent: a comparison of measures of pain intensity and quality in younger and older surgical patients. *Pain* **103**, 11–20.

Gagliese L and Melzack R 2003: Age-related differences in the qualities but not the intensity of chronic pain. *Pain* **104**, 597–608.

Gagliese L, Weizblit N, Ellis W, Chan VW 2005: The measurement of postoperative pain: a comparison of intensity scales in younger and older surgical patients. *Pain* **117**, 412–420.

Gerdle B, Björk J, Henriksson C, Bengtsson A 2004: Prevalence of current and chronic pain and their influences upon work and healthcare-seeking: a population study. *J Rheumatol* **31**, 1399–1406.

Gibson SJ and Helme RD 2001: Age-related differences in pain perception and report. *Clin Geriatr Med* **17**, 433–456.

Gupta S, Hawker GA, Laporte A, Croxford R, Coyte PC 2005: The economic burden of disabling hip and knee osteoarthritis (OA) from the perspective of individuals living with this condition. *Rheumatology* **44**, 1531–1537.

Hadjistavropoulos T, Herr K, Turk DC, Fine PG, Dworkin RH et al. 1997: An interdisciplinary expert consensus statement on assessment of pain in older people. *Clin J Pain* **23**, S1–S43.

Harris L 2004: Review of prevalence of pain in older adults. MMedSci Thesis, Keele University.

Harris T, Cook DG, Victor C, DeWilde S, Beighton C 2006: Onset and persistence of depression in older people-results from a 2-year community follow-up study. *Age Ageing* **35**, 25–32.

Hasselström J, Liu-Palmgren J, Rasjö-Wrååk G 2002: Prevalence of pain in general practice. *Eur J Pain* **6**, 375–385.

Hindley NJ, Jobst KA, King E, Barnetson L, Smith A, Haigh AM 1995: High acceptability and low morbidity of diagnostic lumbar puncture in elderly subjects of mixed cognitive status. *Acta Neurol Scand* **91**, 405–411.

Hootman JM and Helmick CG 2006: Projections of US prevalence of arthritis and associated activity limitations. *Arthritis Rheum* **54**, 226–229.

Horgas A and Tsai P-F 1998: Analgesic drug prescription and use in cognitively impaired nursing home residents. *Nurs Res* **47**, 235–242.

Huffman JC and Kunik ME 2000: Assessment and understanding of pain in patients with dementia. *Gerontologist* **40**, 574–581.

Hunt IM, Silman AJ, Benjamin S, McBeth J, Macfarlane GJ 1999: The prevalence and associated features of chronic widespread pain in the community using the 'Manchester' definition of chronic widespread pain. *Rheumatology (Oxford)* **38**, 275–279.

International Association for the Study of Pain 1986: Classification of chronic pain: Descriptions of chronic pain syndromes and definitions of pain terms. *Pain* **3**, S1–S226.

Jagger C, Matthews R, Lindesay J, Robinson T, Croft P, Brayne C 2009: The effect of dementia trends and treatments on longevity and disability: a simulation model based on the MRC Cognitive Function and Ageing Study (MRC CFAS). *Age Ageing* **38**, 319–325.

Jinks C, Jordan K, Ong BN, Croft P 2004: A brief screening tool for knee pain in primary care (KNEST). 2. Results from a survey in the general population aged 50 and over. *Rheumatol* **43**, 55–61.

Jordan K, Sawyer S, Coakley P, Smith H, Cooper C, Arden N 2004: The use of conventional and complementary treatments for knee osteoarthritis in the community. *Rheumatology* **43**, 381–384.

Kamel HK, Phlavan M, Malekgoudarzi B, Gogel P, Morley JE 2001: Utilizing pain assessment scales increases the frequency of diagnosing pain among elderly nursing home residents. *J Pain Symptom Management* **21**, 450–455.

Landi F, Onder G, Cesari M, Russo A, Barillaro C, Bernabei R; SILVERNET-HC Study Group 2005: Pain and its relation to depressive symptoms in frail older people living in the community: an observational study. *J Pain Symptom Manage* **29**, 255–262.

Leveille SG, Bean J, Ngo L, McMullen W, Guralnik JM 2007: The pathway from musculoskeletal pain to mobility difficulty in older disabled women. *Pain* **128**, 69–77.

Loeser JD and Treede RD 2008: The Kyoto protocol of IASP Basic Pain Terminology. *Pain* **137**, 473–477.

Mallen CD and Peat G 2008: Screening older people with musculoskeletal pain for depressive symptoms in primary care. *Br J Gen Pract* **58**, 688–693.

Mäntyselkä P, Hartikainen S, Louhivuori-Laako K, Sulkava R 2004: Effects of dementia on perceived daily pain in home-dwelling elderly people: a population-based study. *Age Ageing* **33**, 496–499.

Mäntyselkä P, Kumpusalo E, Ahonen R, Kumpusalo A, Kauhanen J, Viinamäki H, et al. 2001: Pain as a reason to visit the doctor: a study in Finnish primary health care. *Pain* **89**, 175–180.

Mäntyselkä PT, Turunen JH, Ahonen RS, Kumpusalo EA 2003: Chronic pain and poor self-rated health. *JAMA* **290**, 2435–2442.

McAlindon TE, Cooper C, Kirwan JR, Dieppe PA 1992: Knee pain and disability in the community. *Br J Rheumatol* **31**, 189–192.

McBeth J, Macfarlane GJ, Hunt IM, Silman AJ 2001: Risk factors for persistent chronic widespread pain: a community-based study. *Rheumatol* **40**, 95–101.

Melding PS 1996: Is there such a thing as geriatric pain? *Pain* **46**, 119–121.

Milton JC, Hill-Smith I, Jackson SHD 2008: Prescribing for older people. *BMJ* **336**, 606–609.

Mossey JM, Gallagher RM, Tirumalasetti F 2000: The effects of pain and depression on physical functioning in elderly residents of a continuing care retirement community. *Pain Med* **1**, 340–350.

Mossey JM and Gallagher RM 2004: The longitudinal occurrence and impact of comorbid chronic pain and chronic depression over two years in continuing care retirement community residents. *Pain Med* **5**, 335–348.

Office for National Statistics 2006: Key population and vital statistics. http://www.statistics.gov.uk/downloads/theme_population/KPVS33_2006/FINAL_KPVS2006-web.pdf [accessed 24 August 2009]

O'Reilly SC, Muir KR, Doherty M 1998: Knee pain and disability in the Nottingham community: association with poor health status and psychological distress. *Br J Rheumatol* **37**, 870–873.

Papageorgiou AC, Silman AJ, Macfarlane GJ 2002: Chronic widespread pain in the population: a seven year follow up study. *Ann Rheum Dis* **61**, 1071–1074.

Porter F, Malhotra K, Wolf C, Morris J, Miller J, Smith M 1996: Dementia and response to pain in the elderly. *Pain* **68**, 413–421.

Rao A and Cohen HJ 2004: Symptom management in the elderly cancer patient: fatigue, pain, and depression. *J Natl Cancer Inst Mongr* **32**, 150–157.

Reyes-Gibby CC, Aday L, Cleeland C 2002: Impact of pain on self-rated health in the community-dwelling older adult. *Pain* **95**, 75–82.

Reynolds KS, Hanson LC, DeVellis RF, Henderson M, Steinhauser KE 2008: Disparities in pain management between cognitively intact and cognitively impaired nursing home residents. *J Pain Symptom Management* **35**, 388–396.

Roberts C, Adebajo A, Long S 2002: Improving the quality of care of musculoskeletal conditions in primary care. *Rheumatol*, **41**, 503–508.

Rollason V and Vogt N 2003: Reduction of polypharmacy in the elderly: a systematic review of the role of the pharmacist. *Drugs Aging* **20**, 817–832.

Rosemann T, Backenstrass M, Joest K, Rosemann A, Szecsenyi J, Laux G 2007: Predictors of depression in a sample of 1,021 primary care patients with osteoarthritis. *Arthritis Rheum* **57**, 415–422.

Scudds RJ and Østbye T 2001: Pain and pain-related interference with function in older Canadians: the Canadian study of health and aging. *Disabil Rehabil* **23**, 654–664.

Schmader KE 2002: Epidemiology and impact on quality of life of post-herpetic neuralgia and painful diabetic retinopathy. *Clin J Pain* **18**, 350–354.

Schwartz JB, Gibb WJ, Tran T 1991: Aging effects on heart rate variation. *J Gerontol* **46**, M99–M106.

Sengstaken EA and King SA 1993: The problems of pain and its detection among geriatric nursing home residents. *J Am Geriatr Soc* **41**, 541–544.

Sufka KJ 2000: Chronic pain explained. *Brain Mind* **1**, 155–179.

Thomas E, Peat G, Harris L, Wilkie R, Croft PR 2004: The prevalence of pain and pain interference in a general population of older adults: Cross-sectional findings from the North Staffordshire Osteoarthritis Project (NorStOP). *Pain* **110**, 361–368.

Thomas E, Mottram S, Peat G, Wilkie R, Croft PR 2007: The effect of age on the onset of pain interference in a general population of older adults: Prospective findings from the North Staffordshire Osteoarthritis Project (NorStOP). *Pain* **129**, 21–27.

Thomas T, Robinson C, Champion D, McKell M, Pell M 1998: Prediction and assessment of the severity of post-operative pain and of satisfaction with management. *Pain* **75**,177–185.

US Census Bureau 2008: International Programe Centre, International Data Base – http://www.census.gov/ipc/www/idb/worldpopinfo.php [access 24 August 2009].

Washington LL, Gibson SJ, Helme RD 2000: Age-related differences in the endogenous analgesic response to repeated cole water immersion in human volunteers. *Pain* **89**, 89–96.

Weinberg JM 2007: Herpes zoster: Epidemiology, natural history, and common complications. *J Am Acad Dermatol* **57**, S130–S135.

Weiner DK 2002: Improving pain management for older adults: an urgent agenda for the educator, investigator and practitioner. *Pain* **97**, 1–4.

Westoby CJ, Mallen CD, Thomas E 2009: Cognitive complaints in a general population of older adults: prevalence, association with pain and the influence of concurrent affective disorders. *Eur J Pain* **13**, 970–976.

Wolfe F, Smythe HA, Yunus MB, Bennett RM, Bombardier C, Goldenberg DL et al 1990: The American College of Rheumatology 1990 Criteria for the Classification of Fibromyalgia. Report of the Multicenter Criteria Committee. *Arthritis Rheum* **33**, 160–172.

Woolf AD and Akesson K 2001: Understanding the burden of musculoskeletal conditions. The burden is huge and not reflected in national health priorities. *BMJ* **322**, 1079–1080.

Zheng Z, Gibson SJ, Khalil Z, Helme RD, McMeeken JM 2000: Age-related differences in the time course of capsaicin-induced hyperanalgesia. *Pain* **85**, 51–58.

Pain and disease

Chapter 17

Disease-related pain: an introduction

Peter Croft

One idea discussed in Chapter 1 was to move from a traditional medical textbook approach to pain, which seeks mainly to ascribe it to an underlying disease, towards an approach that considers chronic pain as a problem in its own right.

However, primary prevention of pathologies that precipitate chronic pain in vulnerable people is still potentially a crucially important public health contribution to population prevention of chronic pain. The size of such a potential contribution will depend on the proportion of chronic pain in the population directly attributable to underlying preventable 'triggering' diseases.

There are remarkably few studies which compare the incidence and prevalence of chronic pain between persons exposed to specific diseases or injuries and unexposed controls, in order to estimate how much pain is linked specifically to the disease or injury in question. By contrast, many uncontrolled studies estimate the incidence and prevalence of pain in relation to a particular disease, with the entirely reasonable purpose of highlighting chronic pain as an important issue in the health care of people with that disease. The problem is that such studies do not help to assess whether chronic pain is any more common in the presence of the disease than in its absence. Chapters that follow in this section consider the evidence about diseases or injuries which might give rise to chronic pain.

Once again we have been selective in the topics chosen for this section. Musculoskeletal conditions might have dominated here – why not discuss shoulder, back, neck, or joint pain in terms of their underlying regional pathology? One reason is that the link between underlying pathology and chronic pain is particularly unclear in that group of conditions. The relationship between magnetic resonance imaging (MRI) changes in the spine and back pain, at the population level, has generally been observed to be weak (e.g. Jensen et al., 1994), although more recent studies comparing symptomatic and asymptomatic persons suggest stronger associations than previously (e.g. Cheung et al., 2009). Depression, for example, is more strongly and consistently predictive of new onset of back-pain episodes than structural changes in the spine (Jarvik et al., 2005). In the case of joint pain in older people, the pathological model of osteoarthritis seems to provide a more clear-cut story: X-ray changes of bony sclerosis and cartilage loss reflecting underlying joint pathology. Despite this, there are many older people with radiographic changes of osteoarthritis who do not have joint pain, and many with joint pain who have minimal osteoarthritic change (Bedson and Croft, 2008). This may of course reflect inadequate imaging, and recent work by Duncan and colleagues on the knee suggest that the link between osteoarthritic pathology and pain in that joint might be stronger than previously thought (Duncan et al., 2007). Furthermore, joint replacement can relieve pain and improve functioning in persons with advanced disease. Even so, the impact of chronic knee pain on daily functioning in older people in the general population is more closely associated with pain severity, co-morbidity, psychological distress, and muscle strength than it is with the degree of radiographic osteoarthritis in the joint (Jordan et al., 1997; Wood et al., 2008; O'Reilly et al., 1998).

Hemingway and his colleagues, in Chapter 20, discuss an example of a regional pain traditionally associated with a specific underlying pathology, namely chronic chest pain and its subcategory of chronic angina. They come to the conclusion that the extent to which the syndrome of chronic chest pain is an indicator of both cardiovascular disease (distinct and separate from acute myocardial events) and risk of premature death has been underestimated. However, they also point to the lack of rigorous studies of pain relief in angina and chest pain, and to observational studies which indicate that substantial proportions of people have persistent pain despite treatment, i.e. the problem is the chronic pain as well as the cardiovascular risk. They urge more studies of the phenomenology and clinical meaning of this symptom, and highlight how prevention studies have concentrated on measuring reduction of heart attacks rather than of chest pain. They lay down two big public health challenges: how to identify the so far unattributed burden and nature of the disease underlying chronic angina and chest pain, and how to manage the extensive burden of chronic pain outside the comforting box of the classic angina history.

Blyth and Boyle spot a different challenge in the case of cancer, discussed in Chapter 21. Here it would seem obvious that there must be a high prevalence of pain directly attributable to the underlying disease among cancer sufferers; and there is certainly evidence that cancer survivors do have more pain overall than unaffected controls. In a paper by Mao et al., data from the US National Health Interview Survey was used to identify a population sample of 1904 cancer survivors and 29 092 controls. (Mao et al., 2007). The rate of 'ongoing pain' was double in the cancer group (34%) compared with controls (18%). Psychological distress (26%) and insomnia (30%) were also higher in frequency, indicating the presence of the amplified syndrome of chronic pain. Pain was 3 times more likely in cancer survivors under 50 than over 64 years, which means that, although cancer overall increases in frequency with age, cancer in young people may be contributing as much as cancer in older people to the frequency of chronic pain in the total population.

Blyth and Boyle highlight the changing population picture, as successful treatment of cancer becomes increasingly available, and there is a shift from end-of-life care to long-term care of chronic symptoms. With respect to the public health significance of chronic pain in cancer patients, their chapter points out that the prevalence of treated or cured disease is such that cancer pain now presents issues similar to other causes of chronic pain in populations and that the non-cancer component of the pain is increasing in importance. However, given the low incidence of cancer relative to common syndromes such as chronic musculoskeletal pain, cancer only contributes a small proportion of the total population burden of chronic pain, whatever the attributable proportion among cancer sufferers with chronic pain.

Chapters 18 (Smith and Torrance) and 19 (Bruce) investigate the particular phenomenon of diseases, injuries or interventions that might injure nerves and give rise to neuropathic pain. This is a potentially unifying mechanism across a range of diseases, such as diabetes or Herpes zoster, or nerve trauma such as might occur during surgery. The two chapters provide persuasive evidence for distinctive types of pain arising from this mechanism, and the likely contribution it might make to population levels of chronic pain. However these authors also point out that pre-existing factors prior to the injury, including psychological and social characteristics, are important in determining the outcome of neuropathic and post-surgical pain.

Other conditions contributing to population levels of chronic pain

Chronic pain is considered to be an important but under-recognized component of diseases such as renal failure, heart failure, and diabetes. Butchart and colleagues surveyed chronic pain in three groups of primary care patients: 184 with heart failure, 221 with diabetes, and 219 general primary care users (Butchart et al., 2009). Similarly, high proportions (over 60%) reported chronic pain in each group. Most of this pain related to the back, hip, or knee in all three groups, suggesting that the dominant nature of chronic pain in patients with heart disease or diabetes may be no different to the population attending primary care in general (i.e. it is mostly musculoskeletal). In a study of hospital outpatients with chronic kidney disease, pain was also common (69%), but this prevalence was no different to other general medical outpatients, and showed similar associations with disordered sleep and depression in the two groups (Cohen et al., 2007).

Globally, diseases such as HIV/AIDS (discussed by Smith and Torrance in Chapter 18 as a source of neuropathic pain) and haemoglobinopathies may be important causes of chronic pain in populations because of their frequency.

Pain is reported to be a significant component of the clinical picture of HIV/AIDS, both overall and in relation to many of the conditions that can complicate the disease. In one controlled study, Lolekha et al. compared 61 children with HIV infection in the age range of 4–15 years in Thailand with an equal number of age-matched control children who had no chronic disease (Lolekha et al., 2004). Chronic pain was reported by 44% of cases compared with 13% of their controls. The emerging story here is similar to that for cancer. Pain levels in advanced disease are high and the benefits of effective pain relief are clear. However, life span in this disease is increasing and longer term quality-of-life is becoming important to the public health picture. Long-term management of chronic pain in patients with an HIV/AIDS diagnosis is the clinical challenge rather than exclusively end-of-life palliation of pain.

Although acute pain and pain during sickle cell 'crises' are well documented, the extent of chronic pain in persons with haemoglobinopathies and the proportion of that pain attributable to that group of diseases has received little systematic epidemiological study. However, there is some suggestion that chronic pain prevalence may be higher than general population rates. In the Pain in Sickle Cell Epidemiology Study in the USA, McClish et al. found that pain scores, as measured on the Short Form-36, were worse in their sample of 308 patients with sickle cell disease than national norms or scores in patients with cystic fibrosis or asthma (McClish et al., 2005).

Injuries, particularly road traffic accidents, represent in total one of the most important triggers for chronic pain in populations globally. They provide an acute unexpected trigger for pain and they are common. Severe injuries appear to be associated with persisting pain. Castillo et al, for example, reported on a group of persons with severe lower limb injury 7 years after the event (Castillo et al., 2006). They found pain scores (measured on the Chronic Pain Grade and therefore relating to the broader or amplified "chronic pain syndrome") to be higher than national norms. In a recent analysis of birth-cohort data, Jones et al. found that children who had been hospitalized following a road traffic accident were at increased risk of developing chronic widespread pain by the age of 45, a finding not explained by adult psychosocial factors (Jones et al., 2009). This may be a specific risk related to trauma at a crucial developmental stage and may be contributing to a longer term propensity for chronic pain through the life-course (see Chapters 14 and 15).

However, even with severe injuries, pre-existing factors appear to influence who will develop chronic pain after an accident. Rivara and colleagues reported on a sample of 3047 persons drawn from a US national sample of 10 371 major trauma sufferers in the age range of 18–84 years (Rivara et al., 2008). Twelve months after the precipitating injury, pain was more likely if there had been untreated depression prior to injury. The complexity of the inter-relation between pain and psychological aspects of injury was highlighted by another analysis from this same study, which found an association between symptoms of post-traumatic stress disorder at 12 months and baseline pain severity in the period immediately following the injury (Zatzick et al., 2007).

A more common exposure (and therefore potentially a bigger contributor to the population burden of chronic pain) is minor trauma following road traffic and other accidents. Follow-up studies suggest that pre-accident factors (propensity) are important determinants of who does and does not develop chronic pain. In one study of persons sampled from the registers of a UK insurance company and followed up for 1 year after road traffic accidents, not only were pre-collision symptoms and use of health care strong predictors of incident widespread pain at 1-year post-accident follow-up, but so also was the presence of early post-collision physical symptoms (Wynne-Jones et al., 2006).

Other injuries may be important on a population scale, notably non-accidental trauma and violence. Chapters 9 (Jones, McBeth, and Power), 14 (Jones and Botello), and 15 (Macfarlane) consider the evidence for higher rates of chronic pain in persons with a previous history of physical and sexual abuse. There is a growing body of literature from large-scale national surveys that pain is more common in persons who report a previous history of abuse and violence at all ages, in both domestic and public settings (e.g. Ellsberg et al., 2008; Sachs-Ericsson et al., 2007; Chartier et al., 2007; Davis et al., 2005). Much of this evidence is cross sectional and relies on retrospective recall of abuse or violence. However, a limited number of prospective studies suggest that psychological distress and widespread pain, in particular, in adults may be linked with abuse in childhood or previous exposure to violence.

The causal pathway here has more than one dimension, and Jones et al. in Chapter 9 have summarized the underlying biological mechanisms which might mediate this link. There is the potential for physical injuries to result in chronic pain, but the particular circumstances of domestic or criminal or political violence mean that such violence is also a component of the 'propensity to chronic pain' via links to long-term mental ill-health and post-traumatic stress. The literature on non-accidental injury, and violence particularly, includes studies from many different countries, indicating the universality of this experience especially in women and the poor [e.g. the World Health Organisation Surveys (Ellsberg et al., 2008)]. The precise contribution to population levels of chronic pain remains to be clarified.

Impact of pain on chronic disease outcome

Finally, it is likely that the experience of pain in the context of disease will add to poor physical and psychological health. Suggestive evidence for this component of health status comes from prospective studies, such as Zatzick et al.'s from the US national study of trauma, in which the risk of post-traumatic stress disorder in patients who had experienced major trauma was higher in those who had experienced higher levels of pain in the immediate aftermath of the injury (Zatzick et al., 2007).

The overall evidence from primary care populations suggests, however, that the specific disease does not add much to the picture provided already by the presence of chronic pain. In the study of Butchart et al. of chronic pain in different groups of primary care patients, persons with chronic pain had worse health than persons without pain in each of the disease groups including the general consulters (Butchart et al., 2009). The only thing that differed about people with pain in the two specific disease groups (i.e. heart failure and diabetes), as compared with those reporting pain in the general consulters group, was that people with pain in those two groups were less likely to be working because of their health.

In a prospective study following up primary health care use among cohorts of pain patients, Von Korff and colleagues showed that among pain patients who were frequent users of the health care system, those with 'lower priority' conditions were no different in terms of pain severity, chronicity, or somatization than those with 'higher priority' conditions, suggesting that chronic pain for which health care is sought is similar regardless of cause. Lower health care use in pain patients was associated with less severe pain and better psychosocial function, again regardless of cause (Von Korff et al., 2007).

Summary

The paucity of controlled data means this is an area in need of stronger epidemiological evidence to construct the population picture. However, the need for a public health perspective should not divert attention from the substantial evidence that attention to chronic pain is needed as part of the care of people across a wide range of chronic diseases, and that triggering events, such as trauma or sickle cell crises, are important causes of acute pain. Therefore, the following observations seem reasonable on the basis of available evidence:

(i) The presence of many chronic diseases is linked to a prevalence of chronic pain higher than in the general population. Whether this is a selection effect or not is unclear, although in the case of cancer survivors and sickle cell disease, controlled evidence suggests it is unlikely to be due to selection alone.

(ii) Prevalence estimates of chronic pain in relation to specific diseases vary from study to study and are likely to reflect differences in definition. However, in studies which have compared people with different diseases, and used a single instrument to do so, prevalence estimates are generally reported to be similar between conditions.

(iii) The predictors of chronic pain in specific diseases are rarely linked strongly or exclusively to disease characteristics, with the possible exception of the importance of severity of acute pain early after an event in predicting future outcome. Social, psychological, and pre-morbid characteristics are generally important associations with the probability of chronic pain.

So the public health conclusion must be that primary prevention of these diseases will contribute to the reduction of population levels of chronic pain but how much that contribution will achieve depends on

a. the prevalence of the disease

b. more precise effect estimates, from controlled follow-up studies, of the size of the contribution of the disease to population burden (the population-attributable proportion).

The evidence also suggests that, in these diseases, secondary prevention of chronic pain and tertiary prevention of its consequences will be concerned more with the general features of the chronic pain syndrome and the presence of propensity for developing chronic pain than with characteristics of the underlying disease.

References

Bedson, J. and Croft, P.R. 2008: The discordance between clinical and radiographic knee osteoarthritis: a systematic search and summary of the literature. BMC Musculoskelet Disord **9**, 116.

Butchart, A., Kerr, E.A., Heisler, M., Piette, J.D., Krein, S.L. 2009: Experience and management of chronic pain among patients with other complex chronic conditions. Clin J Pain **25**, 293–298.

Castillo, R.C., MacKenzie, E.J., Wegener, S.T., Bosse, M.J., LEAP Study Group. 2006: Prevalence of chronic pain seven years following limb threatening lower extremity trauma. Pain **124**, 321–329.

Chartier, M.J., Walker, J.R., Naimark, B. 2007: Childhood abuse, adult health, and health care utilization: results from a representative community sample. Am J Epidemiol **165**, 1031–1038.

Cheung, K,M., Karppinen, J., Chan, D., Ho, D.W., Song, Y.Q., Sham, P., et al. 2009: Prevalence and pattern of lumbar magnetic resonance imaging changes in a population study of one thousand forty-three individuals. Spine **34**, 934–940.

Cohen, S.D., Patel, S.S., Khetpal, P., Peterson, R.A., Kimmel, P.L. 2007: Pain, sleep disturbance, and quality of life in patients with chronic kidney disease. Clin J Am Soc Nephrol **2**, 919–925.

Davis, D.A., Luecken, L.J., Zautra, A.J. 2005: Are reports of childhood abuse related to the experience of chronic pain in adulthood? A meta-analytic review of the literature. Clin J Pain **21**, 398–405.

Duncan, R., Peat, G., Thomas, E., Hay, E., McCall, I. and Croft, P. 2007: Symptoms and radiographic osteoarthritis: not as discordant as they are made out to be? Ann Rheum Dis **66**, 86–91.

Ellsberg, M., Jansen, H.A., Heise, L., Watts, C.H., Garcia-Moreno, C., Campbell, J., et al. 2008: Intimate partner violence and women's physical and mental health in the WHO multi-country study on women's health and domestic violence: an observational study. Lancet **371**, 1165–1172.

Jarvik, J.G., Hollingworth, W., Heagerty, P.J., Haynor, D.R., Boyko, E.J., Deyo, R.A. 2005: Three-year incidence of low back pain in an initially asymptomatic cohort: clinical and imaging risk factors. Spine **30**, 1541–1548.

Jensen, M.C., Brant-Zawadzki, M.N., Obuchowski, N., Modic, M.T., Malkasian, D., Ross, J.S. 1994: Magnetic resonance imaging of the lumbar spine in people without back pain. N Engl J Med **331**, 69–73.

Jones, G.T., Power, C., Macfarlane, G.J. 2009: Adverse events in childhood and chronic widespread pain in adult life: Results from the 1958 British Birth Cohort Study. Pain **143**, 92–96.

Jordan, J., Luta, G., Renner, J., Dragomir, A., Hochberg, M., Fryer, J. 1997: Knee pain and knee osteoarthritis severity in self-reported task specific disability: the Johnston County Osteoarthritis Project. J Rheumatol **24**, 1344–1349.

Lolekha, R., Chanthavanich, P., Limkittikul, K., Luangxay, K., Chotpitayasunodh, T., Newman, C.J. 2004: Pain: a common symptom in human immunodeficiency virus-infected Thai children. Acta Paediatr **93**, 891–898.

Mao, J.J., Armstrong, K., Bowman, M.A., Xie, S.X., Kadakia, R., Farrar, J.T. 2007: Symptom burden among cancer survivors: impact of age and comorbidity. J Am Board Fam Med. **20**, 434–43.

McClish, D.K., Penberthy, L.T., Bovbjerg, V.E., Roberts, J.D., Aisiku, I.P., Levenson, J.L., et al. 2005: Health related quality of life in sickle cell patients: the PiSCES project. Health Qual Life Outcomes **29**, 50.

O'Reilly, S.C., Muir, K.R., Doherty, M. 1998: Knee pain and disability in the Nottingham community: association with poor health status and psychological distress. Br J Rheumatol **37**, 870–873.

Rivara, F.P., Mackenzie, E.J., Jurkovich, G.J., Nathens, A.B., Wang, J., Scharfstein, D.O. 2008: Prevalence of pain in patients 1 year after major trauma. Arch Surg **143**, 282–287.

Sachs-Ericsson, N., Kendall-Tackett, K., Hernandez, A. 2007: Childhood abuse, chronic pain, and depression in the National Comorbidity Survey. Child Abuse Negl **31**, 531–547.

Von Korff, M., Lin, E.H., Fenton, J.J., Saunders, K. 2007: Frequency and priority of pain patients' health care use. Clin J Pain **23**, 400–408.

Wood, L.R., Peat, G., Thomas, E., Duncan, R. 2008: The contribution of selected non-articular conditions to knee pain severity and associated disability in older adults. Osteoarthritis Cartilage **16**, 647–653.

Wynne-Jones, G., Jones, G.T., Wiles, N.J., Silman, A.J., Macfarlane, G.J. 2006: Predicting new onset of widespread pain following a motor vehicle collision. J Rheumatol **33**, 968–974.

Zatzick, D.F., Rivara, F.P., Nathens, A.B., Jurkovich, G.J., Wang, J., Fan, M.Y., et al. 2007: A nationwide US study of post-traumatic stress after hospitalization for physical injury. Psychol Med **37**, 1469–1480.

Chapter 18

Neuropathic pain

Blair H. Smith and Nicola Torrance

Introduction

'Neuropathic pain' (NeuP) is defined by the International Study for the Association of Pain (IASP) as 'pain arising as a direct consequence of a lesion or disease affecting the somatosensory system' (Loeser and Treede, 2008). Most articles or chapters that describe NeuP begin with a version of this definition, for good reason, as will be demonstrated.

Challenges in the epidemiology of neuropathic pain

Epidemiological study of NeuP is not straightforward, being, at best, challenging and, at worst, controversial. The main reason for this is a lack of agreement on the definition, classification, and ascertainment. Even the IASP definition, which seems at first uncomplicated, lacks clarity. What, for example, constitutes a 'lesion' and a 'disease', and can we diagnose NeuP if we are not equipped to identify these incontrovertibly? There are overlaps between this IASP definition and others in its classification of chronic pain (Merskey and and Bogduk, 1994). NeuP is a sub-group of 'neurogenic pain' ('pain initiated or caused by a primary lesion, dysfunction or transitory perturbation in the peripheral or central nervous system'), with the implication that NeuP is the irreversible sub-group. NeuP itself has sub-groups: 'central neuropathic pain' ('pain arising as a direct consequence of a lesion or disease affecting the central somatosensory system'; Loeser and Treede, 2008), and 'peripheral neuropathic pain' ('pain arising as a direct consequence of a lesion or disease affecting the peripheral somatosensory system'; Loeser and Treede, 2008), with the implication that there are important differences dictated by the site of the nerve dysfunction.

Common characteristics and causes

Nevertheless, despite this lack of absolute clarity or agreement, it is clear that a distinct entity roughly equating to NeuP exists, in which abnormal activation of neurological pain pathways produces persistent clinical features that are different from other types of pain. There is good reason to study it epidemiologically with a view to understanding its occurrence, and optimizing treatment and prevention. Traditionally, NeuP is distinguished from 'nociceptive pain' (with the somewhat circular formal definition of 'pain arising from activation of nociceptors' (Loeser and Treede, 2008), but referring to pain caused by actual or potential non-neurological tissue damage). This distinction is a recommended starting point for many treatment algorithms and much decision-making (Finnerup et al., 2007). NeuP has characteristic signs and symptoms that render it a demonstrably different disease condition (Box 18.1). More importantly, the different underlying mechanisms mean that treatment needs and responses to treatments, particularly pharmaceutical, are also distinct. It is, however, important not to take the distinction too far, for many of

Box 18.1 Neuropathic pain descriptors

- Electric shocks, shooting, or stabbing
- Pain evoked by light touch (allodynia)
- Increased pain in response to a normally painful stimulus (hyperalgesia)
- Hot or burning pain
- Dysaethesias and paraesthesias such as tingling, numbness, prickling, itching, pins and needles sensations
- Painful cold or freezing pain

the associated symptoms and biopsychosocial risk markers, and treatment needs, are the same, irrespective of pain type or cause.

Spectrum rather than a binary phenomenon

These similarities between neuropathic and nociceptive pain have attracted recent research attention, raising the question of whether there is a true dichotomy. Some conditions, such as post-herpetic neuralgia (PHN), may be considered almost entirely neurogenic, whilst others, such as osteoarthritis, almost entirely nociceptive. However, many causes of chronic pain, notably low back pain, have both tissue- and nerve-damage contributions. Some nociceptive pain conditions may produce sufficiently potent stimuli to cause secondary neuroplastic changes in the nociceptive system (Treede et al., 2008); in contrast, some neurological disorders, such as multiple sclerosis, are associated with nociceptive pain (O'Connor et al., 2008). Pain in neither of these circumstances should strictly be regarded as neuropathic pain (Treede et al., 2008), yet it has many similar features. In many other cases there may be no demonstrable cause of pain but features characteristic of both nociceptive and neuropathic pain types; such idiopathic pain needs to be addressed in a global way.

For these reasons, the concept of 'mixed pain', has been proposed, with the idea that NeuP is a spectrum and pain can be more or less neuropathic (Rasmussen et al., 2004; Attal and Bouhassira, 2004; Bennett et al., 2006). This needs further testing, comparing broad with narrow classifications (Cruccu et al., 2004), and binary with mixed definitions (Attal and Bouhassira, 2004). Meanwhile, a consensus of international experts, assembled in collaboration with the IASP, proposes to augment the definition of NeuP with a grading system, allowing 'Possible', 'Probable', and 'Definite' NeuP (Treede et al., 2008). The latter two require detailed clinical assessment, while the former can be based on symptoms alone. This system is helpful clinically as it allows treatment to proceed pragmatically on the basis of probability. It is also helpful for research as it will allow case definitions for epidemiological research that do not rely on intensive assessments of participants.

Common neuropathic pain conditions

Some of the common causes of NeuP are shown in Box 18.2 (Dworkin, 2002; Smith and Torrance, 2006). The clinical features of NeuP reflect the underlying nerve disorder, and are summarized as sensory deficit and paradoxical pain sensations (Hansson, 2002). The area of sensory deficit is anatomically logical, representing the dermatome of the disordered nerve. Within this area, symptoms such as paraesthesiae, hypersensitivity, spontaneous shooting pains, burning sensations, and other unfamiliar or unexpected manifestations are characteristic.

Box 18.2   Some common causes of neuropathic pain

Peripheral nerve lesion or dysfunction
   Painful diabetic neuropathy (PDN)
   Post-herpetic neuralgia (PHN)
   Post-surgical pain
   Trigeminal neuralgia
   Complex regional pain syndrome
   Chemotherapy-induce neuropathy
   Neuropathy secondary to tumour infiltration
   HIV-related neuropathy
Central nerve lesion or dysfunction
   Central post-stroke pain
   Multiple sclerosis pain

Treatment challenges

Treatment of NeuP is challenging, and often unsatisfactory. Regardless of the initiating condition, neuropathic pain is widely recognized as one of the most difficult pain syndromes to treat and presents a significant challenge to clinicians as it often does not respond well to conventional analgesic therapies such as nonsteroidal anti-inflammatory drugs (NSAIDs; Dworkin et al., 2003; Rise and Hill, 2006). By contrast, there is good evidence from systematic reviews for the effectiveness of non-conventional painkillers including anti-epileptics (e.g. carbamazepine and gabapentin) or anti-depressants (particularly amitriptyline; Saarto and Wiffen, 2005; Wiffen et al., 2005). Treatment algorithms for neuropathic pain (Finnerup et al., 2007) and painful diabetic neuropathy (PDN) have recently been proposed (Jensen et al., 2006), and recommend the initial use of either a tricyclic antidepressant, selective serotonin noradrenaline re-uptake inhibitor, or alpha-2-delta agonist (e.g. gabapentin or pregabalin), depending on co-morbidities and contraindications. If the pain is still inadequately controlled despite a change in first-line therapy, then combination therapy with the addition of an opioid (including tramadol) may be required (Finnerup et al., 2007).

Evidence suggests that drugs are used sub-optimally in the treatment of NeuP (Torrance et al., 2007; Dieleman et al., 2008), perhaps because of under-recognition of the contribution of neuropathy to pain that presents in primary care.

Responses to non-pharmacological treatment may also be different, with recent evidence suggesting some differences between pain types in psychological and physical functioning, relevant to the design of pain-management programmes (Daniel et al., 2008). These differences are why early recognition of NeuP is important clinically, and why an epidemiological distinction is important to make. New treatments are under development, new biological understandings of pain mechanisms are constantly being derived, and trials of existing treatments are being targeted according to areas of need, and all of this informs and is informed by epidemiological science.

Population estimates

There is no accurate estimate of the population prevalence of NeuP available. Traditionally, the prevalence has been estimated at between 1% and 2%, based on summed estimates of the prevalence in the USA (Bennett, 1997) and the UK (Bowsher et al., 1991) of conditions of which NeuP is a characteristic feature. Overall, these estimates of population prevalence, arising from a number of heterogeneous studies of variable validity, and with the possibility of counting individuals with multiple NeuP conditions more than once, are likely to be inaccurate and are certainly inconsistent. In fact, it is likely that they underestimate the overall prevalence of NeuP (Dworkin, 2002) by including only those cases whose pain is the result of one of the traditionally recognized clinical diagnoses which has been formally diagnosed. Individuals who have pain with neuropathic characteristics but without such a diagnosis (through lack of appropriate clinical assessment, because they have a mixed pain type, or because investigation of the pain has not found one of these causes) will not be included in these estimates. Unfortunately, the number of these individuals in the population remains unknown, and this is the subject of ongoing research, which we describe here.

More recently, the annual incidence of NeuP in the general population has been estimated from a systematic medical records review to be 1% (Dieleman et al., 2008). An important main strength of this study is its scale; the authors examined the computerized records of 362 693 primary care patients in the Netherlands, the total amount of follow-up time was over 1 million person-years, and 9135 new cases of NeuP were identified by employing a search algorithm, followed by a manual records review. However, there are a number of weaknesses in this approach. This methodology only detects those who have presented to primary care. The identification of the cases relies on accurate diagnoses of NeuP (conditions), an accurate coding system, and a method of these being identified through the computerized search and case-notes review. Case ascertainment relied on specialist and general practitioner (GP) diagnoses and the recording of symptoms without objective diagnostic evidence. Cases that did not fall within the identified range of neuropathies included in this study will have been missed, leading to an underestimate of overall incidence. On the other hand, they may have included cases (e.g. some patients with carpal tunnel syndrome, the second commonest NeuP condition identified in this study), where pain was not the primary reason for presentation to their GP. The commonest NeuP condition found in this study was 'mononeuropathy of upper/lower limb', the neuropathic nature of which may be difficult to assess. Neither of these (i.e. carpal tunnel or mononeuropathy) feature strongly in other estimates of the incidence or prevalence of NeuP conditions (Hall et al., 2006; Sadosky et al., 2008; Taylor, 2006), and this discrepancy may be an effect of the data-collection method.

Descriptive epidemiology of neuropathic pain

It is, we suppose, relatively unusual for a chapter in an epidemiology book to begin with such a detailed review of the definition of the condition under consideration. In the case of NeuP, however, such a review is central to any discussion about its epidemiology. Even in the presence of rigorously agreed clinical parameters, an accurate and unarguable diagnosis of NeuP could only be made after a detailed clinical history and examination by a pain specialist or neurologist. Given the impracticality of this in a population sample large enough from which to extrapolate findings meaningfully, it is not surprising that such estimates of incidence and prevalence as we do have are based on proxy measures, less than ideal clinical assessment, or screening tools with variable specificity and sensitivity in comparison with clinical assessment.

Diagnosis

This is where NeuP presents its next challenge to epidemiologists. If (and it remains a big 'if') a definition of NeuP can be agreed, how can we apply this in the field? Despite ongoing discussions in the neurology and pain-specialist communities, there is no 'gold standard' for diagnosing NeuP. Consensus does exist (Treede et al., 2008; Cruccu et al., 2004), but suggests that while a detailed assessment in a clinical setting, by a specialist, including an accurate sensory examination, is 'often enough to reach a diagnosis' (Cruccu et al., 2004), further assessment, including nerve conduction studies and quantitative sensory testing, may be required. While this, and even more detailed assessment, is a good aspiration for the specialist clinic, it is clearly inappropriate for any but the most richly funded epidemiological study. Specialist assessment of individuals with pain has been used epidemiologically in NeuP, e.g. to determine the proportion of various clinic attenders who have this, rather than another, pain type; or in an attempt to validate other, simpler case identification instruments. Such an instrument would have great potential benefit: clinically it might facilitate early diagnosis, e.g. in primary care, and consequent appropriate progress along a treatment algorithm. Academically it would allow case definition for population-based epidemiological studies and clinical trials

Case-identification instruments

Case-identification instruments for NeuP epidemiology need to detect features of pain that are characteristically neuropathic in an efficient, valid, and reliable way. Although pain descriptors used by patients with NeuP are commonly recognized by clinicians, they have rarely been studied formally (Bennett, 2001; Krause and Backonja, 2003). One of the first studies to critically evaluate sensory pain-description terms was conducted by Boureau and colleagues (Boureau et al., 1990). Using a French reconstructed McGill Pain Questionnaire (MPQ), they demonstrated significant differences for 10 sensory words and seven affective words between patients with peripheral neuropathic and nociceptive pain. The six sensory descriptors more frequently used by NeuP pain patients were: 'electric shock', 'burning', 'cold', 'pricking', 'tingling', and 'itching', and these descriptive terms feature in a number of the case-identification instruments.

One of the earliest and first pain measures, specifically designed to identify and quantify patients' neuropathic pain experience, was developed by Galer and Jensen (1997). The Neuropathic Pain Scale (NPS) was developed based on the clinical experience of the authors who 'identified the most frequent words used by NeuP patients to describe their pain'. In addition to two items that assess the global dimensions of pain intensity and pain unpleasantness, it also includes eight items that assess specific qualities of NeuP: 'sharp', 'hot', 'dull', 'cold', 'sensitive', 'itchy', 'deep', and 'surface' pain. Each of these NeuP characteristics is measured using an 11-point numerical rating scale. The NPS was validated by comparing responses to its preliminary and final versions with subsequent, blinded, specialist clinician assessment of pain based on medical history, physical examination, and laboratory tests when indicated. The NPS composite score has been further validated within groups of patients with neuropathic pain and is sensitive to treatment changes (Galer et al., 2002)

The NPS was not designed to discriminate between NeuP and nociceptive pain symptoms. Recently, however, based on the NPS and the work by Boureau and colleagues (Boureau et al., 1990), several simple clinical tools have been designed to distinguish neuropathic symptoms and signs from those arising through nociceptive pain, for research purposes (Bennett and Bouhassira, 2007). They use simple questionnaires that inquire about the presence of pain with features that make it likely to have a neuropathic origin, and include simple clinical examination or self-examination tests. They include the Leeds assessment of neuropathic symptoms and signs (LANSS) Pain Scale (Bennett, 2001), the Neuropathic Pain Questionnaire (NPQ; Krause and Backonja, 2003), and the DN4 which stands for *'douleur neuropathique en 4 questions'* (i.e. neuropathic pain in four questions; Bouhassira et al., 2005).

The LANSS Pain Scale is a tool for identifying patients in whom neuropathic mechanisms dominate their pain experience. The LANSS was developed in two populations of chronic pain patients. In the first ($n = 60$), the use of sensory descriptors and questions was compared in patients with nociceptive and NeuP pain, combined with an objective assessment of sensory function. The clinical diagnosis of the participants was classified by a pain specialist based on clinical features, known pathology, and radiological or electrophysical evidence. These data were used to derive a seven-item pain scale, consisting of grouped sensory description and examination with a simple scoring system. The LANSS was then validated in a second group of patients ($n = 40$; Bennett, 2001). Further research led to the development and validation of the S-LANSS score, a self-report, self-examination version of the LANSS (Bennett et al., 2005).

In developing the NPQ, 32 pain-clinic patients were initially categorized into pain type by medical record review, coded for diagnoses provided by the treating physician. Each patient was then given a preliminary questionnaire containing 32 items. Factor analysis led to the development of the 12-item NPQ which is able, through a complex scoring system, to differentiate NeuP patients from non-NeuP with 66.6% sensitivity and 74.4% specificity (Krause and Backonja, 2003).

For the DN4, the French NeuP Group compiled an initial list of symptoms and signs associated with NeuP, from which was derived a list of questions consisting of both sensory descriptors and signs related to bedside examination (Bouhassira et al., 2005). Each of 160 pain-clinic patients was assessed by two investigators, specialists in pain medicine and neurology, within an interval of 3 days, and their findings compared in a blinded manner. A relatively small number of items was found to be sufficient to discriminate NeuP, and the DN4 consists of four questions (subdivided into seven items related to symptoms and three related to clinical examination). The DN4 has also been further developed and validated to modify the clinician examination forms to a self-administered version (Bouhassira et al., 2008).

Similar processes have been used to develop other recent screening instruments, such as 'painDetect' (Freynhagen et al., 2006) and 'ID Pain' (Portenoy, 2006). Crucially, while these instruments can all identify pain with features suggestive of neuropathy, and have been validated against clinical assessment in pain-clinic populations, they do not in themselves diagnose NeuP. They have been used as the basis for a number of epidemiological studies (Bouhassira et al., 2008; Freynhagen et al., 2006; Torrance et al., 2006), but the entity that they identified has been variously termed 'pain with neuropathic characteristics' (Bouhassira et al., 2008), 'pain of predominantly neuropathic origin' (Bennett et al., 2005), and 'predominantly neuropathic pain' (Freynhagen et al., 2006). Before an epidemiological understanding beyond these ill-defined concepts can be reached, we need to know how responses to these questionnaires are related to specialist clinical examination in a general population sample. Nonetheless, they provide interesting interim estimates, and further work is in progress. They may correspond with the more recent concept of 'possible neuropathic pain' (Treede et al., 2008).

Apart from these broad and imprecise instruments, other approaches to population-based epidemiology of NeuP focus on specific clinical conditions. The two most widely studied NeuP conditions are PHN and painful diabetic neuropathy (PDN); post-surgical pain and lumbar radiculopathy, both mixed pain types with neuropathic features, are also widely researched. Some of these studies have used direct case-ascertainment methods, such as survey or clinical examination, while others rely on indirect methods, such as medical or prescribing records or disease registries.

Systematic search and structured review of the literature of neuropathic pain in the general population and methods of ascertainment

It is informative to review the published research literature reporting the epidemiology of NeuP conditions. A systematic search on Medline, from 1996 to July 2008, using the search strategy in Appendix 1, demonstrates the range of case definitions, case-ascertainment methods, and

Box 18.3 Criteria for including and excluding studies identified by the systematic search

Inclusion criteria

1. Studies that report the incidence or prevalence either (a) of neuropathic-type pain as a single entity, or (b) of specific condition(s) with neuropathic pain as a clinical feature

2. Studies with a study sample either representing the general population or making a reasonable attempt to include all those in the population with the potential to develop the neuropathic pain condition under research (e.g. a sample of all diabetics in a study of painful diabetic neuropathy; not a sample of pain-clinic attenders). Samples corresponding to AAN Classes I and II (general population and non-referral clinic population samples respectively, see below).

3. For review papers, those that used and reported a systematic approach to identifying relevant studies with inclusion criteria corresponding to the above.

Exclusion criteria

1. Studies reporting the proportion of a specific (clinical or demographic) sub-group who experience pain with neuropathic characteristics (e.g. the proportion of those with chronic back pain who have neuropathic features), unless the population proportion of the specific sub-group is also assessed.

2. Studies from which the estimated prevalence or incidence cannot be extrapolated to the general population

3. For review papers, those that did not report a systematic approach to identifying studies to be included in the review, or included only or mainly studies with the above exclusion criteria.

resultant estimates of incidence and prevalence of NeuP. This review includes epidemiological studies in general population samples of conditions in which NeuP is commonly recognized as a main feature, or of neuropathic-type pain as a single, global entity. At least one of the objectives of included studies was to estimate the population prevalence or incidence of the condition in question. Inclusion and exclusion criteria are listed in Box 18.3. Study samples were classified according to the American Academy of Neurology evidence-classification scheme for determining the yield of established diagnostic and screening tests (Edlund et al., 2004; Appendix 2). Although this scheme is designed for the assessment of intervention studies, its classification of population samples is helpful for epidemiological studies of NeuP.

This review identified 159 titles, with 15 original studies of neuropathic pain prevalence in the general population. Of these, four studied NeuP as a single entity, and 11 studied specific NeuP conditions, or groups of conditions. There were also two review papers examining NeuP prevalence in a systematic way (Table 18.1). Information relating to case identification, ascertainment, incidence, and prevalence is shown in Table 18.2.

Prevalence estimates in individual studies

Three of the four studies of neuropathic pain as a single global entity used brief questionnaire screening instruments (DN4, S-LANSS, and a combination of these), purporting to identify pain

Table 18.1 Categories of papers identified in the systematic search and structured review

	Neuropathic pain as a single entity	Specific neuropathic pain diagnoses
Original research	**Category A**	**Category B**
	4 papers	11 papers
	1. Bouhassira	1. Choo (PHN)
	2. Dieleman	2. Davies (PDN)
	3. Gustorff	3. Freynhagen (Back)
	4. Torrance	4. Hall (multi)
		5. Hall (multi)
		6. Helgason (PHN)
		7. Opstelten (PHN)
		8. Sjaastad (Supraorbital N)
		9. Wu (PDN)
		10. Younes (Back)
		11. Yawn (PHN)
Review	**Category C**	**Category D**
	No papers	2 papers
		1. Sadosky
		2. Taylor

'with neuropathic characteristics' or of 'predominantly neuropathic origin' (Bouhassira et al., 2008; Torrance et al., 2006; Gustorff et al., 2008). The fourth study (Dieleman et al., 2008) conducted a search of general practice databases and a manual review of electronic patient records to confirm a NeuP diagnosis. The prevalence in these studies ranged from 3.3% to 8.2%. Although these instruments had been tested by comparing scores with specialist clinical examination, demonstrating reasonable sensitivity and specificity, this had only been done on patients attending a pain clinic, and their ability to detect neuropathic pain in a general population sample (where the prevalence of neuropathic pain is likely to be much lower) remains uncertain. Such a relatively low prevalence would produce a low positive predictive value in a screening instrument, and these studies may therefore have produced overestimates of the population prevalence. On the other hand, these instruments are theoretically capable of detecting neuropathic pain related to causes that would be missed using condition-specific instruments, and some of this potential overestimation may be appropriate. It is of interest to note the similar prevalence estimated by the two studies using the screening instruments as they were designed (6.9% and 8.2%, respectively; Torrance et al., 2006). A review of screening instruments for NeuP highlights their potential value in epidemiological and clinical research, but also some of the limitations (Bennett and Bouhassira, 2007). A comparison of the items found in NeuP screening tools is shown in Table 18.3.

The 11 original general population studies of specific neuropathic diagnoses identified included four of PHN (Choo et al., 1997; Helgason et al., 2000; Opstelten et al., 2002; Yawn et al., 2007), two relating to NeuP originating in the back (Freynhagen et al., 2006; Younes et al., 2006), two of PDN (Davies et al., 2006; Wu et al., 2007), one of supra-orbital neuralgia (Sjaastad et al., 2005), and two of multiple NeuP conditions (Hall et al., 2006; Hall et al., 2008).

In studies of primary care populations, the prevalence of PHN (persistent pain 3 months after herpes zoster (HZ) diagnosis) was reported in the medical records of 2.6–10% of HZ patients

Table 18.2 Information on case identification and ascertainment from papers identified in the systematic search and structured review of the literature

First Author, Year	Sample size	Study method	AAN Class	NeuP Case-ascertainment method/instrument	Diagnosis/es	Overall prevalence/ incidence	Comments on case ascertainment
				Category A – Original research, neuropathic pain as a single entity			
Bouhassira, 2008	23 712	Postal survey, general population sample	I	DN4 questionnaire	'Chronic pain with neuropathic characteristics'	Prevalence 6.9%	Daily pain, ≥3 months; score ≥3 in 7-item screening instrument, previously validated in pain clinic population (but not in general population)
Dieleman, 2008	9311	General practice research database	I	Search using free text and ICPC codes, then manual review of the electronic patient records.	'Neuropathic pain'	Annual incidence of 0.8%	Did not include cases of mixed nociceptive and neuropathic pain. Date and diagnosis of NeuP confirmed by medically trained persons who reviewed patient records. List of NeuP conditions selected by expert panel.
Gustorff, 2008	7707	Interview survey 'performed via internet inquiry' – pre-registered pool, representative of general population	I	Selected items from LANSS and DN4	'Neuropathic pain'	Prevalence 3.3%	Ongoing chronic pain ≥3 months. See above and below for DN4 and LANSS respectively. Unclear how questions were administered or sample selected. No indication of response rate.
Torrance, 2006	3002	Postal survey, general population sample	I	S-LANSS	'Pain of predominantly neuropathic origin'	Prevalence 8.2%	Pain or discomfort ≥ 3 months. Score ≥12 on 7-item screening instrument, previously validated in pain clinic population (but not in general population).

Category B – Original research, specific neuropathic pain diagnosis

First Author, Year	Sample size	Study method	AAN Class	NeuP Case-ascertainment method/instrument	Diagnosis/es	Overall prevalence/ incidence	Comments on case ascertainment
Choo, 1997	250 000	Automated medical records review, general population sample	II	Clinical diagnosis (recorded or likely)	Post-herpetic neuralgia	Incidence 0.003%(8.0% of HZV)	Screening: coded diagnosis of herpes zoster, coded receipt of possible neuralgia treatment. Diagnosis: full-text review of medical records by 2 reviewers: "sensory symptoms in the zoster dermatome more than 30 days after onset of HZV, for which no other cause more likely"
Davies, 2006	353	Postal survey and clinical assessment	I	One item from the Diabetic Neuropathy Symptom (DNS) score; Toronto Clinical Scoring System (TCSS)	Painful diabetic peripheral neuropathy	Prevalence 20.1% of those with Type 2 Diabetes (26.4% of those with Type 2 Diabetes responding positively to DNS score question and attending for assessment)	The four-item DNS score was validated for diagnosing distal diabetic polyneuropathy in clinical practice. TCSS score ≥6, based on 6 symptoms, 5 sensory tests, lower limb reflexes; validated against sural nerve morphology and electrophysiology.
Freynhagen, 2006	7772	Computer-administered survey of primary care attenders with chronic low back pain	II	painDETECT questionnaire	Low back pain with a predominantly neuropathic component	Population prevalence 14.5% of women, 11.4% of men (37.0% of those with chronic low back pain)	Score ≥19 on 9-item screening questionnaire, validated in pain clinic population (but not general population)

Study	N	Method	Diagnosis	Conditions	Incidence/Prevalence	Level	Comments
Hall, 2006	6 800 800	Computerized medical records review	Coded diagnosis of conditions in medical records (Read codes)	Post-herpetic neuralgia, Trigeminal neuralgia, Phantom limb pain, Painful diabetic neuropathy	Incidence per 100,000 person years: PHN 40.2, TN 26.8, PLP 1.5, PDN 15.3. Prevalence unknown	I	Case identification dependent on accurate diagnosis and coding by general practitioner. Prevalence could not be calculated by this method
Hall, 2008	2 900 000	Computerized database of primary care records	Coded diagnosis of conditions in medical records (Read codes)	Post-herpetic neuralgia, Trigeminal neuralgia, Phantom limb pain, Painful diabetic neuropathy	Age standardized incidence per 100,000 person years: PHN 27.3, TN 26.7, PLP 0.8, PDN 26.7. Prevalence unknown	I	As above. Similar to previous study in 2006 but using a different primary care database.
Helgason, 2000	421	Prospective cohort telephone interview study	Non-standard questions to individuals diagnosed with HZV	Post-herpetic neuralgia	Prevalence 7.2% three months after onset of HZV	II	"Discomfort" connected to the dermatome, ranked as none, mild, moderate or severe. Questions repeated at 1, 3, and 12, and follow-up lasted up to 7.6 years after HZV onset
Opstelten, 2002	837	Computerized medical records review	Coded and free text diagnosis of HZV and PHN	Postherpetic neuralgia	Prevalence 2.6% three months after onset of HZV	II	PHN defined as "any pain that persisted at least 1 month after HZ diagnosis"; recorded at 1 month and 3 months. Not clear how identified pain was related to HZV site. Accuracy depends on this, and on accuracy of recorded diagnoses.

First Author, Year	Sample size	Study method	AAN Class	NeuP Case-ascertainment method/instrument	Diagnosis/es	Overall prevalence/ incidence	Comments on case ascertainment
Category B – Original research, specific neuropathic pain diagnosis (continued)							
Sjaastad, 2004	1838	Interview survey	I	Standardized headache questions and clinical examination	Supra-orbital neuralgia	Prevalence 0.5%	Questions sought presence of characteristic headache, detailed clinical examination based on clinical experience only. Very good test-retest agreement.
Wu, 2007	1023	Computer-aided telephone survey	I	Portion of the Michigan Neuropathy Screening Instrument (MNSI), Brief Pain Inventory (BPI)	Pain associated with diabetic peripheral neuropathy (pDPN)	Prevalence 8%	Self-reported diabetes, survey sample, does not include participants with undiagnosed diabetes, bias towards elderly participants.Lack of validation for administering only a portion of the MNSI to estimate prevalence of DPN.
Yawn, 2007	1669	Database records from health care systems	I	Diagnostic or procedure code that might indicate a new case of HZ (ICD-8 codes 052.xx)	Postherpetic neuralgia	Incidence rate of 3.4 per 1000 person-years	Overall 10% of adults had PHN at 90 days Case identification dependent on accurate diagnosis and coding. Only included those who sought care within defined area. Prevalence could not be calculated.
Younes, 2005	4380	Interview survey (not clear whether face-to-face or telephone)	I	Standardized questionnaire and clinical examination	Disc-related sciatica (DRS)	Annual prevalence 2.2% Point prevalence 0.75%	DRS defined as "past or present history of pain in L5 or S1 distribution extending below the knee, with or without low back pain". Questionnaire developed for the study, validation not described. Examination not described.

		Reviews		
Research question	Review type Databases used Time period covered	Study inclusion/ exclusion criteria	Number/type of studies, Definitions of NeuP pain, Total sample number	Main findings
Sadosky, 2008 Summarize what is currently known regarding the incidence and/or prevalence of DPN, PHN and other less common neuropathic pain conditions	Literature review Medline No dates available	Inclusion:Population- based studies or large case series in instances where no population-based studies were identified. English language papers were the primary source although relevant studies were translated. Searched for epidemiology papers in combination with appropriate terms identifying the syndrome or condition	No concise information given on the number of papers/ studies included in review, or of sample size. Summary table of incidence and prevalence estimates (where available) includes data from general population and diagnostic groups samples. Difficult to identify the source of the original data.	GP denotes general population, D denotes disease specific popn **Incidence :** Painful PDN: 15.3/100,000 (D) PHN: 11-40/100,000 (GP) Trigeminal Neuralgia: 4.7-26.8/100,000 (GP) Glosspharyngeal neuralgia: 0.8/100,000 (GP) Cervical radiculopathy 83.2/100,00 (GP) Carpal tunnel syndrome: 105-276/100,000 (GP) **Prevalence:** Painful PDN: 11%-26% (D) PHN: 7-27% (D) HIV-associated polyneuropathy: 30-63% (D) Phantom limb pain: 53-85% (D) Carpal Tunnel syndrome: 2-16% (GP) Central post-stroke pain: 8-11% (D) MS Central NeuP pain: 23-58% (D) Spinal cord injury-assoc NeuP pain; 10-80% (D)

Reviews

Research question	Review type Databases used Time period covered	Study inclusion/ exclusion criteria	Number/type of studies, Definitions of NeuP pain, Total sample number	Main findings
Taylor, 2006 To identify studies investigating the occurrence (incidence and prevalence) of neuropathic pain, its natural history, and its health and economic burden	Review Medline (Pubmed) Up to February 2005	Searched terms were epidemiology OR incidence OR prevalence AND Neuropathic pain OR conditions (named)	12 studies of incidence and prevalence estimates: USA (6), UK (2), Sweden (2), Iceland (1), Spain (1). Design: 4 prospective database studies, 3 surveys, 5 not stated	**Incidence:** PHN: N/A DN: N/A Neuropathic back & leg pain: N/A CRPS I: 5.5/ 100,000 CRPS II: 0.8/100,000 **Prevalence:** PHN: 6.8–38.3/ 100,000 (Iceland), 185/100,000 (USA) DN: 54/ 100,000 (UK), 1140/ 100,000 (USA), 222/100,000 (USA) Note: **Diabetic neuropathy not necessarily pain** Neuropathic back & leg pain: 778/100,000 (USA, care sought for 3 months or more); 7,600/100,000 (pain intense, disabling & chronic), 5,800/100,000 (UK, disability pension), 6,500/100,000 (Spain) CRPS I: 20.6/ 100,000 (Sweden) CRPS II: 4.2/100,000 (Sweden), 48/100,000 (USA)

Abbreviations/Glossary

Screening tools

DN4 = Douleur Neuropathique en 4 questions

DNSS – Diabetic Neuropathy Symptom Score

LANSS= Leeds Assessment of Neuropathic Symptoms & Signs

S-LANSS = Self-complete Leeds Assessment of Neuropathic Symptoms & Signs

TCSS = Toronto Clinical Scoring System

MNSI = Michigan Neuropathy Screening Instrument

Neuropathic pain conditions

CRPS = Complex regional pain syndrome

DRS = Disc-related sciatica

HZV = Herpes Zoster Virus

PHN = Post-herpetic neuralgia

PLP = Phantom limb pain

PDN = Painful diabetic neuropathy

TN = Trigeminal neuralgia

Classification/coding

ICPC = The International Classification of Primary Care (ICPC) has been in use for 10 years. It classifies the broad range of symptoms and problems which make up the work of primary care. Codes can be mapped to the International Classification of Diseases (ICD) for comparison with other controlled vocabularies. ICPC lacks complexity and detail and differs substantially from Read Codes.

Read codes = Read Codes are a coded thesaurus of clinical terms which enable clinicians to make effective use of computer systems for use in General Practice. The codes include terms relating to observations (signs and symptoms), diagnosis, procedures and investigations which map to other coding systems including The International Classification of Diseases Ninth Revision (ICD-9) and the Classification of Surgical Operations & Procedures Fourth Revision (OPCS-4). Read coding covers all areas of clinical practice, including such areas as nursing, physiotherapy and health visiting.

ICD codes = The International Classification of Diseases provides the ground rules for coding and classifying cause-of-death data. Diseases listed on death certificates are assigned specific codes according to this system. The ICD is developed collaboratively between the World Health Organization (WHO) and 10 international centres. This system allows mortality (death) data to be collected and compared among different areas. Since the beginning of the century, the ICD has been modified about once every 10 years in order to stay abreast with advances in medical science. New revisions usually introduce major disruptions in time series of mortality statistics due to changes in classification and rules for selecting underlying cause of death.

Table 18.3 Comparison of items within five self-complete neuropathic pain screening tools *(shaded boxes highlight features shared by two or more tools)*. Reproduced from Bennett et al., 2007a. This table has been reproduced with permission of the International Association for the Study of Pain® (IASP®). The table may not be reproduced for any other purpose without permission.

	LANSS*	DN4*	NPQ	Pain *DETECT*	ID Pain
Symptoms					
Pricking, tingling, pins and needles	√	√	√	√	√
Electric shocks or shooting	√	√	√	√	√
Hot or burning	√	√	√	√	√
Numbness		√	√	√	√
Pain evoked by light touch	√		√	√	√
Painful cold or freezing pain	√	√			
Pain evoked by mild pressure				√	
Pain evoked by heat or cold				√	
Pain evoked by changes in weather			√		
Pain limited to joints**					√
Itching		√			
Temporal patterns				√	
Radiation of pain				√	
Autonomic changes	√				
Clinical examination items					
Brush allodynia	√	√			
Raised soft-touch threshold		√			
Raised pin-prick threshold	√	√			

LANSS = Leeds Assessment of Neuropathic Symptoms & Signs, DN4 = Douleur Neuropathique en 4 questions, NPQ = Neuropathic Pain Questionnaire

* Self-complete versions also available

** Used to identify non-neuropathic pain

(Yawn et al., 2007). This ranged from 5% in those <60 years of age, to 10% in those in the age range of 60–69 years, and to 20% in those in the age group ≥80 years (Yawn et al., 2007). For PDN, prevalence in included studies was reported between 8% and 20% (Davies et al., 2006; Wu et al., 2007) of those with Type 2 diabetes. In addition, for NeuP originating in the back, prevalence ranged from 2.2% (Younes et al., 2006) to 13%. (Freynhagen et al., 2006) of back-pain patients. Differences in study populations, data-collection methods, and whether or not a clinical examination was carried out may explain some of the variability in these population prevalences.

Case identification and ascertainment in individual studies

Five of these studies used interview surveys as the method of case ascertainment (Gustorff et al., 2008; Helgason et al., 2000; Younes et al., 2006; Wu et al., 2007; Sjaastad et al., 2005), although there were differences in the use of standardized instruments. Two of the interview surveys also included a clinical examination (Yoiunes et al., 2006; Sjaastad et al., 2005); one of these was to ascertain the presence of supra-orbital neuralgia and the other was for disc-related sciatica.

Six studies based their case identification and ascertainment on a review of computer-held primary care medical records, using diagnostic codes (Dieleman et al., 2008; Hall et al., 2006; Choo et al., 1997; Opstelten et al., 2002; Yawn et al., 2007; Hall et al., 2008), with two of these checking the validity of the diagnosis by examination of the full-text medical records (Dieleman et al., 2008; Choo et al., 1997). Medical record review in primary care allows relatively simple access to large general population samples. However, as noted above, the accuracy of case ascertainment is entirely dependent on three factors: accuracy of diagnosis by the attending physician (usually the primary care physician), the comprehensiveness of data entry, and the proportion of affected individuals attending a primary care consultation in the first place. In a clinical (rather than a research) setting, these are generally <100% complete.

Review papers

Two review papers that fulfilled the inclusion and exclusion criteria were identified (Sadosky et al., 2008; Taylor, 2006). Search strategies used in these reviews included, in addition to terms relating to epidemiology studies, criteria for specific medical conditions known to be associated with neuropathic pain. Therefore, there was some discrepancy between studies identified by these reviews and those identified in our review, compounded by differing inclusion and exclusion criteria (particularly the time period covered by the searches).

Sadosky et al. (2008) provided estimates of incidence for six neuropathic conditions (i.e. painful peripheral diabetic neuropathy, PHN, trigeminal neuralgia, glossopharyngeal neuralgia, cervical radiculopathy, and carpal tunnel syndrome), and prevalence for eight neuropathic conditions (i.e. painful peripheral diabetic neuropathy, PHN, human immunodeficiency virus (HIV)-associated polyneuropathy, carpal tunnel syndrome, central post-stroke pain, multiple sclerosis central NeuP, and spinal cord injury-associated pain). Although incidence rates for five of the conditions were applicable to the general population, prevalences for all but carpal tunnel syndrome were only found for disease-specific populations. The information relating the figures presented and the original sources was not always clear, and it is difficult to assess case-identification and -ascertainment methods used, and the validity of the estimates presented.

Taylor (2006) identified prevalence estimates for five conditions (i.e. PHN, diabetic neuropathy (although not necessarily painful), neuropathic back and leg pain, and complex regional pain syndrome (CRPS) types I and II) in five countries (Iceland, Spain, Sweden, the UK, and the USA). Incidence estimates were only identified for CRPS I and II. These studies used prospective databases or surveys to derive their estimates, but in five studies, case ascertainment was not clear. Information about case identification in the included studies was not presented.

In summary, the considerable variability in prevalence and incidence of NeuP conditions estimated by general population studies is likely to be due to differences in definitions of NeuP, methods of assessment, and patient selection. There is a need for the development and standardization of valid definitions and assessment for the purposes of general population research, in order that accurate estimates may be made. Good epidemiological studies using these will be informative in understanding the distribution of NeuP and risk factors for its development, and thus informing the development and targeting of treatment and prevention strategies and the resources required to apply these with maximum benefit.

Association with health-related quality of life

There is strong evidence that NeuP is associated with severely reduced functioning in all aspects of daily activities and life, and on every dimension of health-related quality of life (HRQL; Smith et al., 2007; Jensen et al., 2007; Schmader, 2002). The extent of this has been found to be greater than in other types of chronic pain (Smith et al., 2007). In the general population, individuals with NeuP report significant impairment of general health across all dimensions (i.e. physical, psychological, and social), with HRQL scores found to be as low as in patients with clinical depression, coronary artery disease, recent myocardial infarction, or poorly controlled diabetes (Smith et al., 2007). The evidence showing the negative effects of NeuP on HRQL suggests that psychosocial treatments geared towards improving these outcome domains may be helpful (in addition to pharmacological treatments). Such treatments can provide patients with a sense of control over their pain management (Jensen et al., 2007).

Public health implications

The prevalence of NeuP can be expected to increase in the future as the population ages. In addition to the association with age found in a several studies (Dieleman et al., 2008; Bouhassira et al., 2008; Torrance et al., 2006), a number of causes of NeuP are found to be more common in the elderly, including HZ and diabetes. Patients with chronic disease that are associated with NeuP – e.g. cancer, HIV, and diabetes – are also surviving longer due to improved medical care.

Population burden

Given the challenges of agreeing a case identification and with case ascertainment, as well as for very strong practical reasons, an accurate global estimate of the prevalence of NeuP is impossible. It can be seen, however, that in countries such as the UK and USA somewhere between 6% and 8% of the adult population are likely to have a painful neuropathic condition (Dieleman et al., 2008; Bouhassira et al., 2008; Torrance et al., 2006). Internationally, HIV-associated neuropathy may present a particularly prevalent challenge. According to estimates by the World Health Organization (WHO) and UNAIDS (http://www.who.int/hiv/data/en/index.html), 33.2 million people were living with HIV at the end of 2007. That same year, some 2.5 million people became newly infected, and 2.1 million died of AIDS, including 330 000 children. Two-thirds of those infected live in sub-Saharan Africa. It was estimated that 35% of individuals infected with HIV will also suffer from painful distal symmetrical polyneuropathy (Sadosky et al., 2008). The number of individuals with HIV-related NeuP may therefore be as high as 11 million worldwide, and increasing. In developed countries, one of the biggest sources of NeuP is likely to be associated with the high and increasing prevalence of diabetes. The WHO estimates that >180 million people worldwide have diabetes, and that this number is likely to more than double by 2030. In a diabetic population, prevalence estimates for PDN range from 11% to 26% (Sadosky et al., 2008), which translates to between 20 million and 47 million individuals.

Such global estimates are, however, imprecise, and are likely to suffer the same inaccuracies as the longstanding prevalence estimates described above (Bennett, 1997; Bowsher et al., 1991). More precise and detailed epidemiological work would be required to estimate a global burden of painful neuropathies arising from endemic conditions such as HIV and diabetes, and of the overall prevalence of NeuP. However, it is clear that NeuP is therefore increasingly common and debilitating in our community. This, and the resulting high impact on the health services, means that we should be looking at preventing NeuP, as well as improving its detection and management. This requires a good understanding of risk factors for its development, and identification of those that are modifiable.

Risk factors for neuropathic pain and possible preventive measures

General risk factors

Ideally, information on risk should come from prospective cohort studies collecting detailed information on potential risk factors and outcomes (e.g. decreasing or increasing pain, resolution). There are few such studies specific to NeuP in the general population available to review, and such information as we have tends to come from cross-sectional studies, from which it is impossible to determine causation.

There are several common risk factors for NeuP or pain with neuropathic characteristics. Demographic risk factors include gender and age: NeuP is found to be significantly associated with female gender and age >60 years (Dieleman et al., 2008; Bouhassira et al., 2008; Torrance et al., 2006). Employment is also a risk factor: one study found pain with neuropathic features to be twice as prevalent in manual workers or farmers as in managers (Bouhassira et al., 2008), whilst another found significant associations with being unable to work and with having lower educational attainment (Torrance et al., 2006). Location of residence and type of housing were significantly associated with NeuP, with greater prevalence in rural areas than in large urban communities in one study (Bouhassira et al., 2008) and in those living in council-rented accommodation compared with other types of housing in another (Torrance et al., 2006). These suggest that relative deprivation may be a risk factor for NeuP, though more specific information is required.

These associations are not modifiable, or at least not by conventional medical interventions, and are therefore of limited clinical value. The association, described above, between NeuP and poor general health, suggests that managing an individual's health holistically may result in primary, secondary, or tertiary prevention of NeuP. This intuitive approach, however, needs specific testing.

Specific neuropathic conditions

Data on risk factors for specific NeuP conditions is limited although there is some information related to the most common NeuP conditions: PDN, PHN, and post-surgical pain (Dieleman et al., 2008).

Painful diabetic neuropathy (PDN)

The most important PDN is pain associated with chronic sensorimotor polyneuropathy. PDN is estimated to affect between 16% and 26% of the diabetic population (Jensen et al., 2006; Ziegler, 2008). Well-established risk factors for vascular disease in patients with diabetes are also associated with an increased risk of neuropathy; smoking, glycosylated haemoglobin (HbA_{1C}), diabetes duration, and components of the metabolic syndrome (including hypertension, obesity, triglycerides, and cholesterol) were all associated with increased risk of polyneuropathy (Jensen et al., 2006; Tesfaye et al., 2005). In addition, female gender appears to be an independent risk factor for the development of painful neuropathy.

There is some evidence to suggest that neuropathy is associated with impaired glucose tolerance: hyperglycaemia-induced pathways result in nerve dysfunction and damage, which lead to hyper-excitable peripheral and central pathways of pain. In addition to established treatment options (see section on treatment challenges), there is evidence that α-lipoic acid, an antioxidant which prevents experimental diabetic neuropathy, is effective in reducing the chief symptoms of diabetic polyneuropathy, including pain, paraesthesia, and numbness, in randomized trials (Jensen et al., 2006).

Risk factors for PDN (rather than for diabetic neuropathy) have not been extensively studied and the natural course of PDN is variable, with some patients experiencing spontaneous improvement and resolution of pain (Veves et al., 2008). Diabetes screening and early evaluation of nerve function and appropriate intervention may nonetheless be of significant clinical benefit in the primary, secondary, and tertiary prevention of PDN (Veves et al., 2008). Furthermore, long-term management and prevention in patients with PDN should include lifestyle advice and monitoring, glycaemic control, and pharmacological therapy for pain relief.

Of course, the best way of preventing PDN is to prevent diabetes, onset of which is strongly associated with factors such as diet and lifestyle. This would have public health benefits much wider than a reduction in NeuP, but its detailed consideration is beyond the scope of this chapter.

Post-herpetic neuralgia (PHN)

Herpes zoster, or shingles, is characterized by a localized generally painful vesicular rash that is typically unilateral and does not cross the mid-line, and is usually limited to one or two adjacent dermatomes (Harpaz et al., 2008). HZ results from the reactivation of latent Varicella zoster virus (VZV) within the sensory ganglia (Volpi et al., 2008). One of the most frequent complications is PHN, a NeuP syndrome that persists or develops after the rash has healed. Prevalence estimates range from 8% to 19% of those with HZ, when defined as pain at 1 month after rash onset; and 8% when defined as pain at 3 months after rash onset (Schmader, 2002). The most important risk factor for developing HZ and PHN is increasing age. Other known risk factors for PHN include immunocompromise, female gender, the presence of a painful prodrome preceding the rash, greater acute pain intensity, and greater rash severity (Jung et al., 2004). Therefore, for PHN prevention, it is important to treat the acute symptoms of shingles, including pain, aggressively.

Prompt treatment with oral antiviral agents acyclovir, valvacyclovir, and famciclovir decreases the severity and duration of acute pain from zoster (Harpaz et al., 2008), seemingly by attenuating nerve damage (Jung et al., 2004). However, antiviral therapy has been found to have only a limited effect on PHN treatment or prevention (Oxman et al., 2005; Dworkin et al., 2008). The administration of a VZV or 'zoster vaccine' is aimed at boosting cell-mediated immunity to VZV and thus providing protection against HZ and PHN. This zoster vaccine has been shown to reduce the incidence of both HZ and PHN in older adults in a large randomized controlled trial (Oxman et al., 2005). In this study, the administration of the zoster virus reduced the incidence of HZ by 51% and reduced the incidence of PHN by 66%. Recommendations have been made for this vaccine to be made available to all adults >60 years (Harpaz et al., 2008), although it remains uncertain whether this will become public health policy

Chronic post-surgical pain (CPSP)

Considered in detail in chapter 19, the development of chronic pain after surgery is fairly common, with prevalence estimates ranging from 10–50% after many common operations (Shipton, 2008). In 2–10% of these patients, this pain is severe, with many of the clinical features closely resembling NeuP (Jung et al., 2003; Mikkelsen et al., 2004; Kehlet et al., 2006). It has been suggested that this iatrogenic NeuP is probably the most important cause of post-surgical pain, and damage to nerves during surgery is probably a prerequisite for the development of CPSP (Kehlet et al., 2006). Pain before surgery and the intensity of acute postoperative pain are also risk factors; therefore there may be opportunities for prevention around the time of surgery, with good treatment of acute pain and attention to surgical technique.

Central nervous system plasticity that occurs in response to tissue injury may contribute to the development of CPSP. Studies have been conducted using methods to prevent central neuroplastic changes from occurring through the use of pre-emptive or preventive analgesic techniques (Liu and Wu, 2007). These might suggest that effective preventive analgesic techniques may be useful in reducing not only acute pain but also CPSP and resultant disability. Kehlet et al (2006), however, suggests that suppressing the symptom of pain at the time of surgery is probably inadequate to prevent CPSP, and treatment needs to be targeted at the mechanisms of progression, not just the disturbances in sensations that they produce. This would involve neuroprotective treatment incorporating a combination of therapies, directed at both the injured nerve and at the neuroplastic changes subsequently induced in the central nervous system.

Other risk factors for CPSP include female gender and psychosocial factors (such as catastrophizing, perceived social support, and preoperative anxiety) that offer opportunities for trials of preventive intervention (Shipton, 2008; Kehlet et al., 2006). Increasing age at time of surgery seems to reduce the risk of chronic pain (Macrae, 2008). Genetic susceptibility has also been suggested as a risk factor for CPSP.

Future research directions

There is a clear need for standardization and validation of feasible and acceptable questionnaire and clinical assessment methods of case identification in NeuP diagnosis for research purposes, as these either do not exist or are not being used. In addition, further research is required to validate the testing of questionnaire screening instruments in general population samples, including derivation of estimates for positive and negative predictive values of a positive score.

This information should form the basis of more detailed population studies of NeuP prevalence, to inform resource and education requirements. In addition to this research aimed at understanding the distribution of NeuP in the community, clear information on risk factors is required, from prospective longitudinal population studies. These will identify factors associated with its development, and the design of targeted prevention and treatment strategies. However, a broader public health approach to prevention of chronic pain will benefit NeuP sufferers since many risk factors for chronic NeuP are similar to those for other chronic pain conditions

NeuP remains relatively poorly treated, often because of difficulty in its assessment, and because of the challenges associated with successful management, described above. Research is therefore required into methods for wider implementation of effective treatments, and the design of new drug and non-drug treatments. Recent and emerging research into the biological and psychological mechanisms of NeuP should inform these new treatments.

Meanwhile, we need to develop means of increasing the awareness and assessment of NeuP in primary care, and to assess the impact of this in treating and preventing NeuP. Professional education for primary care staff including GPs and other community health care professionals, such as nurses, physiotherapists, and chiropodists, all of whom are likely to encounter patients with common medical conditions (e.g. diabetes and HZ) associated with developing NeuP. Public education may also be effective in reducing NeuP and its impact, e.g. by closer attention to diabetic control.

With the results of this work, trials of early identification and intervention could also be important to determine whether the rapidity and effectiveness of reducing pain severity with appropriate treatment is a factor in long-term prognosis. However, successful management of NeuP at the individual and community level requires, first and foremost, widespread recognition of the condition as it presents to the physician and as an important public health problem. Both of these need to begin with agreement on how to diagnose and assess NeuP, and this is therefore the most important current area of research.

Appendix 1 Search Strategy

Database: Ovid MEDLINE(R) <1996 to April Week 4 2008>
  Search Strategy:

1 central pain.ti,ab. (412)

2 myelopath$.ti,ab. (3345)

3 exp Neuralgia/or exp Trigeminal Neuralgia/ or exp Facial Neuralgia/ or exp Neuralgia, Postherpetic/ (4826)

4 neurogenic pain.ti,ab. (132)

5 neuropathic pain.ti,ab. (4196)

6 peripheral nerve injur$.ti,ab. (1277)

7 peripheral neuropath$.ti,ab. (4982)

8 peripheral sensory neuropath$.ti,ab. (128)

9 polyneuropath$.ti,ab. (3951)

10 polyneuropathies/ or alcoholic neuropathy/ or "hereditary motor and sensory neuropathies"/ or "hereditary sensory and autonomic neuropathies"/ or polyradiculoneuropathy/ (2753)

11 or/1-10 (21970)

12 exp Pain/ (108996)

13 exp Incidence/ (83006)

14 exp Prevalence/ (86068)

15 exp Epidemiology/ (6644)

16 13 or 14 or 15 (167176)

17 11 and 12 and 16 (161)

18 limit 17 to yr="1997 - 2008" (157)

19 limit 18 to humans (155

Appendix 2

American Academy of Neurology evidence classification scheme for determining the yield of established diagnostic and screening tests (Boreau et al., 1990)

  Class I. A statistical, population-based sample of patients studied at a uniform point in time (usually early) during the course of the condition. All patients undergo the intervention of interest. The outcome, if not objective, is determined in an evaluation that is masked to the patients' clinical presentations.

  Class II. A statistical, non-referral-clinic-based sample of patients studied at uniform point in time (usually early) during the course of the condition. Most (>80%) patients undergo the intervention of interest. The outcome, if not objective, is determined in an evaluation that is masked to the patients' clinical presentations.

  Class III. A selected, referral-clinic-based sample of patients studied during the course of the condition. Some patients undergo the intervention of interest. The outcome, if not objective, is determined in an evaluation by someone other than the treating physician.

  Class IV. Expert opinion, case reports, or any study not meeting criteria for classes I–III.

References

Attal, N. and Bouhassira, D. 2004: Can pain be more or less neuropathic? *Pain* **110**, 510–11.

Bennett, G.J. 1997: Neuropathic pain: an overview. In: Borsook D, editor. *Molecular Biology of Pain Seattle, WA: IASP Press* pp. 109–13.

Bennett, M. 2001: The LANSS Pain Scale: the Leeds assessment of neuropathic symptoms and signs. *Pain* **92**, 147–57.

Bennett, M.I., Attal, N., Backonja, M.M., Baron, R., Bouhassira, D., Freynhagen, R., et al. 2007: Using screening tools to identify neuropathic pain. *Pain* **127**, 199–203.

Bennett, M.I. and Bouhassira, D. 2007: Epidemiology of neuropathic pain: can we use the screening tools? *Pain* **132**, 12–13.

Bennett, M.I., Smith, B.H., Torrance, N. and Lee, A.J. 2006: Can pain be more or less neuropathic? Comparison of symptom assessment tools with ratings of certainty by clinicians. *Pain* **122**, 289–94.

Bennett, M.I., Smith, B.H., Torrance, N. and Potter, J. 2005: The S-LANSS score for identifying pain of predominantly neuropathic origin: validation for use in clinical and postal research. *Journal of Pain* **6**, 149–58.

Boureau, F., Doubrere, J.F. and Luu, M. 1990: Study of verbal description in neuropathic pain. *Pain* **42**, 145–52.

Bouhassira, D., Attal, N., Alchaar, H., Boureau, F., Brochet, B., Bruxelle, J., et al. 2005: Comparison of pain syndromes associated with nervous or somatic lesions and development of a new neuropathic pain diagnostic questionnaire (DN4). *Pain* **114**, 29–36.

Bouhassira, D., Lanteri-Minet, M., Attal, N., Laurent, B. and Touboul, C. 2008: Prevalence of chronic pain with neuropathic characteristics in the general population. *Pain* **136**, 380–7.

Bowsher, D., Rigge, M. and Sopp, L. 1991: Prevalence of chronic pain in the British population: a telephone survey of 1037 households. *The Pain Clinic* **4**, 223–30.

Choo, P.W., Galil, K., Donahue, J.G., Walker, A.M., Spiegelman, D. and Platt, R. 1997: Risk factors for postherpetic neuralgia. *Arch Intern Med* **157**, 1217–24.

Cruccu, G., Anand, P., Attal, N., Garcia-Larrea, L., Haanpaa, M., Jorum, E., et al. 2004: EFNS guidelines on neuropathic pain assessment. *Eur J Neurol* **11**, 153–62.

Daniel, H.C., Narewska, J., Serpell, M., Hoggart, B., Johnson, R. and Rice, A.S.C. 2008: Comparison of psychological and physical function in neuropathic pain and nociceptive pain: Implications for cognitive behavioral pain management programs. *Euro J Pain 8*, 12(6), 731–41.

Davies, M., Brophy, S., Williams, R. and Taylor, A. 2006: The prevalence, severity, and impact of painful diabetic peripheral neuropathy in type 2 diabetes. *Diabetes Care* **29**, 1518–22.

Dieleman, J.P., Kerklaan, J., Huygen, F.J., Bouma, P.A. and Sturkenboom, M.C. 2008: Incidence rates and treatment of neuropathic pain conditions in the general population. *Pain* **137**, 681–8.

Dworkin, R.H. 2002: An overview of neuropathic pain: syndromes, symptoms, signs, and several mechanisms. *Clin J Pain* **18**, 343–9.

Dworkin, R.H., Backonja, M., Rowbotham, M.C., Allen, R.R., Argoff, C.R., Bennett, G.J., et al. 2003: Advances in neuropathic pain: diagnosis, mechanisms, and treatment recommendations. *Arch Neurology* **60**, 1524–34.

Dworkin, R.H., Gnann, J.W.,Jr, Oaklander, A.L., Raja, S.N., Schmader, K.E. and Whitley, R.J. 2008: Diagnosis and assessment of pain associated with herpes zoster and postherpetic neuralgia. *J Pain* **9**, S37–44.

Edlund, W., Gronseth, G., So, Y. and Franklin, G. 2004: for the Quality Standard Subcommittee (QSS) and the Therapeutics and Technology Assessment Subcommittee. *Clinical Practice Guideline Process Manual.*

Finnerup, N.B., Otto, M., Jensen, T.S. and Sindrup, S.H. 2007: An evidence-based algorithm for the treatment of neuropathic pain. *MedGenMed* **9**, 36.

Freynhagen, R., Baron, R., Gockel, U. and Tolle, T.R. 2006: painDETECT: a new screening questionnaire to identify neuropathic components in patients with back pain. *Curr Med Res Opin* **22**, 1911–20.

Galer, B.S. and Jensen, M.P. 1997: Development and preliminary validation of a pain measure specific to neuropathic pain: the Neuropathic Pain Scale. *Neurology* **48**, 332–8.

Galer, B.S., Jensen, M.P., Ma, T., Davies, P.S. and Rowbotham, M.C. 2002: The lidocaine patch 5% effectively treats all neuropathic pain qualities: results of a randomized, double-blind, vehicle-controlled, 3-week efficacy study with use of the neuropathic pain scale. *Clin J Pain* **18**, 297–301.

Gustorff, B., Dorner, T., Likar, R., Grisold, W., Lawrence, K., Schwarz, F., et al. 2008: Prevalence of self-reported neuropathic pain and impact on quality of life: a prospective representative survey. *Acta Anaesthesiol Scand* **52**, 132–6.

Hall, G.C., Carroll, D. and McQuay, H.J. 2008: Primary care incidence and treatment of four neuropathic pain conditions: a descriptive study, 2002-2005. *BMC Fam Pract* **9**, 26.

Hall, G.C., Carroll, D., Parry, D. and McQuay, H.J. 2006: Epidemiology and treatment of neuropathic pain: the UK primary care perspective. *Pain* **122**, 156–62.

Hansson, P. 2002: Neuropathic pain: clinical characteristics and diagnostic workup. *Euro J Pain* **6**(Supplement 1), 47–50.

Harpaz, R., Ortega-Sanchez, I.R. and Seward, J.F. 2008: Advisory Committee on Immunization Practices (ACIP) Centers for Disease Control and Prevention (CDC). Prevention of herpes zoster: recommendations of the Advisory Committee on Immunization Practices (ACIP). *MMWR Recomm Rep* **57**(RR-5), 1, 30.

Helgason, S., Petursson, G., Gudmundsson, S. and Sigurdsson, J.A. 2000: Prevalence of postherpetic neuralgia after a first episode of herpes zoster: prospective study with long term follow up. *BMJ* **321**, 794–6.

Jensen, M.P., Chodroff, M.J. and Dworkin, R.H. 2007: The impact of neuropathic pain on health-related quality of life: review and implications. *Neurology* **68**, 1178–82.

Jensen, T.S., Backonja, M.M., Hernandez Jimenez, S., Tesfaye, S., Valensi, P. and Ziegler, D. 2006: New perspectives on the management of diabetic peripheral neuropathic pain. *Diabetes & Vascular Dis Res* **3**, 108–19.

Jung, B.F., Ahrendt, G.M., Oaklander, A.L. and Dworkin, R.H. 2003: Neuropathic pain following breast cancer surgery: proposed classification and research update. *Pain* **104**, 1–13.

Jung, B.F., Johnson, R.W., Griffin, D.R. and Dworkin, R.H. 2004: Risk factors for postherpetic neuralgia in patients with herpes zoster. *Neurology* **62**, 1545–51.

Kehlet, H., Jensen, T.S. and Woolf, C.J. 2006: Persistent postsurgical pain: risk factors and prevention. *Lancet* **367**, 1618–25.

Krause, S.J. and Backonja, M.M. 2003: Development of a neuropathic pain questionnaire. *Clin J Pain* **19**, 306–14.

Liu, S.S. and Wu, C.L. 2007: The effect of analgesic technique on postoperative patient-reported outcomes including analgesia: a systematic review. *Anesth Analg* **105**, 789–808.

Loeser, J.D. and Treede, R.D. 2008: The Kyoto protocol of IASP Basic Pain Terminology. *Pain* **137**, 473–7.

Macrae, W.A. 2008: Chronic post-surgical pain: 10 years on. *Br J Anaesth* **101**, 77–86.

Merskey, H. and Bogduk, N. 1994: *Classification of chronic pain: descriptions of chronic pain syndromes and definitions of pain terms.* 2nd edn. Seattle: IASP Press.

Mikkelsen, T., Werner, M.U., Lassen, B. and Kehlet, H. 2004: Pain and sensory dysfunction 6 to 12 months after inguinal herniotomy. *Anesth Analg* **99**, 146–51.

O'Connor, A.B., Schwid, S.R., Herrmann, D.N., Markman, J.D. and Dworkin, R.H. 2008: Pain associated with multiple sclerosis: systematic review and proposed classification. *Pain* **137**, 96–111.

Opstelten, W., Mauritz, J.W., de Wit, N.J., van Wijck, A.J., Stalman, W.A. and van Essen, G.A. 2002: Herpes zoster and postherpetic neuralgia: incidence and risk indicators using a general practice research database. *Fam Pract* **19**, 471–5.

Oxman, M.N., Levin, M.J., Johnson, G.R., Schmader, K.E., Straus, S.E., Gelb, L.D., et al. 2005: A vaccine to prevent herpes zoster and postherpetic neuralgia in older adults. *N Engl J Med* **352**, 2271–84.

Portenoy, R. 2006: Development and testing of a neuropathic pain screening questionnaire: ID Pain. *Curr Med Res Opin* **22**, 1555–65.

Rasmussen, P.V., Sindrup, S.H., Jensen, T.S. and Bach, F.W. 2004: Symptoms and signs in patients with suspected neuropathic pain. *Pain* **110**, 461–9.

Rice, A.S. and Hill, R.G. 2006: New treatments for neuropathic pain. *Annu Rev Med* **57**, 535–51.

Saarto, T. and Wiffen, P.J. 2005: Antidepressants for neuropathic pain. *Cochrane Database Syst Rev* **20**;(3) (3):CD005454.

Sadosky, A., McDermott, A.M., Brandenburg, N.A. and Strauss, M. 2008: A review of the epidemiology of painful diabetic peripheral neuropathy, postherpetic neuralgia, and less commonly studied neuropathic pain conditions. *Pain Practice* **8**, 45–56.

Schmader, K.E. 2002: Epidemiology and impact on quality of life of postherpetic neuralgia and painful diabetic neuropathy. *Clin J Pain* **18**, 350–4.

Shipton, E. 2008: Post-surgical neuropathic pain. *ANZ J Surg* **78**, 548–55.

Sjaastad, O., Petersen, H.C. and Bakketeig, L.S. 2005: Supraorbital neuralgia. Vaga study of headache epidemiology. *Cephalalgia* **25**, 296–304.

Smith, B.H. and Torrance, N. 2006: Epidemiology. In: Bennett MI, ed. *Neuropathic Pain*. Oxford: Oxford University Press. pp. 17–23.

Smith, B.H., Torrance, N., Bennett, M.I. and Lee, A.J. 2007: Health and quality of life associated with chronic pain of predominantly neuropathic origin in the community. *Clin J Pain* **23**, 143–9.

Taylor, R.S. 2006: Epidemiology of refractory neuropathic pain. *Pain Practice* **6**, 22–6.

Tesfaye, S., Chaturvedi, N., Eaton, S.E., Ward, J.D., Manes, C., Ionescu-Tirgoviste, C., et al. 2005: Vascular risk factors and diabetic neuropathy. *N Engl J Med* **352**, 341–50.

Torrance, N., Smith, B.H., Bennett, M.I. and Lee, A.J. 2006: The epidemiology of chronic pain of predominantly neuropathic origin. Results from a general population survey. *J Pain* **7**, 281–9.

Torrance, N., Smith, B.H., Watson, M.C. and Bennett, M.I. 2007: Medication and treatment use in primary care patients with chronic pain of predominantly neuropathic origin. *Fam Pract* **24**, 481–5.

Treede, R.D., Jensen, T.S., Campbell, J.N., Cruccu, G., Dostrovsky, J.O., Griffin, J.W., et al. 2008: Neuropathic pain: redefinition and a grading system for clinical and research purposes. *Neurology* **70**, 1630–5.

Veves, A., Backonja, M. and Malik, R.A. 2008: Painful diabetic neuropathy: epidemiology, natural history, early diagnosis, and treatment options. *Pain Med* **9**, 660–74.

Volpi, A., Gatti, A., Pica, F., Bellino, S., Marsella, L.T. and Sabato, A.F. 2008: Clinical and psychosocial correlates of post-herpetic neuralgia. *J Med Virol* **80**, 1646–52.

Wiffen, P., Collins, S., McQuay, H., Carroll, D., Jadad, A. and Moore, A. 2005: Anticonvulsant drugs for acute and chronic pain. *Cochrane Database Syst Rev* Jul **20**;(3)(3):CD001133.

Wu, E.Q., Borton, J., Said, G., Le, T.K., Monz, B., Rosilio, M., et al. 2007: Estimated prevalence of peripheral neuropathy and associated pain in adults with diabetes in France. *Current Medical Research & Opinion* **23**, 2035–42.

Yawn, B.P., Saddier, P., Wollan, P.C., St Sauver, J.L., Kurland, M.J. and Sy, L.S. 2007: A population-based study of the incidence and complication rates of herpes zoster before zoster vaccine introduction. *Mayo Clin Proc* **82**, 1341–9.

Younes, M., Bejia, I., Aguir, Z., Letaief, M., Hassen-Zrour, S., Touzi, M., et al. 2006: Prevalence and risk factors of disk-related sciatica in an urban population in Tunisia. *Joint, Bone, Spine: Revue Du Rhumatisme* **73**, 538–42.

Ziegler, D. 2008: Painful diabetic neuropathy: treatment and future aspects. *Diabetes Metab Res Rev* **24** Suppl 1, S52–7.

Chapter 19

Post-surgical pain

Julie Bruce

Introduction

Until the early 1980s, persistent postoperative pain was considered a rare adverse surgical event, with only the occasional case study or case series appearing in the anaesthesia literature. Chronic post-surgical pain (CPSP) was largely underreported and there was little mention of this iatrogenic event in surgical textbooks or journals. Over the last 30 years or so, the huge increase in literature, particularly epidemiological studies reporting prevalence and risk factors for CPSP, has improved both clinical and patient awareness of this postoperative condition. Up to one-third of patients undergoing common surgical procedures report persistent or intermittent pain of varying severity at 1 year postoperatively (Kehlet et al., 2006). CPSP is mostly, but not entirely, neuropathic in character, with loss of sensory function and hypersensitivity often initiated by innocuous stimuli (Gottrup et al., 2000). Patients experience burning, shooting, or stabbing pains, often paroxysmal and of varying intensity and duration. Chronic pain is difficult and costly to treat, with wider costs associated with increased health service use, reduced quality of life, and economic productivity. The burden of disease from CPSP is potentially enormous if we consider the volume of surgical procedures performed annually. The aim of this textbook is to consider pain from a wider public health perspective, thus focusing on the impact and consequent disability caused by chronic pain in the population. This chapter provides a short overview of chronic pain associated with surgery and presents findings from epidemiological studies, mostly using examples from hernia, breast, and thoracic surgery. Persistent pain has been reported after many other procedures, including thoracic, abdominal, gynaecological, orthopaedic, and amputation surgery. Finally, this chapter concentrates on the epidemiology of CPSP, and thus focuses on aetiological factors and population burden rather than clinical interventions evaluating the efficacy of treatment or management of intractable pain.

Defining chronic pain after surgery

As with all clinical conditions, prevalence estimates vary depending upon the case definition used, sampling method, and timing of postoperative assessment. There is no standardized definition for chronic pain after surgery; most epidemiological studies use the International Association for the Study of Pain (IASP) definition for chronic pain: 'pain which persists past the normal time of healing'. The IASP Subcommittee on Taxonomy recommend that for non-malignant pain, 'three months is the most convenient point of division between acute and chronic pain, but for research purposes six months will often be preferred'. In addition, IASP published two surgery-specific pain definitions: [a] post-mastectomy pain syndrome, 'chronic pain immediately or soon after mastectomy or removal of lump, affecting the anterior thorax, axilla, and/or medial arm'; and [b] post-thoracotomy pain, defined as 'an aching or burning pain that persists or recurs along a thoracotomy scar at least two months following the surgical procedure'. Macrae and

Davies (1999) were the first to propose that specific criteria should be satisfied in order for chronic pain to be defined as post-surgical:

(1) The pain must develop after a surgical procedure;
(2) The pain is of at least two months duration;
(3) Other causes for the pain have been excluded;
(4) The possibility that the pain is from a pre-existing condition has been excluded. There is an obvious grey area here in that surgery may simply exacerbate a pre-existent condition, but attributing escalating pain to the surgery is clearly not possible as natural deterioration cannot be ruled out.

The first two criteria are straightforward, although pain duration of 2 months is shorter than the IASP recommendation. These definitions assume a constant pain experience, whereby acute postoperative pain continues on for several weeks or months to eventually become chronic. However, empirical studies show that a proportion of patients are pain free or have mild pain in the acute postoperative period, with new-onset pain and/or altered sensations developing after several weeks or months (Smith et al., 1999; Poobalan et al., 2003). The two latter criteria proposed by Macrae and Davies are the more challenging, particularly when using survey methods of large populations to determine whether or not pain is attributable to preceding surgery. Assurance that other causes for the pain have been excluded cannot be completely satisfied and there is some margin for error during case-ascertainment. Excluding pre-existing conditions and disentangling indeterminate pains can be difficult, particularly if pain was present preoperatively, e.g. prolapsed painful hernia or angina. Chronic post-sternotomy pain, for example, usually localized over the incision area or diffuse over the chest wall, has been described as a burning, stabbing, or sharp pain, and can be easier to differentiate from anginal pain as it is often non-radiating, unrelated to exercise, and can be affected by posture (Conacher et al., 1993; Bruce et al., 2004). Patients report pain or altered sensations in the area supplied by damaged nerves or sensitive areas around the incision site, exacerbated by touch, clothing, or other benign stimuli, indicative of hyperalgesia and allodynia (Smith et al., 1999; Poobalan et al., 2003; Conacher et al., 1993; Bruce et al., 2004). Pain distribution is likely to follow nerve pathways, e.g. after inguinal hernia repair, altered sensations can be experienced in the groin, testicles, and down the front or inner thigh (Poobalan et al., 2003). Despite some limitations, the additional criteria for CPSP are specific to surgery and provide a more useful working definition than the generic IASP definition for chronic pain.

Prevalence

Numerous primary studies and secondary reviews have reported on CPSP prevalence. Estimates from epidemiological studies vary widely but overall, between 10% and 30% of surgical patients will report some degree of persistent pain at 1 year postoperatively, with higher rates (>40%) observed after major thoracic surgery (Steegers et al., 2008; Macrae and Bruce, 2008; Macrae, 2008). A smaller proportion, up to 5% of all surgical patients, reports severe, disabling pain at 1 year (Alfieri et al., 2006; Poobalan et al., 2001). In general, estimates of CPSP prevalence are derived from postoperative cross-sectional studies, prospective surgical cohorts, and clinical trials. One UK study considered frequency and cause of pain from the secondary care perspective: a survey of 5000 patients attending outpatient pain clinics revealed that 22% of patients attributed surgery as the main or major contributory cause of their chronic pain (Crombie et al., 1998).

Two systematic reviews summarized the frequency of CPSP after inguinal herniorrhaphy: the first included data from 40 epidemiological studies and randomized controlled trials, concluding that moderate-to-severe chronic pain occurred in 10% of patients at 1 year (Poobalan et al., 2003). Meta-analysis was not possible due to heterogeneity and poor quality of reporting in the primary studies. An updated review included an additional 35 publications published over 2 years, with inclusion criteria restricted to studies with sample sizes >100 patients and follow-up at or beyond 6 months (Aasvang and Kehlet, 2005). The authors concluded that 12% of patients will suffer CPSP and 6% persistent testicular pain after inguinal herniorrhaphy. These systematic reviews of post-herniorrhaphy pain highlight the recent increase in published literature and recognition of CPSP and other adverse surgical complications. In addition to persistent groin pain, a national registry-based Norwegian study found that 7% of males suffered from moderate-to-severe pain during sexual activity after hernia repair (Aasvang et al., 2006). Dysejaculation and sexual dysfunction was a clinically significant problem in 3% of younger men. Few patients had sought help from their physician, but 9% of those surveyed wanted to speak to a psychologist or physician about these problems when asked.

A review of chronic pain after breast cancer surgery reported prevalence estimates ranging from 13% to 69%, although not all of the primary studies included within this systematic review assessed patients beyond 6 months postoperatively (Jung et al., 2003). These authors proposed a classification system for different pain syndromes after breast cancer surgery: phantom breast pain; intercostobrachial neuralgia; neuroma and scar pain; and pain from other nerve injury. Although potentially useful for research purposes, this classification fails to account for variation or potential misclassification within the study samples, given that primary studies mostly used postal methodology rather than detailed clinical assessment. Kudel and colleagues (Kudel et al., 2007) found that women reporting multiple pains after breast surgery (e.g. phantom breast pain, scar pain, or 'other pain as a result of mastectomy') were more likely to have a greater degree of disability and distress, suggesting an additive negative impact from concurrent postoperative pain syndromes.

Most studies of pain after breast surgery focus on patients undergoing mastectomy or breast-conservation surgery, with or without axillary sampling/biopsy. In an early study, Wallace et al. (1996) assessed women 1–5 years after mastectomy with or without breast reconstruction and also included women having cosmetic breast augmentation. Rates of CPSP were higher after mastectomy with reconstruction (49%) and breast augmentation (38%) compared with women having mastectomy (31%). The term 'post-mastectomy pain' syndrome encompasses a range of pain and altered sensations in the chest, arm, axilla, and shoulder region (Kudel et al., 2007; Baron et al., 2007; Macdonald et al., 2005). Common descriptors reported by women include stabbing pain, tenderness, tightness, pulling/dragging sensations, and numbness (Smith et al., 1999; Baron et al., 2007; Macdonald et al., 2005). Despite changes in surgical practice whereby radical mastectomy has mostly been replaced with less invasive breast-conservation surgery (e.g. wide local excision/lumpectomy) plus axillary surgery and adjuvant treatment, rates of CPSP and other postoperative symptoms remain remarkably high. A study of 187 women, having either sentinel lymph node biopsy (SNLB) or axillary lymph node dissection (ALND), found that 22% and 55%, respectively, had postoperative numbness at 5 years after surgery (Baron et al., 2007). A follow-up study of women with post-mastectomy pain at 3 years postoperatively found that half continued to suffer from persistent or intermittent pain and arm morbidity for up to 12 years after surgery (Macdonald et al., 2005). This was the first study to investigate long-term prognosis and changes in pain and quality of life over time.

Mechanisms for development

Persistent postoperative pain is predominantly, but not always, neuropathic in character as a consequence of intra-operative nerve damage (Kehlet et al., 2006; Gottrup et al., 2000). Patients are broadly subjected to a similar surgical insult but mechanisms and processes contributing to pain onset may vary, e.g. nociceptive or neuropathic pain from peripheral or central lesions, neuralgia from nerve entrapment, and ongoing inflammatory processes rather than neuropathic injury, all of which may be mediated by variation in underlying individual susceptibility. It is entirely plausible that duration of surgery, associated with persistent surgical nociception and sustained peripheral injury, could trigger changes in the central nervous system. Yet there is relatively little data to support the theory that the more severe the surgical insult or tissue damage, the greater the risk of persistent pain (Caumo et al., 2002). Rates of severe acute postoperative pain and chronic pain are higher after major thoracic surgery but can also occur after minimally invasive surgery, including laparoscopic procedures and vasectomy (Macrae, 2008; Granet et al., 2004; Manikandan et al., 2004). However, in a heterogeneous sample of patients having minor, intermediate, and major surgery, Peters and colleagues (2007) found that surgery lasting >3 h predicted increased pain, poor functional outcome, and poor global recovery at 6 months postoperatively. Severe acute postoperative pain (odds ratio (OR): 3.2, 95% confidence interval (CI): 1.6–6.3) also predicted increased pain at 6 months.

Mechanisms for pain development are likely to be similar to processes for neuropathic pain, whereby sensitization of neurones in the dorsal horn of the spinal cord, secondary to prolonged peripheral injury or prolonged post-stimulus sensory disturbances, can lead to allodynia and hyperalgesia (Woolf and Mannion, 1999). More than one mechanism can operate within an individual and also these mechanisms may change over time. Prolonged central sensitization can lead to alterations and excitability in the central nervous system, contributing to chronic pain which can persist long after withdrawal of the acute painful stimuli (Woolf and Mannion, 1999; Melzack et al., 2001). Central sensitization has been reported in patients with abnormal sensitivity associated with post-mastectomy pain but sensitization was absent in those who were pain-free (Gottrup et al., 2000). In order to correlate preoperative pain intensity and sensory function in men waiting for hernia surgery, assessment of pain hypersensitivity was conducted using quantitative sensory testing(QST) (Aasvang et al., 2009). There was no evidence of pain-induced altered sensory or nociceptive function in the groin area. Pain thresholds in other body regions (e.g. arm) were not assessed nor were pain-free controls included as a comparator in this small study. Aasvang and colleagues concluded that mechanisms other than preoperative pain-mediated neuroplastic changes must contribute to the development of CPSP after herniorrhaphy, e.g. genetic predisposition. It is reasonable to assume that, as with many other diseases, there are both genetic and environmental component factors in every causal mechanism. Our study of patients undergoing median sternotomy and venous saphenectomy found a higher than expected proportion of patients with CPSP at both operative sites, suggesting a constitutional predisposition for chronic pain (Bruce et al., 2003; Devor, 2004). Pain sensitivity varies widely; increased susceptibility has been demonstrated in animals and more recently, in humans (Diatchenko et al., 2005). Pain susceptibility is known to be influenced by several genes, and human genetic studies have mostly focused on polymorphisms in candidate genes. Further research on the genetics of CPSP is currently being undertaken at several centres and is likely to be illuminating (Katz and Seltzer, 2009).

Risk factors

The application of epidemiological methods has been important for identifying risk factors thought to contribute to the development of CPSP. Putative risk factors include presence of preoperative chronic pain, younger age, surgical technique/approach, intra-operative nerve handling, genetic predisposition, increased body mass index (BMI), psychological distress and resilience, intensity of acute postoperative pain, type of anaesthesia, and postoperative management. A discussion of findings from selected studies is presented below.

Preoperative pain

In a sample of patients having elective abdominal surgery, higher levels of pain immediately before surgery (OR: 2.96; 95%CI: 1.32–6.60) and presence of chronic pain before surgery (lasting >6 months; OR: 1.75; 95%CI: 1.03–2.98) independently predicted moderate-to-intense pain in the acute postoperative period (Caumo et al., 2002). Preoperative pain at or near to the surgical site has also been found to predict chronic pain in patients having hernia and amputation surgery (Liem et al., 2003; Wright et al., 2002). Patients with chronic post-herniorrhaphy pain were more likely to have presented with a painful hernia and have had a history of another chronic pain syndrome: headache, backache, or irritable bowel syndrome (Wright et al., 2002). A multicentre Dutch randomized controlled trial found higher risk of CPSP in patients with preoperative inguinal pain (adjusted HR: 1.7; 95% CI: 1.1–2.6), independent of procedural approach and age (Liem et al., 2003). Cross-sectional studies report a two- to threefold increased risk of CPSP among patients with preoperative pain, although these estimates are based on patient recall of preoperative pain status (Poobalan et al., 2001). Methodologically, it is important to measure pain status preoperatively, as retrospective recall of preoperative pain may be biased by presence and intensity of pain. In a Scandinavian study investigating postoperative stump and phantom pain after amputation, presence and intensity, but not duration, of pre-amputation pain was predictive of phantom limb pain at 3 months postoperatively (Nikolajsen et al., 1997). Patients had distorted recall about the level of their preoperative pain; pre-amputation pain intensity was significantly overestimated after 6 months with more exaggerated estimates as time elapsed (Nikolajsen et al., 1997). In addition to current pain intensity, pain memory is affected by emotion, expectation of pain, and recall of peak intensity of previous pain (Kalso, 1997). Interestingly, recent research has investigated pain ratings provided by healthy subjects who had not undergone surgery: these subjects provided accurate estimates of the likely qualitative characteristics of postoperative pain, comparable to the actual pain ratings experienced by patients having vascular surgery. Terry and colleagues speculated that when asked to recall pain, people may provide estimates based on general knowledge of pain descriptions rather than actual memory or recollections (Terry et al., 2008).

In addition to preoperative pain, higher levels of pain in the acute postoperative period are known to predict pain weeks and months after surgery; this association has been replicated in different surgical cohorts, including studies of hernia, breast, thoracic, and laparoscopic cholecystectomy surgeries (see reviews Kehlet et al., 2006; Gottrup et al., 2000; Macrae and Bruce, 2008). Whilst the data on severe acute pain predicting chronic pain are relatively consistent, the precise nature of the mechanisms involved and whether these relationships are associative or causal has yet to be determined (Katz and Seltzer, 2009).

Age

Younger patients are more likely to develop CPSP (Smith et al., 1999; Steegers et al., 2008; Poobalan et al., 2001; Bruce et al., 2003) but this finding is inconsistent across studies (Liem et al., 2003; Page et al., 2002). Younger women are more likely to have chronic pain, axillary pain, and other persistent sensory symptoms after surgery for breast cancer, although younger patients are also more likely to have a higher histopathological tumour grade and undergo more aggressive adjuvant treatment (Kroman et al., 2000). In a comprehensive prospective study of women undergoing breast cancer surgery, the probability of CPSP incidence decreased by 5% with each 1-year increase in age (OR: 0.95; 95% CI: 0.91–0.99) (Poleschuck et al., 2006). These data correlate with a Scottish study of CPSP after hernia surgery, where a 5% reduction in odds of developing pain was found per 1-year increase in age (Poobalan et al., 2001). Mechanisms explaining the increased incidence of chronic pain in younger patients are unknown, but may relate to reduction in peripheral nociceptive function with increased age. Potential confounding factors, such as physical activity, motivation to return to usual activity/type of employment (e.g. whether self-employed) and other factors should be considered when investigating the inverse relationship between age and CPSP.

Psychological factors

Studies investigating risk factors for CPSP have mostly assessed demographic, somatic, and perioperative biomedical factors, although there has been recent interest in the role of psychological factors, particularly vulnerability and resilience, in predicting late surgical outcome. Psychological vulnerability has been defined as 'a reaction readiness defined by a low threshold for being influenced and a risk of inexpedient reactions in social interactions and health-related behaviour' (Hinrichs-Rocker et al., 2009). Psychological distress is known to predict acute postoperative pain, but less is known about the interrelationship between psychological distress, acute pain and the processes involved in the transition from acute to chronic pain after surgery. Individuals with high trait or dispositional anxiety are thought to be more hypersensitive and psychologically more reactive to threatening stimuli (Caumo et al., 2002; Johnston and Voegle, 1993). State-trait anxiety and depression are predictive of acute postoperative pain; preoperative anxiety is correlated with high postoperative anxiety, postoperative pain intensity, analgesic requirements, and longer length of hospital stay (Caumo et al., 2002). A systematic review by Johnston and Vogele (1993) investigated the role of psychological preparation for surgery, whereby procedural information, behavioural instruction, and cognitive interventions were found to significantly reduce postoperative pain and the use of analgesics postoperatively. However, of the 35 studies included in this systematic review, none assessed patients beyond the second postoperative week.

Orthopaedic studies of patients undergoing spinal surgery for chronic low back pain report high preoperative depression scores compared with the general population. These patients already have chronic pain and thus are more likely to be chronically stressed and have established emotional and cognitive pain-coping mechanisms (Hinrichs-Rocker et al., 2008). Research has widened from measurement of affect to include other constructs of distress, including catastrophizing. Pain catastrophizing, defined as a 'tendency to exaggerate negative responses and perceived inability to control pain', comprises elements of rumination, magnification, and helplessness (Sullivan et al., 1995). Catastrophizing, argued to be a stable, trait-like variable, has mostly been assessed in non-surgical chronic pain populations or surgical patients assessed within the acute postoperative period (Sullivan et al., 1995; Granot and Ferber, 2005). One small Canadian study found that preoperative catastrophizing and co-morbidities independently predicted pain ratings 2 years after knee arthroplasty (Forsythe et al., 2008). Sullivan and colleagues (2009) recently reported that pain catastrophizing independently predicted postoperative pain at 6 weeks after knee arthroplasty; long-term follow-up of this cohort is required.

Dispositional optimism, psychological 'robustness', expectation of pain control, and expectations about functional recovery before surgery have also been assessed in surgical cohorts and are associated with acute pain and, more recently, CPSP. Emotional distress (i.e. anxiety, depression, illness behaviour, somato-sensory amplification, etc.) were significant risk factors for clinically meaningful acute pain (defined as visual analogue scale (VAS) scores >5) at 1 month after breast cancer surgery, but made no independent contribution to persistent pain at 3 months postoperatively (Poleshuck et al., 2006; Katz et al., 2005). A large prospective surgical cohort of 625 patients undergoing minor, intermediate, and major operative procedures found that fear of the long-term consequences of surgery (OR: 1.9; 95% CI: 1.1, 3.3) predicted increased pain at 6 months postoperatively, independent of type of surgical procedure and other somatic factors (Peters et al., 2007). Fear related to surgery was the most consistent psychological predictor of unfavourable outcome, whereas dispositional optimism was related to better long-term functional recovery after surgery. It is unclear whether psychological factors predict 'type' of pain (e.g. neuropathic) or whether the pathway for surgically induced chronic pain is mediated by psychological factors.

Intra-operative nerve injury

Nerves are at risk of injury during surgery from partial or complete division, stretching, contusion, crushing, electrical damage from diathermy, entrapment, or compression (e.g. from rib retraction; Wantz, 1993; Ravichandran et al., 2000). Additional risks occur during prosthetic implantation, where damage or kinking may occur, e.g. when stapling or suturing mesh into position during hernia repair. Chronic irritation can occur, or hypersensitive reactions to non-absorbable material or implants (e.g. staples, sternal bone wires) or neuroma formation following entrapment of fibres in scar tissue. Relatively few studies have assessed whether intra-operative nerve handling, or elective preservation or division of major sensory nerves, contributes to the development of chronic pain and/or numbness. The major sensory nerve often severed during breast and axillary surgery is the intercostobrachial nerve (ICBN), which branches from the second intercostal nerve, the sensory nerve supplying the inferior aspect of the arm and posterior aspect of the axilla. The ICBN can be sacrificed to achieve full axillary clearance and reduce risk of tumour recurrence. Evidence regarding optimal ICBN management is contradictory; early reports suggested that careful preservation would significantly reduce incidence of CPSP (Stevens et al., 1995). Other trials found no difference in rates of chronic pain, sensory deficit or functional outcome after ICBN preservation or dissection (Salmon et al., 1998). Contradictory findings are possibly due to methodological shortcomings as these studies are often very small and underpowered to detect statistically significant differences in persistent pain. A trial comparing SNLB versus axillary node dissection reported significantly reduced numbness and parasthaesia (chronic pain not recorded) 1 year after SNLB; findings were attenuated when adjusted for ICBN preservation (Purushotham et al., 2005).

With regard to hernia surgery, the nerves in the inguinal canal most often implicated in the genesis of post-herniorrhaphy neuralgia include the ilioinguinal, iliohypogastric, and genitofemoral nerves. Division of the ilioinguinal nerve is thought to increase risk of chronic pain but some surgeons have argued for intentional but careful severance of all sensory nerves (Wantz, 1993). Much is based on expert opinion and again, there is lack of consensus over current surgical management (Ravichandran et al., 2000; Mui et al., 2006). Chronic pain and groin numbness is half as likely to occur after laparoscopic compared to open hernia surgery, although testicular pain is more common after laparoscopic repair (Wright et al., 2002; Grant et al., 2004). A recent systematic review pooled data from three small randomized controlled trials and concluded that there was no difference in pain at 6 months after identification and division (or resection) of the ilioinguinal nerve compared to identification and preservation (incidence CPSP 21% vs. 23%; Wijsmuller et al., 2007). Studies included in the systematic review used different pain scales; therefore, the pooled estimate was calculated using a random effects model to account for methodological and clinical heterogeneity. Interestingly, the process of just identifying the nerve structures in the inguinal canal appears to be beneficial in open hernia repair (Wijsmuller et al., 2007).

The largest study to investigate intra-operative nerve handling and CPSP has been an Italian multicentre prospective study of 955 patients undergoing open mesh herniorrhaphy (Alfieri et al., 2006). Nerve handling was carefully recorded and patients with moderate-to-severe pain were examined by clinicians after 1 year. Non-identification of nerves was significantly associated with CPSP, as was nerve division, and the prognostic significance of not identifying one or more inguinal nerves was maintained after adjustment for age and sex (Alfieri et al., 2006). This is biologically plausible given that nerves may be inadvertently sectioned, entrapped, or secured to other structures. Unfortunately, our UK survey of 850 general surgeons found significant variation with regard to routine visualization and handling of inguinal nerve structures (Ravindran et al., 2006). Of responding surgeons, 299 (42%) reported they did not routinely visualize the iliohypogastric nerve or the genitofemoral nerves ($n = 396$; 56%). Volume of hernia surgery was related to nerve-handling experience: surgeons who performed high numbers of hernia repairs (>50 per year) were more likely to identify, visualize, and preserve nerves compared to surgeons performing hernia surgery less frequently. Future studies investigating CPSP should endeavour to record data on intra-operative visualization and handling of nerve structures.

Challenges for measurement

Advances in surgical technology over the last 30 years have led to a raft of innovative surgical approaches, including endoscopic, laparoscopic, robotic procedures, and 'natural orifice' surgery (Harrell and Heniford, 2005). Many of these minimally invasive procedures are conducted as day-cases, with earlier patient mobilization, reduced hospitalization, and limited postoperative follow-up by clinical teams. Other surgical advances include the advent of biosurgical glues and sealants, replacing the need for staples or sutures during gastrointestinal procedures, and muscle-sparing techniques used during thoracic surgery. Studies report patient benefit in the short term, but few surgical teams conduct routine postoperative assessment, other than for neoplastic surgery, and therefore late adverse events may well go undetected or underreported. Long-term follow-up can be costly and challenging to conduct but is crucial for determining operative success from the patient's perspective.

The epidemiological approach to assessing postoperative outcome is undertaken using postal questionnaires because detailed clinical examination of large populations is costly and unfeasible. There is no single validated method for distinguishing between pains of somatic, visceral, or neuropathic origin although instruments to assess neuropathic pain have recently been developed and validated using clinical samples (e.g. Neuropathic Pain Scale; PainDetect, Leeds Assessment Scale for Neuropathic Symptoms and Signs (LANSS) (Bennett, 2001; Bouhassira et al., 2005; Freynhagen et al., 2006; see also Chapter 18)). Despite the lack of a gold standard for the diagnosis of neuropathic pain, the common characteristics include partial or complete sensory loss, spontaneous ongoing or paroxysmal pain, and stimulus-evoked pain (Jensen and Hansson, 2006). Many of the earlier studies classify CPSP as 'neuropathic' based on verbal descriptors or the McGill Pain Questionnaire (MPQ) in conjunction with body maps and descriptions about pain distribution (e.g. Boureau et al., 1990; Melzack, 1975; Bruce et al., 2004). Our Scottish regional surveys of postoperative cohorts revealed that patients predominantly reported neuropathic pain after breast, cardiac, and hernia surgeries, based on sensory-discriminative descriptors selected from the MPQ, although some had features of both nociceptive and neuropathic pain (Bruce et al., 2004). Steegers et al. (2008) found that half of patients with CPSP at 2 years after thoracic surgery had visceral pain and half had definite or probable neuropathic pain, classified using the PainDetect screening tool. Some have argued that classifying pain types as nociceptive or neuropathic is an oversimplification, as clinical presentation can vary; Rasmussen and colleagues (2004) found evidence of abnormal sensory phenomena in patients with both definite and likely neuropathic pain and those without neuropathic pain.

Burden of disease

Given the public health approach of this book, it is important to consider the societal burden from persistent surgical pain and the potential future impact on health care services from patients seeking treatment. Data from specialist chronic pain clinics will be an underrepresentation of people in the community living with persistent pain associated with surgery. Approximate burden of disease can be estimated from routine data on volume of surgery conducted in the UK. Inguinal hernia is a common condition, with an incidence of 6–12% among adult males. In 2001, 70 000 surgical repairs were conducted in England and >8000 procedures were performed in Scotland (National Institute for Clinical Excellence, 2004; Macrae and Bruce, 2008). Assuming a conservative figure of severe pain affecting 5% of UK patients gives an estimated 3900 cases of CPSP per annum. In 2003, more than 800 000 groin hernia repairs were conducted in the USA (Rutgow, 2003).

In the UK, the figures for breast cancer surgery are equally sobering; 46 000 new cases of breast cancer were diagnosed in 2005. Incidence of breast cancer has almost doubled in the last 30 years: age-standardized incidence increased from 74 to 123 per 100 000 women between 1975 and 2005 (Cancer Research UK, 2009). Given that the majority of newly diagnosed patients are treated surgically, the burden from persistent pain is potentially enormous. In 1971, the 5-year survival rate after diagnosis was only 52%; by 2003, this had increased to 80% (Cancer Research UK, 2009). Survival has improved, patients live longer, and as a consequence, there is increased emphasis on improving postoperative quality of life and reducing long-term adverse treatment effects. Chronic pain interferes with activities of daily living; patients with mild pain have lower quality-of-life scores compared to those who recover pain free. Unsurprisingly, the more severe the pain intensity, the greater the level and impact of interference; patients with CPSP are significantly less likely to return to work and resume usual social activities (Courtney et al., 2002; Wright et al., 2002).

In the absence of effective treatment for many chronic pain syndromes, it has been argued that a public health approach be adopted to reduce the population at risk of post-surgical pain (Macrae Macrae and Bruce, 2008). A descriptive analysis of all surgeries performed in the USA revealed a staggering 38% increase in the top 10 surgical procedures performed over a 10-year period (1983–94) (Rutgow, 1997). Patients should be discouraged from having unnecessary or inappropriate surgery. Indeed, surgeons themselves now debate whether elective hernia patients who are mostly asymptomatic should be treated surgically, weighing the relatively small risk of incarceration or hernia strangulation against the potentially substantial risk of CPSP (Page et al., 2002). Hernia recurrence is still the primary clinical outcome of interest, but the UK National Institute for Clinical Excellence (NICE) recommend that future research studies should include chronic pain and numbness as patient-reported outcomes. Health care professionals should accept that CPSP is a very likely adverse event for particular patient subgroups and therefore individual blame for its occurrence is inappropriate (National Institute for Clinical Excellence, 2004). The risks should be discussed openly along with preoperative information about other likely events, such as surgical site infection. Many patient and surgical websites now describe CPSP as a possible consequence of surgery, and patients should be fully informed and involved in decisions about treatment options.

Another observation from a population epidemiological perspective is that there are rather few cohort studies that have compared chronic pain rates in post-surgical patients with chronic pain rates in non-surgical population-based control groups. Therefore, the attributable effect of surgery on chronic pain in the general population is difficult to estimate. Estimates of CPSP prevalence, and of the cause-and-effect relationship between surgery and subsequent pain, generally draw on studies using the definitions discussed earlier. The evidence is based on:

a. reports of attribution of the pain to surgery and pain character, drawing on features such
   as the pain being first experienced in the early postoperative period, being different to

preoperative pain, localized to the region of surgery, and being predominantly neuropathic in character; examples of studies include case series, surveys of patients attending chronic pain clinics, and surveys of patients after surgery;

b. internal comparisons of surgical cohorts between those who have CPSP and those who do not, highlighting variation in pain according to characteristics of surgery (i.e. locality, extent, or degree of nerve damage); examples of studies include prospective surgical cohorts, with or without baseline preoperative assessment of pain and other characteristics; and

c. randomized controlled trials of surgery versus other treatments, e.g. conservative management.

Such studies, reviewed in this chapter, represent a convincing body of evidence about the occurrence of specific pains related to individual surgical procedures. However, we must be circumspect about the overall impact of surgery on population pain in the absence of controlled observational studies. In this regard, the randomized controlled trials contribute interesting information. Trials of surgery versus watchful waiting for asymptomatic inguinal hernias (i.e. hernias not causing pain or activity-limiting discomfort) have been done precisely to investigate whether surgical gains (general health improvement and avoidance of mechanical complications of hernias) are outweighed by postoperative onset of chronic pain caused by surgery. Two such trials to date have shown that rates of pain at 12 and 24 months (O'Dwyer et al., 2006; Fizgibbons et al., 2006) after surgery were similar in surgical and control groups, suggesting that overall rates of pain in men with minimal symptoms of inguinal hernia are not affected by the surgical procedure. These findings have to be considered besides the substantial evidence reviewed above about the incidence and prevalence of pain with the specific defining characteristics of CPSP following many operative procedures.

Future directions

Well-designed, prospective, epidemiological studies should be used to unravel the complex inter-relationship among biological, surgical, and psychosocial factors contributing to CPSP. Prospective studies of elective surgery patients should incorporate quantitative and qualitative measures of preoperative pain (e.g. presence, distribution, intensity, and character) and health status to provide an accurate baseline against which subsequent outcomes can be compared. It is beyond the scope of this chapter to provide an overview of current therapeutic modalities or pharmacologic agents for the prevention and management of chronic pain. However, the increase in awareness of CPSP has led to a huge body of research investigating, e.g. pre-emptive analgesia and other preventive strategies. Evidence of prevention is currently limited as trials of pre-emptive (e.g. gabapentin) and perioperative analgesia are either contradictory or inconclusive, possibly due to poor design and small sample sizes that lack statistical power (Macrae and Bruce, 2008; Katz and Seltzer, 2009). Many studies investigating efficacy of perioperative anaesthetic or analgesic agents show an effect in the acute postoperative period, but benefit is often not demonstrated in the long term (for reviews, see Katz and Seltzer, 2009; Joshi et al., 2008). Although there is still much to learn about mechanisms, the relationship between acute postoperative pain and subsequent CPSP has been well demonstrated empirically, and the immediate goal for all extended surgical teams should, therefore, be the control of pain during the acute postoperative period.

Summary

Given the impact and scale of the problem from chronic pain, it is vital that efforts continue in order to understand the aetiology, prevention, and management of pain after surgery. This requires collation of good-quality data at multiple time-points along the health care pathway, including pre-, peri-, and postoperatively. Surgery provides an ideal model for investigation; it is a natural experiment whereby patients undergo a controlled injury, offering an opportunity to investigate mechanisms for pain development and understanding of the transitional pathway from acute to chronic pain. Patients undergoing elective surgery are broadly exposed to similar levels of tissue injury, nerve damage, and nociceptive barrage; most recover uneventfully but, for 5% of patients, severe postoperative pain can persist for months or years after the initial insult. Intra-operative nerve damage may occur but it is not sufficient in itself; other patients may have little or minimal damage to major nerve pathways yet go on to develop chronic neuropathic symptoms or a continuous inflammatory pain (Kehlet et al., 2006). Pain expression is influenced by physiological, genetic, and psychological factors and the challenge for researchers is to accurately predict and identify susceptible patients who are at greatest risk. Relatively few prospective studies investigating CPSP have been of sufficient size or methodological rigour to produce definitive conclusions regarding predictors of outcome. There has been recent impetus for scientists to reach consenssus agreement about the core prognostic factors and outcomes for inclusion within prospective studies of low back pain (Pincus et al., 2008). This collaborative approach could be applied to the investigation of CPSP. Agreement about core domains to be included within future studies, e.g. pain, pain-related physical and emotional functioning, psychological factors, and surgical/intra-operative factors, would provide a framework for researchers to collate minimum datasets across multiple patient cohorts and health care settings. This would allow data aggregation, not only for systematic reviews, but also for providing larger samples sizes for the development and refinement of prognostic models. Further exploration of the complex relationship among biophysical, surgical, and psychological processes along the transitional pathway will aid our understanding both of the aetiology and trajectory of chronic pain after surgery.

References

Aasvang, E.K., Hansen, J.B. and Kehlet, H. 2009: Pre-operative pain and sensory function in groin hernia. *Eur J Pain* **13**, 1018–22.

Aasvang, E. and Kehlet, H. 2005: Chronic postoperative pain: the case of inguinal herniorrhaphy. *Br J Anaesth* **95**, 69–76.

Aasvang, E.K., Mohl, B., Bay-Nielsen, M. and Kehlet, H. 2006: Pain related sexual dysfunction after inguinal herniorrhaphy. *Pain* **122**, 258–63.

Alfieri, S., Rotondi, F., Di Giorgio, A., Fumagalli, U., Salzano, A., Di Miceli, D. et al. 2006: Influence of preservation versus division of ilioinguinal, iliohypogastric, and genital nerves during open mesh herniorrhaphy: prospective multicentric study of chronic pain. *Ann Surg* **243**, 553–8.

Baron, R.H., Fey, J.V., Borgen, P.I., Stempel, M.M., Hardick, K.R. and van Zee, K.J. 2007: Eighteen sensations after breast cancer surgery: a 5-year comparison of sentinel lymph node biopsy and axillary lymph node dissection. *Ann Surg Oncol* **14**, 1653–61.

Bennett, M. 2001: The LANSS Pain Scale: the Leeds assessment of neuropathic symptoms and signs. *Pain* **92**, 147–57.

Bouhassira, D., Attal, N. and Alchaar, H. 2005: Comparison of pain syndromes associated with nervous or somatic lesions and development of a new neuropathic pain diagnostic questionnaire (DN4). *Pain* **114**, 29–36.

Boureau, F., Doubrère, J.F. and Luu, M. 1990: Study of verbal description in neuropathic pain. *Pain* **42**, 145–52.

Bruce, J., Drury, N., Poobalan, A.S., Jeffrey, R.R., Smith, W.C. and Chambers, W.A. 2003: The prevalence of chronic chest and leg pain following cardiac surgery: a historical cohort study. *Pain* **104**, 265–73.

Bruce, J., Poobalan, A.S., Smith, W.C. and Chambers, W.A. 2004: Quantitative assessment of chronic postsurgical pain using the McGill Pain Questionnaire. *Clin J Pain* **20**, 70–75.

Cancer Research UK. Cancer facts and figures. http://www.cancerresearchuk.org/.

Caumo, W., Schmidt, A.P., Schnieder, C.N., Bergmann, J., Iwamoto, C.W., Adamatti, L.C. et al. 2002: Preoperative predictors of moderate to intense acute postoperative pain in patients undergoing abdominal surgery. *Acta Anaesthesiol Scand* **46**, 1265–71.

Conacher, I.D., Doig, J.C., Rivas, L. and Pridie, A.K. 1993: Intercostal neuralgia associated with internal mammary artery grafting. *Anaesthesia* **48**, 1070–1.

Courtney, C.A., Duffy, K., Serpell, M.G. and O'Dwyer, P.J. 2002: Outcome of patients with severe chronic pain following repair of groin hernia. *Br J Surg* **89**, 1310–14.

Crombie, I.K., Davies, H.T.O. and Macrae, W.A. 1998: Cut and thrust: antecedent surgery and trauma among patients attending a chronic pain clinic. *Pain* **76**, 167–71.

Devor, M. 2004: Evidence for heritability of pain in patients with traumatic neuropathy. *Pain* **108**, 200–1.

Diatchenko, L., Slade, G.D., Nackley, A.G. Bhalang, K., Sigurdsson, A., Belfer, I. et al. 2005: Genetic basis for individual variations in pain perception and the development of a chronic pain condition. *Hum Mol Genet* **14**, 135–43.

Forsythe, M.E., Dunbar, M.J., Hennigar, A.W., Sulilvan, M.J. and Gross, M. 2008: Prospective relation between catastrophising and residual pain following knee arthoplastye: two-year follow-up. *Pain Res Manage* **13**, 335–41.

Freynhagen, R., Baron, R., Gockel, U. and Tolle, T.R. 2006: painDETECT: a new screening questionnaire to identify neuropathic components in patients with back pain. *Curr Med Res Opin* **22**, 1911–20.

Gottrup, H., Andersen, J., Arendt-Nielsen, L. and Jensen, T.S. 2000: Psychophysical examination in patients with post-mastectomy pain. *Pain* **87**, 275–84.

Granot, M. and Ferber, S.G. 2005: The roles of catastrophising and anxiety in the prediction of postoperative pain intensity: a prospective study. *Clin J Pain* **21**, 439–45.

Grant, A.M., Scott, N.W., O'Dwyer, P.J. and MRC Laparoscopic Groin Hernia Trial Group. 2004: Five-year follow-up of a randomized trial to assess pain and numbness after laparoscopic or open repair of groin hernia. *Br J Surg* **91**, 1570–4.

Harrell, A.G. and Heniford, B.T. 2005: Minimally invasive abdominal surgery: *lux et veritas* past, present, and future. *Am J Surg* **190**, 239–43.

Hinrichs-Rocker, A., Schulz, K., Jarvinen, I., Lefering, R., Simanski, C. and Neugebauer, E.A.M. 2009: Psychosocial predictors and correlates for chronic post-surgical pain (CPSP) – A systematic review. *Eur J Pain* **13**, 719–30.

Jensen, T.S. and Hansson, P.T. 2006: Chapter 34. Classification of neuropathic pain syndromes based on symptoms and signs. In Cervero, F., Jensen, T.S., eds. *Handbook of Clinical Neurology* Vol. 81, pp. 517–26. Elsevier, Amsterdam.

Johnston, M. and Vöegle, C. 1993: Benefits of psychological preparation for surgery: a meta-analysis. *Ann Behav Med* **15**, 245–56.

Joshi, G.P., Bonnet, F. and Shah, R. 2008: A systematic review of randomized trials evaluating regional techniques for postthoracotomy analgesia. *Anesth Analg* **107**, 1026–40.

Jung, B.F., Ahrendt, G.M., Oaklander, A.L. and Dworkin, R.H. 2003: Neuropathic pain following breast cancer surgery: proposed classification and research update. *Pain* **104**, 1–13.

Kalso, E. 1997: Memory for pain. *Acta Anaesthesiol Scand* **415**, 129–30.

Katz, J., Poleshuck, E.L., Andrus, C.H. Hogan, L.A., Jung, B.F., Kulick, D.I., Dworkin, R.H., et al. 2005: Risk factors for acute pain and its persistence following breast cancer surgery. *Pain* **119**, 16–25.

Katz, J. and Seltzer, Z. 2009: Transition from acute to chronic postsurgical pain: risk factors and protective factors. *Expert Rev Neurother* **9**, 723–44.

Kehlet, H., Jensen, T.S. and Woolf, C.J. 2006: Persistent postsurgical pain: risk factors and prevention. *Lancet* **367**, 1618–25.

Kroman, N., Jensen, M.B., Wohlfahrt, J., Mouridsen, H.T., Andersen, P.K. and Melbye, M. 2000: Factors influencing the effect of age on prognosis in breast cancer: population based study. *BMJ* **320**, 474–8.

Kudel, I., Edwards, R.R., Kozachik, S. Block, B.M., Agarwal, S., Heinberg, L.J. et al. 2007: Predictors and consequences of multiple persistent postmastectomy pains. *J Pain Symptom Manage* **34**, 619–27.

Liem, M.S., van Duyn, E.B., van der Graaf, Y., van Vroonhoven, T.J. and Coala Trial Group. 2003: Recurrences after conventional anterior and laparoscopic inguinal hernia repair: a randomized comparison. *Ann Surg* **237**, 136–41.

Macdonald, L., Bruce, J., Scott, N.W., Smith, W.C.S. and Chambers, W.A. 2005: Long-term follow-up of breast cancer survivors with post-mastectomy pain syndrome. *Brit J Cancer* **92**, 225–30.

Macrae, W.A. 2008: Chronic post-surgical pain: 10 years on. *Br J Anaesth* **101**, 77–86.

Macrae, W. and Bruce, J. 2008: Chronic pain after surgery, in Wilson, P.R., Watson, P.J., Haythornthwaite, J.A., Jensen, T.S., eds. *Clinical Pain Management: Chronic Pain*, pp. 405–14. Hodder Arnold, London.

Macrae, W.A. and Davies, H.T.O. 1999: Chronic postsurgical pain. In Crombie IK ed. *Epidemiology of Pain*, pp. 125–42. IASP Press, Seattle.

Manikandan, R., Srirangam, S.J., Pearson, E. and Collins, G.N. 2004: Early and late morbidity after vasectomy: a comparison of chronic scrotal pain at 1 and 10 years. *BJU Int* **93**, 571–4.

Melzack, R. 1975: The McGill Pain Questionnaire: major properties and scoring methods. *Pain* **1**, 277–99.

Melzack, R., Coderre, T.J., Katz, J. and Vaccarino, A.L. 2001: Central neuroplasticity and pathological pain. *Ann N Y Acad Sci* **933**, 157–784.

Mui, W.L., Ng, C.S., Fung, T.M. et al. 2006: Prophylactic ilioinguinal neurectomy in open inguinal hernia repair: a double-blind randomized controlled trial. *Ann Surg* **244**, 27–33.

National Institute for Clinical Excellence (NICE) 2004: Laparoscopic surgery for inguinal hernia repair. NICE Technology Appraisal Guidance 83, London.

Nikolajsen, L., Ilkær, S., Kroner, K., Christensen, J.H. and Jensen, T.S., et al. 1997: The influence of preamputation pain on postamputation stump and phantom pain. *Pain* **72**, 393–405.

Page, B., Paterson, C., Young, D. and O'Dwyer, P.J. 2002: Pain from primary inguinal hernia and the effect of repair on pain. *Br J Surg* **89**, 1315–18.

Peters, M.L., Sommer, M., de Rijke, J.M., Kessels, F., Heineman, E., Patijn, J. et al. 2007: Somatic and psychologic predictors of long-term unfavourable outcome after surgical intervention. *Ann Surg* **245**, 487–94.

Pincus, T., Santos, R., Breen, A., Burton, K., Underwood, M. and the Multinational Musculoskeletal Inception Cohort Study collaboration. 2008: A review and proposal for a core set of factors for prospective cohorts in low back pain: a consensus statement. *Arthritis Rheum* **59**, 14–24.

Poleshuck, E.L., Katz, J., Andrus, C.H., Hogan, L.A., Jung, B.F., Kulick, D.I. et al. 2006: Risk factors for chronic pain following breast cancer surgery: a prospective study. *J Pain* **7**, 626–34.

Poobalan, A.S., Bruce, J., King, P.M., Chambers, W.A., Krukowski, Z.H. and Smith, W.C.S. 2001: Chronic pain and quality of life following open inguinal hernia repair. *Brit J Surg* **88**, 1122–26.

Poobalan, A.S., Bruce, J., Smith, W.C.S., King, P.M., Krukowski, Z.H. and Chambers, W.A. 2003: A review of chronic pain after inguinal herniorrhaphy. *Clin J Pain* **19**, 48–54.

Purushotham, A.D., Upponi, S., Klevesath, M.B., Bobrow, L., Millar, K., Myles, J.P., et al. 2005: Morbidity after sentinel lymph node biopsy in primary breast cancer: results from a randomised controlled trial. *J Clin Oncol* **23**, 4312–21.

Rasmussen, P.V., Sindrup, S.H., Jensen, T.S. and Bach, F.W. 2004: Symptoms and signs in patients with suspected neuropathic pain. *Pain* **110**, 461–9.

Ravichandran, D., Kalambe, B.G. and Pain, J.A. 2000: Pilot randomized controlled study of preservation or division of ilioinguinal nerve in open mesh repair of inguinal hernia. *Br J Surg* **87**, 1166–7.

Ravindran, R., Bruce, J., Debnath, D., Poobalan, A. and King, P.M. 2006: A United Kingdom survey of surgical technique and handling practice of inguinal canal structures during hernia surgery. *Surgery* **139**, 523–6.

Rutgow, I.M. 1997: Surgical operations in the United States. Then (1983) and now (1994). *Arch Surg* **132**, 983–90.

Rutgow, I.M. 2003: Demographic and socioeconomic aspects of hernia repair in the United States in 2003. *Surg Clin North Am* **83**, 1045–51.

Salmon, R.J., Ansquer, Y. and Asselain, B. 1998: Preservation versus section of intercostal-brachial nerve (IBN) in axillary dissection for breast cancer–a prospective randomized trial. *Eur J Surg Oncol* **24**, 158–61.

Smith, W.C.S., Bourne, D., Squair, J., Phillips, D.O. and Chambers, W.A. 1999: A retrospective cohort study of post mastectomy pain syndrome. *Pain* **83**, 91–5.

Steegers, M.A.H., Snik, D.M., Verhagen, A.F., van der Drift, M.A. and Wilder-Smith, O.H.G. 2008: Only half of the chronic pain after thoracic surgery shows a neuropathic component. *J Pain* **9**, 955–61.

Stevens, P.E., Dibble, S.L. and Miaskowski, C. 1995: Prevalence, characteristics, and impact of postmastectomy pain syndrome: an investigation of women's experiences. *Pain* **61**, 61–8.

Sullivan, M.J.L., Bishop, S.R. and Pivik, J. 1995: The Pain Catastrophizing Scale: development and validation. *Psychol Assess* **7**, 524–32.

Sullivan, M., Tanzer, M., Stanish, W., Fallaha, M., Keefe, F.J., Simmonds, M., et al. 2009: Psychological determinants of problematic outcomes following total knee arthoplasty. *Pain* **143**, 123–9.

Terry, R.H., Niven, C.A., Brodie, C.E., Jones, R.B. and Prowse, M.A. 2008: Memory for pain? A comparison of nonexperiential estimates and patients' reports of the quality and intensity of postoperative pain. *J Pain* **9**, 342–9.

Wallace, M.S., Wallace, A.M., Lee, J. and Dobke, M.K. 1996: Pain after breast surgery: a survey of 282 women. *Pain* **66**, 195–205.

Wantz, G.E. 1993: Testicular atrophy and chronic residual neuralgia as risks of inguinal hernioplasty. *Surg Clin North Am* **73**, 571–82.

Wijsmuller, A.R., van Veen, R.N., Bosch, J.L., Lange, J.F., Kleinrensink, G.J., Jeekel, J., et al. 2007: Nerve management during open hernia repair. *Br J Surg* **94**, 17–22.

Woolf, C.J. and Mannion, R.J. 1999: Neuropathic pain: aetiology, symptoms, mechanisms and management. *Lancet* **353**, 1959–64.

Wright, D., Paterson, C., Scott, N., Hair, A. and O'Dwyer, P.J. 2002: Five-year follow-up of patients undergoing laparoscopic or open groin hernia repair. *Ann Surg* **235**, 333–7.

Chapter 20

Chronic chest pain, myocardial ischaemia, and coronary artery disease phenotypes

Harry Hemingway, Justin Zaman, and Gene Feder

Introduction

Importance

If an overarching goal of management of patients with chronic chest pain thought to be due to angina is to alleviate symptoms and mitigate the increased risk of coronary death, then current strategies are failing. In women and men the incidence of angina remains high – up to 2 per 100 population based on primary care-diagnosed cases in Finland (Hemingway et al., 2006). In older and younger patients, and in those with and without a confirmed test abnormality, the diagnosis of angina is associated with higher coronary mortality rates when compared with the general population, see Figure 20.1 (Hemingway et al., 2006). At 6-years follow-up after coronary angiography, the proportion of patients reporting ongoing angina symptoms was 45%, 58%, and 58% after surgical, percutaneous intervention, or medical therapy, respectively (Griffin et al., 2007). These observations motivate the enquiry in this chapter.

Heterogeneous angina syndromes

Different angina syndromes can be distinguished by different patterns of symptoms of chronic chest pain, evidence of myocardial ischaemia, and evidence of coronary artery atheroma. While angina pectoris is commonly defined as typical chest pain due to myocardial ischaemia caused by coronary atheroma, there are no internationally agreed criteria for defining 'a' case of angina pectoris, and >10 clinical syndromes of angina are recognized by differing patterns of presence and severity of symptoms, myocardial ischaemia, and coronary atheroma. Some of these are summarized in Table 20.1. As biological understanding – principally through new imaging modalities, genomics, proteomics, and metabonomics – increases, we may be able to clarify the extent to which these syndromes represent distinct disease phenotypes. Few, if any, previous reviews have focused on chronic chest pain and chronic coronary syndromes, and have largely concerned their principal complication, of acute myocardial infarction (MI). Figure 20.2 illustrates how different syndromes associated with chronic chest pain may be associated with subsequent fatal and non-fatal cardiovascular events.

Aim

To give an overview of the public health importance – including burden, trends, cause, treatment, and prevention from a population perspective – of chronic stable angina and to assess where distinguishing heterogenous syndromes may be important in future epidemiological research.

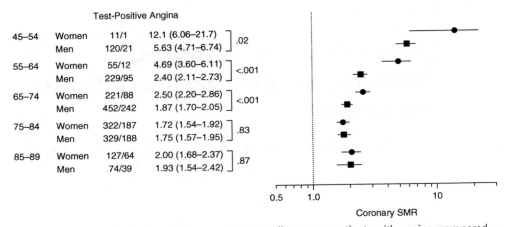

Fig. 20.1 Age standardized ratios for coronary mortality among patients with angina, compared with the general population. Reproduced from Hemingway et al., (2006), with permission. Copyright © (1996) American Medical Association. All rights reserved.
Angina defined in primary care by anti-anginal medication in combination with an abnormal coronary angiogram or exercise ECG.

Structure of chapter

The chapter starts with the symptoms of angina pectoris, then turns to the combination of symptoms with evidence of ischaemia, and lastly their combination with evidence of atheroma. The reason for this structure is that most of the evidence comes from populations defined by, or selected at the point of, having one or other of these dimensions assessed; there are no population studies yet assessing all three dimensions. Such a structure furthermore helps to distinguish possible phenotypes. Within each of these three sections, we begin with historical and social scientific considerations, because the expression of symptoms varies historically and culturally and because hypotheses and models of disease are themselves located in a specific socio-historical context. This is then followed by sections on measurement, epidemiology, and prevention and treatment.

Chronic chest pain symptoms

History

The notion of typical symptoms of angina pectoris has emerged over time – the history of their relation to ischaemia and atheroma is dealt with in later sections. The term 'angina pectoris' was probably first used in a public forum by William Heberden in an oration to the London Royal College of Physicians in 1768, although in a description of 20 cases he mentioned the heart only once and it is unlikely that he considered this to be the source of the pain.

> There is a disorder of the breast with strong and peculiar symptoms, considerable for the kind of danger belonging to it and not extremely rare ... The seat of it and sense of strangling and anxiety with which it is attended, may make it not improperly called Angina pectoris. Those who are afflicted with it are seized, while they are walking and more particularly when they walk soon after eating with a painful and most disagreeable sensation in the breast, which seems as if it would take their life away if it were to increase or to continue; the moment they stand still, all this uneasiness vanishes. (Heberden, 1772)

This description has taken on an iconic identity and no article or textbook chapter on angina seems complete without it. We make no apologies for reproducing it here, partly because of its

Table 20.1 Defining heterogeneous angina syndromes

Name of syndrome	Constellation of findings		
	Chronic chest pain	Evidence of myocardial ischaemia on electrocardiogram or other test	Evidence of coronary atheroma on angiography
Population-based case of angina	Present, based on standard instrument, the Rose questionnaire	Usually confined to resting ECG if any	(Increasingly will include MR angiography and CT calcium findings)
Chronic stable angina	Present	Present	Present
Isolated angina	Present	Present, but no previous infarction	Present
Refractory angina	Present despite revascularization and medical therapy	Present	Present
Variant angina (Prinzmetal)	Present but with some atypical features, e.g. at rest and early morning	Present ST elevation	May be absent
Silent ischaemia	Present but not occurring at the same time as ST changes	ST depression on 24-h recording	±
Symptomatic, non-ischaemic, coronary disease	Present	Absent	Present
Chronic coronary disease	May not be mentioned	±	Present, markers of plaque 'vulnerability' await evaluation
Microvascular angina (Syndrome X)	Present	Present	Absence of flow-limiting stenosis; dipyridamole echo;
'Non-cardiac' chest pain	Yes, but often atypical, or non-specific	Usually negative	Usually not sought

These syndromes are commonly described in the literature; their relative frequency in the general population, causes, and prognosis (in terms of future risk of persistent symptoms or subsequent acute myocardial infarction) are not well understood.

clarity and resonance with our patients' description of angina today and partly because of its emotional and semiotic content, to which we return in the next section.

Whether its description by Heberden reflects the emergence of angina as a new syndrome or the naming of symptoms that were already prevalent before the mid-18th century is debatable. Heberden himself commented that the condition was ignored in medical texts and cited only one previous observation of the symptoms by Erasistratus of Chios, a Greek physician to Seleucus I Nicator of Syria in the 3rd century BC. The medical historian Leon Michaels has found only 6 case reports of exertional chest pain in the 2000 years between Erasistratus' and Heberden's description (Michaels, 2001) and makes a strong case for angina as a new phenomenon in the 18th century, associated with a sharp rise in 'palpitation of the heart' as a cause of death. Michaels attributes the

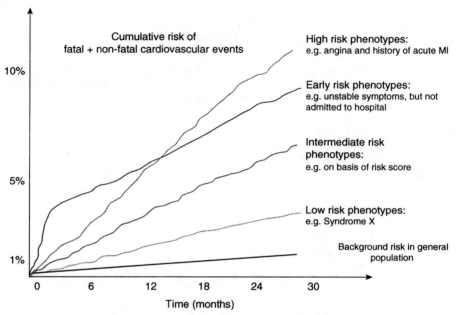

Fig. 20.2 Prognosis of different angina syndromes: hypothetical data.

emergence of angina in Britain before the rest of the world to dramatic alterations in diet after the enclosure acts in the second half of the 18th century.

Anthropological studies

The patterning of chest-pain symptoms is culturally specific, as are explanations for chest pain. It is possible to understand angina as a construction or bodily experience that varies with the cultural context of the patient. For example, in patients presenting to chest pain clinics in England, a higher proportion of south Asians presented with atypical than typical symptoms (Zaman et al., 2008). Interpretation of chest pain and willingness to seek medical advice differs between cultures and may be mediated by aspects of identity, such as masculinity. An interview study of men with a history of angina or MI, found that white, but not south Asian, men were less likely to disclose chest pain because they felt that tolerating pain and discomfort was a masculine attribute (Galdas et al., 2007). Cultural patterning extends to the meaning that patients attribute to their symptoms. In a study of 'heart distress' in an Iranian village, Good found that the term referred to a complex of physical and emotional experiences (Good, 1994). Linking of chest pain and the heart to emotion is ubiquitous across cultures, including European and North American, although its form varies dramatically (Helman, 1984). This is exemplified in religious texts, poetry, and stories. In the context of stable coronary disease, it is also reflected in the association of clinical depression and anxiety with established angina.

Ethnographic studies of doctors and their patients

A more challenging perspective is to include the activity of cardiovascular researchers and clinicians into a model for understanding angina. The ontological premise for this perspective is that all aspects of the human condition, including anatomical structures, physiological processes, diseased organs, as well as mental states, are enacted or performed through human activities. It does not mean that these entities have no independent existence, but that their specific identity only exists in the context of human action. Mol has applied this perspective in an empirical investigation of diagnosis and management of peripheral vascular disease, with the aim of under-standing what that condition is and means, synthesizing the patient's narrative, the doctor's accounts, histopathological findings, the diagnostic use of angiography, and the range of treat-ments offered by doctors (Mol, 2003).

We have used this perspective in an ethnographic study using participant observation of the diagnosis of angina among people with new-onset chest pain (Somerville et al., 2008). This study made direct observations on the nature of the clinical history, finding that the diagnosis is con-structed from a 'canon' of questions which potentially exclude important diagnostic and prog-nostic features. History 'taking' by doctors is relentlessly diagnostic and the principal purpose of eliciting descriptors of a chest pain history is to help with diagnosis, that is to shift the pre-test probability that coronary artery disease or myocardial ischaemia accounts for the symptoms. The clinical history acts as a marker of risk (pre-test probability of coronary artery narrowing) which will help with dichotomous patient-management decisions such as conducting further investiga-tions or not. This study found that patients 'rarely gave a history that, without further interroga-tion, satisfied the doctors, who actively restructured the complex narrative until it fitted a diagnostic canon, detaching it from the patient's interpretation and explanation. A minority of doctors asked about chest pain symptoms outside the canon. Doctors actively re-structured patient accounts into the canonical classification. Patients sometimes resisted this process, con-testing key concepts, such as exertion. Symptom narratives were sometimes unstable, with central features changing on interrogation and re-telling. When translation was required for south Asian patients, doctors considered the history less relevant to the diagnosis. We concluded that diagno-sis and effective treatment could be enhanced by research on the diagnostic and prognostic value of the terms patients use to describe their symptoms'.

Descriptions of chest pain in women and ethnic minorities

In a study of chest-pain narratives elicited by questionnaire from people being investigated for coronary disease with angiography, women described more throat, neck, or jaw pain than men among those with low physical functioning, in the presence of coronary artery disease and in those who were not subsequently revascularized. Women also gave more accounts than men of breathlessness and other symptoms. Thus gender differences in language use do exist and descrip-tion of angina pain may influence subsequent revascularization. Further research is necessary to investigate the nature and consequences of gender differences in language use at this and earlier stages in the referral process (Philpott et al., 2001). Decisions about investigation may be affected, as was found in an interview study of black and white men referred for coronary angiography for suspected angina: black men were more likely than white men to report shortness of breath and the presence of shortness of breath made it less likely that they would be offered revascularization independent of the severity of coronary artery disease (Hravnak et al., 2007).

Measurement and classification

Chronic chest pain does not have simple objectively measured correlates, and there has been little research in using standard pain stimuli (e.g. temperature, pressure, or ischaemia) to predict the patterns and evolution of reported pain among people with suspected angina.

Neural basis

Some of the characteristic symptoms of angina can be attributed to the course of the nerves con-necting the brain to the heart. Sympathetic nerve fibres, which carry nociceptive sensory informa-tion, have endings in the epicardium, with a higher density towards the anterior cardiac wall. Surgical sympathectomy relieves the sensation of neck and jaw discomfort during angina attacks. Denervation of the heart occurs in transplantation, and though atherosclerosis is accelerated, the sensation of angina is absent for a number of years. (Bristow, 1990). The myocardium itself does not demonstrate nerve endings; however, nerve fibres are found traversing it through connective tissue. These fibres originate between cervical level C8 and thoracic level T9 of the spinal cord and it is within this region of the cord that a degree of interaction with somatic sensory fibres from the chest and arms is thought to result in the classical sensation of chest tightness and arm symptoms during angina attacks. In contrast, vagal nerve fibres have been predominantly identified within the endocardium and more so towards the inferior cardiac wall. A similar interaction with somatic fibres is proposed to explain this but the reason for the C1–C3 cervical spinal cord level remains unclear. These nociceptive impulses reach the brain via the spinothalamic tract of the spinal cord, with less clear involvement from other ascending tracts and dorsal columns. The translation of these impulses into the perception of anginal pain has been demonstrated by brain positronic emission tomography (PET) to occur within the hypothalamus, periacqueductal grey, lateral prefrontal cortex, and left inferior anterocaudal cingulate cortex, with the thalamus potentially acting as a pain gateway (Rosen et al., 1994).

Molecular basis

Multiple chemical factors at the tissue level are known to mediate the generation of pain-related nerve impulses, with adenosine and bradykinin playing significant roles. However, the process of chemical release during ischaemia, as well as the sequence and interaction between these factors remains unclear. In a review, Hayashida et al., (2005) summarised: "Characteristic central adenosine A1 receptor-mediated pain-relieving effects have been observed after intravenous adenosine infusion in human inflammation/sensitization pain models and in patients with chronic neuropathic pain. Adenosine compounds, in low doses, can reduce allodynia/hyperalgesia more consistently than spontaneous pain, suggesting that these compounds affect neuronal pathophysiological mechanisms involved in central sensitization. Such pain-relieving effects, which are mostly mediated via central adenosine A1 receptor activation, have a slow onset and long duration of action, lasting usually for hours or days and occasionally for months". Substance P is another chemical factor that has been shown to exacerbate the sensation of pain rather than being causative of pain and may have a role in the explanation of the different experiences of angina severity. Mechanisms explaining symptom diversity are also lacking. Genetic polymorphisms for the reception and interpretation of pain as well as the expression of symptoms may provide a possible explanation and require further research.

Typicality

Notwithstanding the complexities of symptom descriptions, one of the most remarkable, and enduring, observations in clinical medicine is the power of typical anginal symptoms to predict the presence of one or more narrowings at coronary angiography. The symptom of chest pain or discomfort in which myocardial ischaemia is suspected is assessed by clinicians for its typicality, severity, and stability. These adjectives in common parlance have specific technical meanings. The canon of chest pain typicality was developed in 1979 by George Diamond and Duncan Forrester in a paper which brought the categorical assessment of history into a Bayesian perspective which continues to have profound implications for diagnosis (Diamond and Forrester, 1979). There are standardized questionnaires for the assessment of typical angina symptoms in population studies, developed in the 1960s by Geoffrey Rose (Rose, 1962).

Severity

The Canadian Cardiovascular Society angina classification (CCS) classes I–IV gives different grades for the severity of angina. Although the validity, scaling properties, and reliability of this measure have been questioned, it does show a correlation with angiographic disease and subsequent mortality (Hemingway et al., 2004) and has been in widespread clinical use at the time of revascularization. A consequence of the doctor's concern with diagnosis is that features of the symptoms which are important to the patient – such as the severity of symptoms – are given less relevance. An example of this is that in our ethnographic study severity of chest pain was seldom assessed (Somerville et al., 2008). This is particularly odd given that clinical guidelines give symptom severity an important role in directing further treatment, and that a patient's assessment of severity may differ importantly from that of their physician (Nease et al., 1995).

Stability

The 'stability' of symptoms refers to the extent to which symptoms are new, or worsening in frequency or severity, or present at rest. While clinical experience shows that such 'unstable' symptoms are reported in ambulatory populations, a convention has evolved whereby unstable angina is a term exclusively reserved for patients who have been admitted acutely to hospital. Research into the temporal fluctuation of symptoms and their impact on early prognosis is required.

Science of assessing chronic chest pain

Given the undisputed centrality of symptom description in angina, there has been surprisingly little research into refining definitions of typical symptoms, symptom severity or symptom stability. For example, the importance of non-exercise precipitants, non-rest relieving factors, or the time during which symptoms must be relieved (5–15 min vs. other) is not known. The reliability of a clinical history has rarely been investigated; thus two doctors might reach different conclusions on typicality. Important items in the history may be defined in clinical practice guidelines (Fox et al., 2006) but how they should be elicited or recorded or combined with other information is not. Patients and clinicians differ in their assessment of the distress caused by symptoms (Nease et al., 1995). As a global measure of function, patient-defined measures take into account factors such as whether the patient is in employment, their usual physical fitness, and differing levels of anxiety about the implications of having angina that may affect their desired outcomes from treatment (Hlatky, 1995).

Epidemiology

Pyramid of chest-pain populations

A 'pyramid of populations' of chronic chest pain has as its broad base the experience of pain or discomfort over the anterior chest wall which is commonly reported in general population epidemiological surveys. A large proportion of such patients do not seek help (Eslick, 2008). Among those who do seek medical attention (the next level of the pyramid), unspecified chest pain accounts for up to 1.5% of consultations in primary care (Nilsson et al., 2003) and the UK incidence has been estimated at 15.5 per 1000 person-years (Ruigomez et al., 2006). In a UK community survey of chronic pain, Carnes and colleagues found that while 6% of the population had chronic chest pain, <1% had pain confined to the chest (Carnes et al., 2007). Among those consulting with chest pain in primary care, <18% were attributed to a cardiac cause (Ruigomez et al., 2006).

'Non-cardiac' chronic chest pain

The term non-cardiac chest pain is used to denote chest pain for which evidence of ischaemia, coronary disease, or both are lacking (Eslick et al., 2003). Prognostic studies suggest that the 'non-cardiac' label may be misleading. Consider two types of population. First, in primary care: patients ($n = 3028$) who had chest pain but did not have diagnosed angina at baseline were more likely than controls over follow-up to receive a first diagnosis of coronary disease (hazard ratio (HR): 18.2) or to die (HR: 2.3); these patients with chest pain also commonly had a history of, or went on to be diagnosed with, gastro-oesophageal reflux disease (Ruigomez et al., 2009). Second, in chest-pain clinics where patients are assessed by a cardiologist: here about one-third of all coronary deaths and non-fatal acute coronary syndromes over a 3-year follow-up occur among patients in whom the initial diagnosis is non-cardiac (Sekhri et al., 2007). This issue of the diagnosis considered, but not made, has been described as 'The art and science of non-disease' (Meador, 1965). These findings suggest limitations in current methods of diagnosing angina.

Time trends in prevalence

Time trends of the incidence of chronic angina might be expected to mirror the well-documented decline in acute MI, under the assumption that the causes of each are the same. Unfortunately there are no large-scale, reliable data to assess time trends in incidence of chronic stable angina. Time-trend data are, however, available for the prevalence of angina pectoris, as assessed by the Rose angina questionnaire on five occasions between 1991 and 2003 in the Health Survey for England (see Figure 20.4). What these data show is that the prevalence of Rose angina cases did decline, but at a much slower rate than that of MI mortality. Furthermore, the prevalence of self-reported diagnosis of angina showed no evidence of decline (Aitsi-Selmi et al., 2008). This is consistent with the growing importance of chronic angina, relative to acute coronary syndromes, but it is not possible to distinguish differential effects on incidence and case fatality.

International variations in angina prevalence

Symptoms of angina pectoris assessed by the Rose angina questionnaire are common across the globe in women and men (see Figure 20.3; Hemingway et al., 2008). A conundrum in angina pectoris research has been the apparent contradiction between symptom studies reporting a similar prevalence of anginal symptoms in women and men, despite the fact that women are less likely to have obstructive disease of the coronary arteries than men. This might reflect an artefact of reporting on questionnaires in which women are more likely to over-report, or men to under-report, their symptoms. Further, this may be conditioned by cultural factors, prevailing health care systems, and other factors which vary between countries. Recently, a systematic review of 74 reports of sex prevalence ratios from 31 countries (Hemingway et al., 2008) found that this lack of male excess was robust across countries which differed markedly in MI mortality rate and was found at all ages. Among doctor-diagnosed incident cases, incidence is similar in women and men (Hemingway et al., 2006); taken together these findings suggest that angina may not share the same causes as acute MI, with its well-recognized preponderance in men.

Symptoms as prognostic endpoints

The patient presenting with symptoms might reasonably expect their clinician to know their chances of being symptom free under different scenarios. However, there is a lack of data on angina symptoms as outcomes. Indeed in a systematic review of 77 studies investigating the role of C reactive protein in the prognosis of stable coronary disease, none reported whether the patients' symptoms improved (Hemingway et al., 2009). South Asian populations were less likely to experience long-term improvement in angina following coronary revascularization when compared to white populations, despite a similar prognosis for adverse clinical events such as MI and death, even after having taken into account appropriateness for revascularization and differences in clinical characteristics (Zaman et al., 2009).

Prevention and treatment

Treatments aimed primarily at ischaemia or atheroma are considered in later sections. Given the high proportion of patients in whom symptoms persist, or recur, there is a need to identify risk factors for

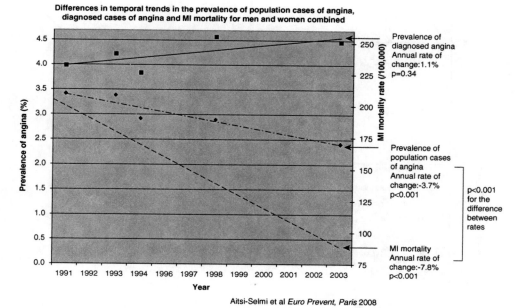

Fig. 20.3 Time trends in diagnosed angina, symptoms of angina, and death from acute myocardial infarction. Reproduced from Hemingway et al., (2008), Prevalence of angina in women versus men: a systematic review and meta-analysis of international variations across 31 countries. Circulation 117, 1526–36 with permission.

Five waves of Health Survey for England 1991 to 2003 n~70,00 participants
Population cases of angina defined by the Rose angina questionnaire.

onset and persistence that might be preventable or that might identify subgroups in the population for targeted interventions or new targets. To reduce the population burden of chronic chest pain, we need to consider primary prevention (stop people getting symptoms in the first place), secondary prevention (pain recurrence or persistence), or tertiary prevention of disability or work loss. It has not been a public health priority *per se* to prevent chronic symptoms of chest pain, because the focus has been on preventing heart attacks. The changes in smoking, obesity, physical activity, and diet known to prevent MI, have seldom been investigated for impact on angina. Symptoms are rarely the primary endpoints in randomized trials, but exceptions do exist (Rapola et al., 1996; Fletcher et al., 1988).

Detection: should more patients with chronic chest-pain consult?

The effectiveness, and cost-effectiveness, of increasing the proportion of people with symptoms who consult their doctor has not been modelled. Public awareness campaigns, so conspicuous for acute chest pain, are lacking for chronic chest pain. Such a campaign for chronic chest pain might promote the message that no woman or man should experience chronic chest tightness without being assessed, and where appropriate, investigated to exclude myocardial ischaemia and coronary artery disease.

Chronic chest pain and myocardial ischaemia

History

Supply–demand hypothesis and early drug development

Pathophysiological understanding of angina through the 20th century focused on the ischaemia resulting from a mismatch between oxygen supply and demand. The first specific treatment for

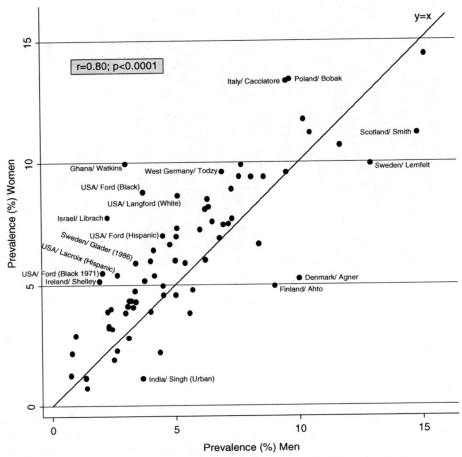

Fig. 20.4 Prevalence of angina symptoms in 31 countries (74 studies) (Hemingway et al., 2008).

Angina defined by the Rose angina questionnaire. Pooled sex-prevalence ratio (women vs. men), from random effects model 1.20 (95% CI: 1.14–1.28).

angina – amyl nitrite, a coronary artery vasodilator – was developed in the 19th century by Brunton (1867). It is one of the few drugs in the 19th-century pharmacopeia that is the basis of current therapy (nitrates). Medical therapy for angina has another distinction: beta-blockers and calcium-channel blockers were among the first drugs designed from a pathophysiological hypothesis and specifically synthesized. Beta-blockers were designed by James Black to decrease oxygen consumption in the heart by slowing its rate, and calcium-channel blockers to increase oxygen supply in the heart through vasodilatation of coronary arteries by Albrecht Fleckenstein. Both became available for clinical use in 1962. Beta-blockers were evidence of the supply–demand model, and had they not worked, this model might have had less enduring success.

Symptoms and the electrocardiogram

The electrocardiogram (ECG; Feil and Siegel, 1928) is the only marker of myocardial ischaemia used in clinical practice and in epidemiological studies. Wolferth and Wood described the use of exercise to provoke attacks of angina pectoris in 1931. They investigated the ECG changes in normal subjects and those with angina but dismissed as too dangerous a technique 'to induce anginal attacks indiscriminately' (Wood et al., 1931). Robert Bruce and colleagues described their multistage treadmill exercise test: 'You would never buy a used car without taking it out for a drive and seeing how the engine performed while it was running . . . and the same is true for evaluating the function of the heart' (Bruce et al., 1963; Bruce and McDonough, 1969). These non-invasive methods were intended to improve on symptom-based diagnoses, although they may only make a small contribution to diagnostic and prognostic accuracy (Sekrhi et al., 2008).

Measurement

Myocardial ischaemia is only indirectly measured in routine clinical practice, with markers such as ST depression on the resting or exercise ECG. More direct measures of ischaemia – coronary sinus oxygen, lactate, and pH – are only used for research purposes. There is intense interest in identifying a circulating biomarker of chronic stable angina, but there is insufficient evidence for individual candidates (such as highly sensitive troponin, or ischaemia-modified albumin) or metabolomic signatures (Brindle et al., 2002).

Ischaemia–pain relations

There is only an oblique relation between evidence of myocardial ischaemia and the presence and severity of angina symptoms. Transient ST depression on the ambulatory ECG commonly occurs without the experience of pain (Chierchia et al., 1983). A threshold of ischaemic activity (duration and severity) may be required before a pain response is initiated, although such relationships show wide inter- and intra-individual variability. So-called 'silent ischaemia' may be more common among people with diabetes and thought to be a result of autonomic dysfunction (Marchant et al., 1993). In patients admitted to the coronary care unit because of unstable angina, the use of diaries of symptoms alongside Holter ambulatory ECG monitoring during the first 24 h of admission reveals that >90% of patients have at least one episode of silent transient myocardial ischaemia (Bugiardini et al., 1995). The duration of ECG ischaemia rather than the presence of recurrent angina was associated with a poorer prognosis in this study.

During ischaemia, a sequence of events is precipitated by an imbalance between myocardial oxygen supply and demand. Studies carried out during coronary angioplasty have shown that this begins with changes in left ventricular compliance, followed by a decreased ejection fraction, increased end-diastolic pressure, ST-segment abnormalities without pain, and finally angina pectoris (Hauser et al., 1985). Newer techniques for the non-invasive assessment of myocardial perfusion such as cardiac magnetic resonance or cardiac computed tomography (CT) may prove to be more sensitive indicators than ECG measurements as they may be able to detect changes at a lower intensity of ischaemia, and thereby precede ECG changes.

Epidemiology

Prevalence and incidence

The prevalence of resting ECG changes of ischaemia are common in developed world populations, with prevalence increasing with age and greater among people with diabetes, obesity and other risk factors (De Bacquer et al., 2000). Women and men with prevalent symptoms of angina (Rose questionnaire) have more ECG abnormalities (ST and T-wave changes) than women and men without angina (Nicholson et al., 1999) and also increased carotid intima–media thickness (Sorlie et al., 1996). In a prospective cohort study of initially healthy civil servants, among first reports of people with angina, 718/970 (74%) did not have a diagnosis. Of the 718, 85 had evidence of ischaemia on the resting ECG carried out as part of the research study (i.e. not for clinical care). Of the 252 with a diagnosis, 80 had evidence of a test abnormality, including tests carried out as part of clinical care. (Hemingway et al., 2003).

Prognosis

Resting ECG changes of ischaemia are associated with coronary heart disease (CHD) mortality (Sekhri et al., 2008), and this association may be stronger among those with concurrent symptoms (Hemingway et al., 2000). Exercise ECG changes of ischaemia are strongly associated with CHD mortality (Lauer et al., 1999), although in ambulatory patients with suspected angina, exercise ECG provided limited incremental value over the clinical history and 47% of all events during follow-up occurred in patients with a negative exercise ECG result (Sekhri et al., 2008).

Prevention and treatment

Primary prevention of onset of ischaemia with drugs

Different classes of anti-anginal medications may not differ in their ability to prevent the onset of angina. The opportunity to investigate this comes from randomized trials of agents used both for lowering blood pressure and for relief of angina symptoms. In one such trial comparing a beta-blocker with a calcium-channel blocker among patients who were hypertensive, the incidence of stable angina (defined as typical symptoms + either ischaemia or evidence of coronary atheroma) was high (4 per 1000 population) and similar in both trial arms (Dahlof et al., 2005). As a growing proportion of the general population are treated with primary preventive medication, Go and colleagues reported that statin use may alter the relative proportions of initial manifestations of coronary disease, decreasing acute MI and increasing chronic stable angina (Go et al., 2006).

Prevention of ischaemic episodes among patients with ischaemia

Current therapies that reduce angina frequency aim to increase the threshold at which demand-induced myocardial ischaemic symptoms become evident. These include drugs (e.g. nitrates, β-blockers, calcium antagonists, nicorandil, and ranolazine), exercise conditioning, enhanced external counterpulsation, and coronary revascularization. The use of anti-anginal drugs improves symptoms but not prognosis for serious adverse clinical events (Heidenreich et al., 1999), whilst a meta-analysis of randomized controlled trials comparing coronary revascularization with drugs alone (including those for secondary prevention such as statins and aspirin) concluded that revascularization led to a reduction in angina but conferred no beneficial effects on risk of MI or death (Bucher et al., 2000).

Chronic chest pain and coronary atheroma

History

Shift in emphasis from symptom to site

The role of atherosclerosis of the coronary arteries in chronic chest pain has evolved markedly since an Italian physician Morgagni (1761) described arteriosclerosis of coronary arteries in 1761 (he did not attribute symptoms to these post-mortem findings). In shifting the emphasis of diagnosis from 'symptom to site' (Porter, 1997), he led the way for English physicians' patho-anatomical investigations. Edward Jenner, before his smallpox research, and Caleb Parry (Parry, 1799) were the first to attribute angina pectoris to obstruction and ossification of the coronary arteries. Parry also suggested that this may be due to myocardial ischaemia. The first page of the first issue of the *New England Journal of Medicine* in 1812 was devoted to angina pectoris (Warren and Bracket, 1812), emphasizing the role of coronary ossification, although there were few case reports from North America, or indeed mainland Europe, until well into the 19th century. Alan Burns, a Scottish scientist without medical qualifications (who nevertheless performed surgery in St Petersburg), experimented with cutting blood supply to limbs, observing loss of function. Early in the 19th century he hypothesized that this was the underlying pathological process in angina: '[T]he supply of energy and expenditure do not balance' (Burns, 1809). A plumbing model of angina emerged narrowing of coronary artery, due to atherosclerosis in the large coronary arteries, leads to myocardial ischaemia, which in turn leads to chest pain. Mason Sones carried out the first coronary angiogram in 1959, allowing visualization of the luminal narrowing of large coronary arteries in live patients. The rate of coronary angiography expanded rapidly with the advent of coronary artery bypass grafting surgery in 1967 and angioplasty in 1974, and the angiographic findings to some extent came to supplant the patient's symptoms in the diagnosis of angina.

Variable relationship between stenoses and angina

In his Lumelian lectures on angina pectoris in 1910, Osler stated: 'We are all united in the acceptance . . . of the close connection of lesions of the coronary arteries with the disease . . . The most remarkable peculiarity is the variation in the extent of the involvement' (Opie, 2004). Osler classified angina into 'true, false, and hysterical' forms, based on its association (or not) with underlying coronary artery pathology, emphasizing that it was a term for a symptom complex, not a disease. James Mackenzie, one of the pioneers of cardiological research, who then moved on to found an institute of general practice research, suffered from angina for decades. He included himself (case No. 23) in his 123 case series in *Angina Pectoris*, a classical text published in 1923. He requested that his heart be submitted to macro- and microscopic examination after his death; this exemplified the relationship between his symptoms and underlying pathology (Waterston et al., 1939). He championed long-term follow-up of patients as a means of studying all stages of disease, especially its predisposing and early phases.

Measurement

Lumen

Coronary atheroma is measured only indirectly in routine clinical care, i.e. there is rarely any direct acquisition of tissue in which the pathognomonic cellular and molecular processes of plaque biology are directly observed. Invasive coronary angiography is currently the only widely performed investigation for assessing coronary atheroma. It measures the inside of the artery – the lumen – identifying the number of vessels involved, and the site and extent of the stenosis (narrowing). Between 20% and 30% of patients with symptoms of angina have no evidence of obstruction at angiography; and this proportion has changed little over the last five decades. There is no clear relationship between degree of luminal stenosis and risk of plaque rupture. Flow-limiting stenoses are present in only 30–40% of cases of MI (Little et al., 1988). Narrowed coronary arteries do not necessarily cause symptoms of chronic chest pain. A patient with narrowing and chest pain, but with a negative non-invasive ischaemic test may derive no symptomatic benefit from revascularization. In such situations the lesion was not a 'culprit' but a 'bystander'. This can create difficult management problems, particularly when the pain is atypical. The processes which make a lesion become symptomatic are poorly understood. Population-based cohorts assessed with computed tomographic or magnetic resonance angiography may help elucidate these factors.

Wall

There are three main limitations of invasive coronary angiography. First, it provides little information about the arterial wall. The coronary artery adapts to the presence of an atherosclerotic plaque by positive remodelling, a process in which the vessel dilates to accommodate the plaque without narrowing the lumen (Glagov et al., 1987). Intravascular ultrasound provides a measure of atherosclerotic plaque and the vessel wall beyond the lumen, but a recent review found no papers correlating findings with chest pain symptoms (Springer and Dewey, 2009). The intracoronary physiologic measurement of fractional flow reserve (the ratio of maximal blood flow in a stenotic artery to normal maximal flow) during percutaneous coronary revascularization is increasingly used to identify ischaemia-causing lesions that might require stenting. In a clinical trial assessing fractional flow reserve for guiding stent placement, the intervention reduced myocardial infarction and revascularisation rates but not angina at 1-year follow-up, compared to conventional angiographic methods (Tonino et al., 2009).

Function

The second limitation of invasive angiography is that it provides no information on morphological and functional aspects of atheroma. Non-invasive CT angiography, coronary artery calcification and magnetic resonance angiography and PET may provide insights into the causes of chronic chest pain. Nuclear medicine myocardial perfusion-imaging techniques can identify the territory of coronary artery involvement, but most research on perfusion scans relates to diagnostic or prognostic (event prediction) performance, rather than any role in understanding symptoms.

Microvascular

Third, invasive angiography images only large arteries, and many patients with chronic chest pain do not have evidence of large artery involvement. The microvascular coronary circulation can be assessed non-invasively by the coronary flow reserve in the left anterior descending artery by dipyridamole echocardiography (Graf et al., 2007). These techniques are, however, seldom applied outside a research context and they do not provide direct evidence that abnormal coronary flow reserve is the cause of chest pain.

Epidemiology

Large-scale clinical record studies based in primary care suggest that new-onset angina defined by both a new filled prescription for anti-anginal medication, and evidence of a test abnormality (such as abnormal exercise ECG or coronary angiography) is common with an incidence of 1–3 per 100 patients per year (Hemingway et al., 2006). This rate is 2–5 times more common than the incidence of MI. The incidence increases with age into the ninth decade of life.

Determinants of onset (aetiologic factors)

The epidemiology of stable coronary atheroma is poorly understood, and has received less attention than the epidemiology of its principal complication, acute MI. Population-based cases of prevalent typical angina symptoms are strongly associated in women and men with the presence and amount of coronary artery calcium (Oei et al., 2004); see Table 20.2. Several lines of evidence suggest that the aetiology of acute coronary syndromes and stable coronary atheroma may differ. First, the Multi Ethnic Study of Atherosclerosis showed that blacks in the general population have a lower prevalence of any coronary artery calcium and a lower mean distribution of calcium scores, after adjustment for risk factors (Bid et al., 2005), yet overall mortality from

Table 20.2 Association between angina symptoms from Rose angina questionnaire and coronary artery calcium distribution

Distribution of coronary artery calcification	Total number	Number with angina	*Odds ratio for association between angina and coronary artery calcification
Men: lowest quartile	233	2	1.0 (reference_
	233	5	1.7
	234	17	7.4
highest quartile	233	32	14.1
Women: lowest quartile	270	8	1.0
	270	12	1.4
	269	10	1.1
highest quartile	271	29	3.6

*Adjusted for age, body mass index, systolic blood pressure, total cholesterol, HDL-cholesterol, diabetes, smoking
Data from Oei et al., 2004.

CHD (which incorporates case fatality) shows a small excess among African Americans. Second, a study of coronary angiography among patients undergoing valvular surgery found that the prevalence of atherosclerosis did not fall during a period of rapid decline in acute MI incidence (Enriquez-Sarano et al., 2007). Third, the Wellcome Trust genome-wide association study (Samani et al., 2007) reported a locus on chromosome 15 which appeared to have a stronger effect for coronary artery disease alone, than for cases with MI, although this awaits replication.

Prognosis of coronary atheroma

The number of diseased vessels at coronary angiography is consistently related to all-cause and cardiovascular mortality. For example, there is about a twofold risk of cardiovascular death among patients with two-vessel disease compared to those with no diseased vessels, among those treated medically. However, it is important to set into context the strength of this association – it is similar in magnitude to other risk factors (such as current vs. never smokers) for cardiovascular disease events. This suggests that, according to current methods of measurement, coronary atheroma is a risk factor for, but not synonymous with, other disease manifestations such as acute MI.

Prognosis of 'normal' coronary angiographic findings

In patients with cardiac syndrome X, typical ST-segment depression on the ECG during exercise suggests myocardial ischaemia, but in the absence of narrowed large coronary arteries. The prognosis (in terms of risk of death or acute MI) of such patients is not as benign as was once thought (Bugiardini et al., 2007). Among 2198 women and 1449 men with 'normal' coronary angiograms, within 1 year of catheterization, 1% died, 0.6% had a stroke, and 0.1% underwent revascularization. Thirty (1.4 %) women were re-hospitalized for acute coronary syndrome or chest pain with repeat cardiac catheterization compared with seven men (0.5%; Humphries et al., 2008). Coronary micro-vascular dysfunction is associated with chest-pain symptoms (Camici and Crea, 2007).

Prevention and treatment

A major focus of the prevention and treatment of chronic chest pain associated with angiographic changes has been anatomical: to identify and 'revascularize' one or more coronary artery lesion with coronary artery bypass grafts or percutaneous coronary intervention (PCI). Whilst each procedure is effective, improving symptom control compared with medication, their relative effectiveness and cost-effectiveness remains unclear. In this regard, the recent Clinical Outcomes Utilizing Revascularization and Aggressive Drug Evaluation (COURAGE) trial (Boden et al., 2007) is a particularly important study for two reasons. First, it suggests that intensive medical management for patients with symptoms and angiographic evidence of disease is associated with similar rates of cardiovascular events alone or in combination with PCI. By contesting the role of PCI, this raises the question of the extent to which imaging of the coronary arteries is required in the first place. Second, it provides 'reverse phenotyping' evidence. If the causal model by which stable coronary disease leads to cardiovascular events involves 'culprit lesions' but removing these specific luminal narrowing does not lower event rates, the model is undermined.

Refractory chronic angina

Treatment 'failure' may occur early after therapy initiation; after 6-years follow-up, 50% of patients are symptomatic regardless of initial therapy. Genetic factors might play a role. The anti-anginal drugs, dihydropyridine calcium-channel blockers, appear to interact with common variants in the *NOS1AP* gene, such that cardiovascular mortality is higher among users with minor G allele (Becker et al., 2009). Angina which is refractory to revascularization, or medical management, has poorly understood causes, and this is one reason for the heterogenous range of potential therapeutic options, including analgesic modalities (e.g. transcutaneous electric nerve stimulation, left stellate ganglion blockade, endoscopic thoracoscopic sympathectomy, thoracic epidural anaesthesia, and spinal cord stimulation), external balloon counter pulsation, stem cell therapy, and myocardial laser revascularization by surgical or percutaneous technique (Mannheimer et al., 2002). There is no evidence that these procedures improve prognosis for future adverse major cardiac events, and only a few of these options have been tested in randomized studies for their effect on reducing pain.

Syndrome X

Whilst the main aim of clinical management is the control of symptoms, there have been few trials. In addition to the usual anti-anginal drugs such as β-blocking agents and calcium antagonists, beneficial effects have been reported from exercise rehabilitation programmes (Asbury et al., 2008). Although there is no evidence that treating depression or anxiety improves angina symptoms in patients with persistent chest pain after optimum medical treatment, one trial of imipramine in women with chest pain despite the absence of coronary stenosis found reduction in symptoms, independent of psychiatric morbidity (Cannon et al., 1994).

Cardiac rehabilitation and behavioural change

Cardiac rehabilitation – typically involving exercise training, education, and counselling – may improve chest pain and mental state, although it is not possible to distinguish which facet of therapy is effective (Asbury et al., 2008). However, rehabilitation is less commonly offered to, or taken up by, patients with chronic stable angina compared with patients post MI. Patients with stable angina randomized to a 12-month exercise training had higher event-free survival and exercise capacity at 1 year compared with patients randomized to PCI (Hambrecht et al., 2004).

The exercise-training group was also associated with lower costs due to lower re-hospitalizations and repeat revascularizations.

Multifaceted, complex interventions

Since the diagnosis and management of chronic angina is a complex process, multifaceted, system-level interventions designed to improve symptomatic and event outcomes are potential targets for evaluation in cluster randomized trials. The first specialist contact may offer a locus for intervention in those countries, such as the UK, where this occurs to a large extent in dedicated clinics in each hospital. Research on improving management decisions early in the trajectory of symptomatic coronary disease has been largely neglected (Mant et al., 2004). Robust cluster-randomized trials are feasible in cardiac care settings to test system-level interventions (Ritchie et al., 2003). Interventions might include clinical decision-support systems, with patient-specific guidance on investigation (Junghans et al., 2007; Hemingway et al., 2008), and early initiation of risk-lowering medication, in relation to formal assessment of prognostic risk (Clayton et al., 2005).

Conclusion

Were it the case that the frequency of diagnosed angina in the general population was declining and people with chronic chest pain were reliably triaged into cardiac and non-cardiac chest pain, and that most patients were free of symptoms over long-term follow-up, and that the risk of cardiovascular death was similar to that of the general population, then there would be grounds for considering angina pectoris a low priority in terms of public health and clinical research. The fact that none of these statements is true suggests the importance of new approaches, identifying novel interventions, as well as better implementation of what is known to be effective.

Understanding chest-pain diagnosis and management in the presence of coronary artery stenosis, as well as the challenge of angina symptoms in the absence of stenosis or after treatment, requires investigation of all the activity that contributes to the performance of angina in primary care and specialist settings. The ultimate goal is to further develop diagnosis and management that is culturally and psychologically competent, recognizes and engages with lay models of chest pain and heart disease, and offers medical and surgical interventions to the right people.

References

Aitsi-Selmi, A., Shipley, M. and Hemingway, H. 2008: Stable angina pectoris: comparison of trends in symptoms and diagnosed cases of angina from 1991 to 2003 with trends in MI mortality. *Euro Prevent, Paris.*

Asbury, E.A., Slattery, C., Grant, A., Evans, L., Barbir, M. and Collins, P. 2008: Cardiac rehabilitation for the treatment of women with chest pain and normal coronary arteries. *Menopause* 15, 454–60.

Becker, M.L., Visser, L.E., Newton-Cheh, C., Hofman, A., Uitterlinden, A.G., Witteman, J.C., et al. 2009: A common NOS1AP genetic polymorphism is associated with increased cardiovascular mortality in users of dihydropyridine calcium channel blockers. *Br J Clin Pharmacol* 67, 61–7.

Bild, D.E., Detrano, R., Peterson, D., Guerci, A., Liu, K., Shahar, E., et al. 2005: Ethnic differences in coronary calcification: the Multi-Ethnic Study of Atherosclerosis (MESA). *Circulation* 111, 1313–20.

Boden, W.E., O'Rourke, R.A., Teo, K.K., Hartigan, P.M., Maron, D.J., Kostuk, W.J., et al. 2007: Optimal medical therapy with or without PCI for stable coronary disease. *N Engl J Med* 356, 1503–16.

Brindle, J.T., Antti, H., Holmes, E., Tranter, G., Nicholson, J.K., Bethell, H.W., et al. 2002: Rapid and noninvasive diagnosis of the presence and severity of coronary heart disease using 1H-NMR-based metabonomics. *Nat Med* 8, 1439–44.

Bristow, M.R. 1990: The surgically denervated, transplanted human heart. *Circulation* 82, 658–60.

Bruce, R.A., Blackmon, J.R., Jones, J.W. and Strait, G. 1963: Exercise testing in adult normal subjects and cardiac patients. *Pediatrics* **32**, Suppl-56.

Bruce, R.A. and McDonough, J.R. 1969: Stress testing in screening for cardiovascular disease. *Bull N Y Acad Med* **45**, 1288–305.

Brunton, T.L. 1867: On the use of nitrite of amyl in angina pectoris. *Lancet* **2**, 97–8.

Bucher, H.C., Hengstler, P., Schindler, C. and Guyatt, G.H. 2000: Percutaneous transluminal coronary angioplasty versus medical treatment for non-acute coronary heart disease: meta-analysis of randomised controlled trials. *BMJ* **321**, 73–7.

Bugiardini, R., Badimon, L., Collins, P., Erbel, R., Fox, K., Hamm, C., et al. 2007: Angina, "normal" coronary angiography, and vascular dysfunction: risk assessment strategies. *PLoS Med* **4**, e12.

Bugiardini, R., Borghi, A., Pozzati, A., Ruggeri, A., Puddu, P. and Maseri, A. 1995: Relation of severity of symptoms to transient myocardial ischemia and prognosis in unstable angina. *J Am Coll Cardiol* **25**, 597–604.

Burns, A. 1809: Observations on some of the most frequent and important diseases of the heart; on aneurysm of the thoracic aorta; on preternatural pulsation in the epigastric region; and on the unusual origin and distribution of some of the large arteries of the human body. Edinburgh: Bryce and Co.

Camici, P.G. and Crea, F. 2007: Coronary microvascular dysfunction. *N Engl J Med* **356**, 830–40.

Cannon, R.O., III, Quyyumi, A.A., Mincemoyer, R., Stine, A.M., Gracely, R.H., Smith, W.B. et al. 1994: Imipramine in patients with chest pain despite normal coronary angiograms. *N Engl J Med* **330**, 1411–17.

Carnes, D., Parsons, S., Ashby, D., Breen, A., Foster, N.E., Pincus, T., et al. 2007: Chronic musculoskeletal pain rarely presents in a single body site: results from a UK population study. *Rheumatology* **46**, 1168–70.

Chierchia, S., Lazzari, M., Freedman, B., Brunelli, C. and Maseri, A. 1983: Impairment of myocardial perfusion and function during painless myocardial ischemia. *J Am Coll Cardiol* **1**, 924–30.

Clayton, T.C., Lubsen, J., Pocock, S.J., Voko, Z., Kirwan, B.A., Fox, K.A., et al. 2005: Risk score for predicting death, myocardial infarction, and stroke in patients with stable angina, based on a large randomised trial cohort of patients. *BMJ* **331**, 869.

Dahlof, B., Sever, P.S., Poulter, N.R., Wedel, H., Beevers, D.G., Caulfield, M., et al. 2005: Prevention of cardiovascular events with an antihypertensive regimen of amlodipine adding perindopril as required versus atenolol adding bendroflumethiazide as required, in the Anglo-Scandinavian Cardiac Outcomes Trial-Blood Pressure Lowering Arm (ASCOT-BPLA): a multicentre randomised controlled trial. *Lancet* **366**, 895–906.

De Bacquer, D., De Backer, G. and Kornitzer, M. 2000: Prevalences of ECG findings in large population based samples of men and women. *Heart* **84**, 625–33.

Diamond, G. and Forrester, J. 1979: Analysis of probability as an aid in the clinical diagnosis of coronary artery disease. *N Engl J Med* **300**, 1350–8.

Enriquez-Sarano, M., Klodas, E., Garratt, K.N., Bailey, K.R., Tajik, A.J. and Holmes, D.R. Jr. 1996: Secular trends in coronary atherosclerosis--analysis in patients with valvular regurgitation. *N Engl J Med* **335**, 316–22.

Eslick, G.D. 2008: Chest pain units. *Dis Mon* **54**, 613–14.

Eslick, G.D., Jones, M.P. and Talley, N.J. 2003: Non-cardiac chest pain: prevalence, risk factors, impact and consulting--a population-based study. *Aliment Pharmacol Ther* **17**, 1115–24.

Feil, H. and Siegel, M.L. 1928: Electrocardiographic changes during attacks of angina pectoris. *Am J Med Sciences* **175**, 255–60.

Fletcher, A., McLoone, P. and Bulpitt, C. 1988: Quality of life on angina therapy: a randomised controlled trial of transdermal glyceryl trinitrate against placebo. *Lancet* **2**, 4–8.

Fox, K., Garcia, M.A., Ardissino, D., Buszman, P., Camici, P.G., Crea, F., et al. 2006: Guidelines on the management of stable angina pectoris: executive summary: the Task Force on the Management of Stable Angina Pectoris of the European Society of Cardiology. *Eur Heart J* **27**, 1341–81.

Galdas, P., Cheater, F. and Marshall, P. 2007: What is the role of masculinity in white and South Asian men's decisions to seek medical help for cardiac chest pain? *J Health Serv Res Policy* **12**, 223–9.

Glagov, S., Weisenberg, E., Zarins, C.K., Stankunavicius, R. and Kolettis, G.J. 1987: Compensatory enlargement of human atherosclerotic coronary arteries. *N Engl J Med* **316**, 1371–5.

Go, A.S., Iribarren, C., Chandra, M., Lathon, P.V., Fortmann, S.P., Quertermous, T., et al. 2006: Statin and beta-blocker therapy and the initial presentation of coronary heart disease. *Ann Intern Med* **144**, 229–38.

Good, B.J. 1994: Medicine, Rationality and Experience: An Anthropological Perspective. Cambridge: Cambridge University Press.

Graf, S., Khorsand, A., Gwechenberger, M., Novotny, C., Kletter, K., Sochor, H., et al. 2007: Typical chest pain and normal coronary angiogram: cardiac risk factor analysis versus PET for detection of microvascular disease. *J Nucl Med* **48**, 175–81.

Griffin, S.C., Barber, J.A., Manca, A., Sculpher, M.J., Thompson, S.G., Buxton, M.J. and Hemingway H. 2007: Cost effectiveness of clinically appropriate decisions on alternative treatments for angina pectoris: prospective observational study. *BMJ* **334**, 624.

Hambrecht, R., Walther, C., Mobius-Winkler, S., Gielen, S., Linke, A., Conradi, K., et al. 2004: Percutaneous coronary angioplasty compared with exercise training in patients with stable coronary artery disease: a randomized trial. *Circulation* **109**, 1371–8.

Hauser, A.M., Gangadharan, V., Ramos, R.G., Gordon, S. and Timmis, G.C. 1985: Sequence of mechanical, electrocardiographic and clinical effects of repeated coronary artery occlusion in human beings: echocardiographic observations during coronary angioplasty. *J Am Coll Cardiol* **5**, 193–7.

Hayashida, M., Fukuda, K., and Fukunaga, A. 2005: Clinical application of adenosine and ATP for pain control. *J Anaesth* **19**, 225–35.

Heberden, W. 1772, Some account of a disorder of the breast. *Medical Transactions of the Royal College of Physicians* **2**, 59–67.

Heidenreich, P.A., McDonald, K.M., Hastie, T., Fadel, B., Hagan, V., Lee, B.K., et al. 1999: Meta-analysis of trials comparing beta-blockers, calcium antagonists, and nitrates for stable angina. *JAMA* **281**, 1927–36.

Helman, C.G. 1984: Disease and pseudo-disease: a case history of pseudo-angina. In: Hahn RA, Gaines AD, eds. *Physicians of Western Medicine: Anthropological Perspectives on Theory and Practice*. Dordrecht: D. Reidel Publishing Company; pp. 293–331.

Hemingway, H., Chen, R., Junghans, C., Timmis, A., Eldridge, S., Black, N., et al. 2008: Appropriateness criteria for coronary angiography in angina: reliability and validity. *Ann Intern Med* **149**, 221–31.

Hemingway, H., Fitzpatrick, N.K., Gnani, S., Feder, G., Walker, N., Crook, A.M., et al. 2004: Prospective validity of measuring angina severity with Canadian Cardiovascular Society class: The ACRE study. *Can J Cardiol* **20**, 305–9.

Hemingway, H., Philipson, P., Chen, R., Fitzpatrick, N.K., Damant, J., Shipley, M. et al. 2010: Evaluating the Quality of Research into a Single Prognostic Biomarker: A Systematic Review and Meta-analysis of 83 Studies of C-Reactive Protein in Stable Coronary Artery Disease. PLoS Medicine www.plosmedicine.org 7, e100028

Hemingway, H., Langenberg, C., Damant, J., Frost, C., Pyorala, K. and Barrett-Connor, E. 2008: Prevalence of angina in women versus men: a systematic review and meta-analysis of international variations across 31 countries. *Circulation* **117**, 1526–36.

Hemingway, H., McCallum, A., Shipley, M., Manderbacka, K., Martikainen, P. and Keskimäki, I. 2006: Incidence and prognostic implications of stable angina pectoris among women and men. *JAMA* **295**, 1404–11.

Hemingway, H., Shipley, M., Britton, A., Page, M., MacFarlane, P. and Marmot, M. 2003: Prognosis of angina with and without a diagnosis: 11 year follow up in the Whitehall II prospective cohort study. *BMJ* **327**, 895.

Hemingway, H., Shipley, M., MacFarlane, P. and Marmot, M. 2000: Impact of socioeconomic status on coronary mortality in people with symptoms, electrocardiographic abnormalities, both or neither: the original Whitehall study 25 year follow up [In Process Citation]. *J Epidemiol Community Health* **54**, 510–16.

Hlatky, M.A. 1995: Patient preferences and clinical guidelines. *JAMA* **273**, 1219–20.

Hravnak, M., Whittle, J., Kelley, M.E., Sereika, S., Good, C.B., Ibrahim, S.A., et al. 2007: Symptom expression in coronary heart disease and revascularization recommendations for black and white patients. *Am J Public Health* **97**, 1701–8.

Humphries, K.H., Pu, A., Gao, M., Carere, R.G. and Pilote, L. 2008: Angina with "normal" coronary arteries: sex differences in outcomes. *Am Heart J* **155**, 375–81.

Junghans, C., Feder, G., Timmis, A.D., Eldridge, S., Sekhri, N., Black, N., et al. 2007: Effect of patient-specific ratings vs conventional guidelines on investigation decisions in angina: Appropriateness of Referral and Investigation in Angina (ARIA) Trial. *Arch Intern Med* **167**, 195–202.

Lauer, M.S., Francis, G.S., Okin, P.M., Pashkow, F.J., Snader, C.E. and Marwick, T.H. 1999: Impaired chronotropic response to exercise stress testing as a predictor of mortality. *JAMA* **10**, 281, 524–9.

Little, W.C., Constantinescu, M., Applegate, R.J., Kutcher, M.A., Burrows, M.T., Kahl, F.R., et al. 1988: Can coronary angiography predict the site of a subsequent myocardial infarction in patients with mild-to-moderate coronary artery disease? *Circulation* **78**, 1157–66.

Mannheimer, C., Camici, P., Chester, M.R., Collins, A., DeJongste, M., Eliasson, T., et al. 2002: The problem of chronic refractory angina; report from the ESC Joint Study Group on the Treatment of Refractory Angina. *Eur Heart J* **23**, 355–70.

Mant, J., McManus, R.J., Oakes, R.A., Delaney, B.C., Barton, P.M., Deeks, J.J., et al. 2004: Systematic review and modelling of the investigation of acute and chronic chest pain presenting in primary care. *Health Technol Assess* **8**, iii, 1–158.

Marchant, B., Umachandran, V., Stevenson, R., Kopelman, P.G. and Timmis, A.D. 1993: Silent myocardial ischemia: role of subclinical neuropathy in patients with and without diabetes. *J Am Coll Cardiol* **22**, 1433–7.

Meador, C.K. 1965: The art and science of nondisease. *N Engl J Med* **272**, 92–5.

Michaels L. 2001: The eighteenth century origins of Angina Pectoris : predisposing causes, recognition and aftermath. London: Wellcome Trust Centre.

Mol, A. 2003: The Body Multiple: Ontology in Medical Practice. Durham: Duke University Press.

Morgagni, G.B. 1761. De Sedibus et Causis Morborum per Anatomen Indagatis (On the Seats and Causes of Diseases Investigated by Anatomy). Venice: Folio

Nease, R.F., Jr., Kneeland, T., O'Connor, G.T., Sumner, W., Lumpkins, C., Shaw, L., et al. 1995: Variation in patient utilities for outcomes of the management of chronic stable angina. Implications for clinical practice guidelines. Ischemic Heart Disease Patient Outcomes Research Team. *JAMA* **273**, 1185–90.

Nicholson, A., White, I.R., MacFarlane, P., Brunner, E. and Marmot, M. 1999: Rose questionnaire angina in younger men and women: gender differences in the relationship to cardiovascular risk factors and other reported symptoms. *J Clin Epidemiol* **52**, 337–46.

Nilsson, S., Scheike, M., Engblom, D., Karlsson, L.G., Molstad, S., Akerlind, I., et al. 2003: Chest pain and ischaemic heart disease in primary care. *Br J Gen Pract* **53**, 378–82.

Oei, H.H., Vliegenthart, R., Deckers, J.W., Hofman, A., Oudkerk, M. and Witteman, J.C. 2004: The association of Rose questionnaire angina pectoris and coronary calcification in a general population: the Rotterdam Coronary Calcification Study. *Ann Epidemiol* **14**, 431–6.

Opie, L.H. 2004: Angina pectoris: the evolution of concepts. *J Cardiovasc Pharmacol Ther* **9**, Suppl 1:S3–S9.

Parry, C. 1799: Inquiry into the Symptoms and Causes of the Syncope Anginose, commonly called Angina Pectoris.London: Cadell and Davis

Philpott, S., Boynton, P.M., Feder, G. and Hemingway, H. 2001: Gender differences in descriptions of angina symptoms and health problems immediately prior to angiography: the ACRE study. Appropriateness of Coronary Revascularisation study. *Soc Sci Med* **52**, 1565–75.

Porter, R. 1997: *The Greatest Benefit to Mankind: A Medical History of Humanity from Antiquity to the Present.* London: Harper Collins.

Rapola, J.M., Virtamo, J., Haukka, J.K., Heinonen, O.P., Albanes, D., Taylor, P.R., et al. 1996: Effect of vitamin E and beta carotene on the incidence of angina pectoris. A randomized, double-blind, controlled trial. *JAMA* **275**, 693–8.

Ritchie, V., Spencer, L. and O'Connor, W. 2003: carrying out qualitative analysis. In: Ritchie, J., Lewis, J., eds. *Qualitative Research Practice*. London: Sage.

Rose, G. 1962: The diagnosis of ischaemic heart pain and intermittent claudication in field surveys. *Bull WHO* **27**, 645–58.

Rosen, S.D., Paulesu, E., Frith, C.D., Frackowiak, R.S., Davies, G.J., Jones, T., et al. 1994: Central nervous pathways mediating angina pectoris. *Lancet* **344**, 147–50.

Ruigomez, A., Masso-Gonzalez, E.L., Johansson, S., Wallander, M.A. and Garcia-Rodriguez, L.A. 2009: Chest pain without established ischaemic heart disease in primary care patients: associated comorbidities and mortality. *Br J Gen Pract* **59**, e78–86.

Ruigomez, A., Rodriguez, L.A., Wallander, M.A., Johansson, S. and Jones, R. 2006: Chest pain in general practice: incidence, comorbidity and mortality. *Fam Pract* **23**, 167–74.

Samani, N.J., Erdmann, J., Hall, A.S., Hengstenberg, C., Mangino, M., Mayer, B., et al. 2007: Genomewide association analysis of coronary artery disease. *N Engl J Med* **357**, 443–53.

Sekhri, N., Feder, G.S., Junghans, C., Eldridge, S., Umaipalan, A., Madhu, R., et al. 2008: Incremental prognostic value of the exercise electrocardiogram in the initial assessment of patients with suspected angina: cohort study. *BMJ* **337**, a2240.

Sekhri, N., Feder, G.S., Junghans, C., Hemingway, H. and Timmis, A.D. 2007: How effective are rapid access chest pain clinics? Prognosis of incident angina and non-cardiac chest pain in 8762 consecutive patients. *Heart* **93**, 458–63.

Sekhri, N., Timmis, A., Chen, R., Junghans, C., Walsh, N., Zaman, J., et al. 2008: Inequity of access to investigation and effect on clinical outcomes: prognostic study of coronary angiography for suspected stable angina pectoris. *BMJ* **336**, 1058–61.

Somerville, C., Featherstone, K., Hemingway, H., Timmis, A. and Feder, G. 2008: Performing stable angina: an ethnographic study. *Soc Sci Med* **66**, 1467–508.

Sorlie, P.D., Cooper, L., Schreiner, P.J., Rosamond, W. and Szklo, M. 1996: Repeatability and validity of the Rose questionnaire for angina pectoris in the Atherosclerosis Risk in Communities Study. *J Clin Epidemiol* **49**, 719–25.

Springer, I. and Dewey, M. 2009: Comparison of multislice computed tomography with intravascular ultrasound for detection and characterization of coronary artery plaques: A systematic review. *Eur J Radiol* **71**, 275–82.

Tonino, P.A., De, B.B., Pijls, N.H., Siebert, U., Ikeno, F., Veer, M., et al. 2009: Fractional flow reserve versus angiography for guiding percutaneous coronary intervention. *N Engl J Med* **360**, 213–24.

Warren, J. and Bracket, J. 1812: Remarks on angina pectoris. *N Engl J Med Surg* **1**, 1–11.

Waterston, D., Orr, J. and Cappell, D.F. 1939: Sir James Mackenzie's Heart. *Br Heart J* **1**, 237–48.

Wood, F.C., Wolferth, C.C. and Livezey, M.M. 1931: Angina Pectoris: the clinical and electrocardiographic phenomena of the attack and their comparison with the effects of experiemental temporary coronary occlusion. *Arch Intern Med* **47**, 339–65.

Zaman, M.J., Crook, A.M., Junghans, C., Fitzpatrick, N.K., Feder, G., Timmis, A.D., et al. 2009: Ethnic differences in long-term improvement of angina following revascularization or medical management: a comparison between south Asians and white Europeans. *J Public Health* **31**, 168–74.

Zaman, M.J., Junghans, C., Sekhri, N., Chen, R., Feder, G.S., Timmis, A.D., et al. 2008: Presentation of stable angina pectoris among women and South Asian people. *CMAJ* **179**, 659–67.

Chapter 21

Cancer and chronic pain

Fiona M. Blyth and Frances Boyle

Introduction

Population prevalence studies of chronic pain from different countries suggest that cancer is an uncommon cause of persistent pain in the community. As cancer is common, and most people with cancer experience pain, it would seem that mortality from cancer minimizes the contribution of cancer pain to the community burden of persistent pain. However, as cancer incidence rates increase and mortality rates decline, an increasingly large long-term cancer-survivor cohort has emerged in most developed countries.

Both cancer and persistent pain (e.g. due to musculoskeletal diseases) are conditions associated with ageing, so that the same segment of the population is at risk of experiencing disease burden attributable to both conditions. This observation, taken together with the increased survivorship from cancer, should lead us to challenge existing thinking about persistent pain and cancer. In the context of increasingly long survival, the distinction between cancer pain and non-cancer pain perhaps becomes less useful. If people are developing cancer at the same age as experience of persistent pain is most common, what might the impact of pre-existing non-cancer persistent pain be on the experience of new pain from cancer? And what is the persistent pain experience of long-term cancer survivors, irrespective of the underlying cause?

Trends in cancer incidence, mortality, and survival

Cancer survival rates are increasing, due to a combination of factors including earlier detection of cancer (when cancer is at an earlier phase of development) and better therapeutic interventions. The changing landscape of cancer survival has led to calls for cancer to be thought of as a chronic disease [Centre for Disease Control and Prevention (CDC), 2004]. Less than half of those currently diagnosed with cancer will die of the disease (CDC, 2004). Predicting future trends in cancer incidence (i.e. new cases of cancer) is difficult because of the many factors which may influence it, particularly when making comparisons between or across countries. However, the impact of a growing world population and increasing longevity on global cancer incidence rates is clear – there will be more people living longer, and it is older people who are most at risk of developing cancer. In other words, the ageing of populations in many countries will drive cancer incidence rates in years to come. On this basis, the estimated number of new cancers of all types worldwide is expected to rise from 10.06 million in 2000 to 15.35 million in 2020 and to 23.83 million in 2050 (Parkin, 2001).

Overview of cancer-related pain

While the focus of this chapter is not on the many causes of cancer-related pain, this section provides a brief overview of this complex topic as context for the following sections. Broadly speaking,

Table 21.1 Overview of causes of pain in people with cancer

Direct effects of tumour (primary and metastatic disease) e.g. mechanical pressure, infiltration of neural structures
Indirect effects of tumour (primary and metastatic disease) e.g. pathological fractures
Treatment-related e.g. invasive diagnostic procedures, post-surgical pain (acute and persistent), radiation therapy, chemotherapy, other therapies (e.g. immunotherapies, hormonal therapies)
Pre-existing non-cancer pain conditions e.g. osteoarthritis

pain can be due to the direct and indirect effects of tumours themselves, invasive diagnostic procedures, and also from cancer treatments (Table 21.1). These causes of pain act through a complex array of pathological mechanisms (sometimes co-occurring) and are expressed through a wide range of clinical presentations (e.g. as neuropathic pain, musculoskeletal pain, or inflammation-related pain).

Two recent systematic reviews have highlighted the extent of cancer-related pain (van den Beuken-van Everdingen et al., 2007; Deandra et al., 2008). In a systematic review of 52 studies conducted between 1966 and 2005 that met methodological quality criteria, van den Beuken-van Everdingen and colleagues (2007) estimated pooled prevalence rates for pain during different phases of cancer treatment. In studies of persons after curative treatment, the pooled prevalence estimate was 33%; the corresponding estimates for those undergoing 'anticancer treatment' and for those in the advanced/metastatic/terminal stages of cancer were 59% and 64%, respectively (although these latter two groups were not uniformly defined across studies). The overall pooled estimate across all groups was 53%. There was significant heterogeneity across studies included in the review, but this did not appear to be due to study-specific factors such as when the studies were carried out or where they were set.

In the following year, Deandra et al. (2008) examined the prevalence of under-treatment for cancer pain in a systematic review of studies that used Pain Management Indices to measure the adequacy of analgesic medication relative to reported pain. The weighted mean value for the prevalence of under-treatment was 43%; in other words, almost one in two patients with cancer pain was undertreated in cancer care settings. It should be noted that there were variations by setting in these findings. To our knowledge, there are no equivalent studies that examine under-treatment using non-pharmacological interventions.

Persistent pain also has an effect on providers of care to people with cancer, although this has been less well documented (Ferrell et al., 1991): concerns about recurrence, impaired quality of life, anxiety, and depression which result from pain also take their toll on carers, who may often function as gatekeepers and managers of analgesia.

The combined effects of increasing length of survival with diagnosis at earlier stages of disease (when tumours are smaller and less invasive), and evolving diagnostic techniques and better treatments for cancer, might be expected to reduce the incidence and prevalence of cancer-related pain in the future. However, under-treatment of cancer pain, as described in this section, and the co-occurrence of non-cancer pain at the time of cancer diagnosis (as discussed subsequently) may both be important determinants of the experience of pain in cancer patients in the future.

The concept of survivorship in cancer

In recent times, the emergence of the concept of cancer survivorship has resulted in calls for a public health agenda that addresses a range of needs that are currently not being met adequately

(CDC, 2004). These needs include strategies to maximize long-term health and functional capacity, and to optimize quality of life. Pain and symptom management are identified as key objectives within this framework. It has been recognized by care providers that this is a growing population with often complex needs (Ferrell and Winn, 2006).

The concept of cancer survivorship has been redefined recently, so that survivorship starts with initial diagnosis (Mullan, 1985). Events in the acute survivorship stage (characterized by intensive investigations, treatment, and monitoring) may be important in contributing to subsequent experience of persistent pain (see previous section). It is during the subsequent extended and permanent stages that troublesome persistent pain is more likely to manifest itself. More generally, research has been urged to identify which characteristics of longer term cancer survivors (both in terms of their cancer experience and other characteristics) either predispose them to, or prevent them from, developing subsequent health problems (CDC, 2004). This would be a more appropriate framework to use in the context of persistent pain.

Pain experience in longer-term cancer survivors: implications for population burden of persistent pain

While there have been calls to develop an assessment and treatment framework for persistent pain in cancer survivors that incorporates concepts, principles, and tools from the field of persistent non-cancer pain, the focus has generally been on causes of persistent pain arising from the cancer itself or from the related treatments (Burton et al., 2007). However, this represents at least a partial shift in thinking away from the current position that places cancer pain and non-cancer pain in separate self-contained silos. This 'silo effect' discourages cross-thinking about pain.

With increasing long-term survival, persistent and troublesome pain will need to be considered and treated in its own right, irrespective of which 'silo' it belonged to originally. It will also require us to reframe questions about the population burden of chronic pain.

Historically, studies of the population burden of chronic pain have tried to ascertain what underlying causes contribute to this burden ('What is your chronic pain due to?'). The answer to this question would appear to be 'Not much' in relation to cancer (Fig. 21.1).

However, when the question is framed as 'How much chronic pain occurs in those who have had a diagnosis of cancer?', a different picture emerges (Reyes-Gibby et al., 2006), as the latter question implicitly accepts the combined impact of cancer and non-cancer pain (Fig. 21.2).

Prior pain experience in people diagnosed with cancer: implications of central sensitization for subsequent pain experience related to cancer

In the Introduction, it was pointed out that cancer and persistent pain are both largely conditions associated with ageing, and tend to occur in the same population subgroups. However, the

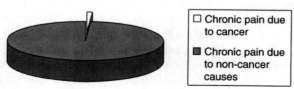

Fig. 21.1 Proportion of population burden of chronic pain due to cancer, based on estimates from Elliot et al., (1999); Català et al., (2002); Breivik et al., (2006).

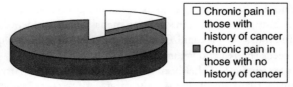

Fig. 21.2 Proportion of chronic pain experienced by those with and without a history of cancer, based on estimates from Reyes-Gibby et al., (2006).

possibility that prior pain experience (typically from musculoskeletal conditions that manifest in mid-life) may influence pain experience related to a subsequent cancer diagnosis is rarely explored. Current thinking about persistent pain as a condition with a distinct pathology (Siddall and Cousins, 2004) would make it reasonable to recognize the potential for people who have already experienced troublesome or intrusive persistent pain that has affected daily life to be potentially at higher risk of experiencing similar difficulties when exposed to the new pain challenges of cancer. However, the magnitude and nature of this effect is rarely explored in cancer research.

There is research on prognostic factors for persistent non-cancer pain that suggests there may be risk factors that are common for different clinical diagnoses (e.g. different types of regional musculoskeletal pain; Mallen et al., 2007; Von Korff and Dunn, 2008). In prognostic studies of this type, prior troublesome pain experience predicts, to some extent, subsequent pain experience. This would fit with the distinct central nervous system pathology of persistent pain as described by Siddall and Cousins (2004).

Few studies in the cancer literature have examined the prior pain experience of those diagnosed with cancer. Early studies provided a range of estimates of prior non-cancer pain experience in patient-based cancer cohorts (ranging from 8% to 26%; Portnoy et al., 1992; Twycross et al., 1996; Zeppetella et al., 2000). However, these relatively small studies provided few insights into the role that prior non-cancer pain experience might play in the subsequent experience of cancer pain. Valeburg et al. (2008) studied this in a group of 217 cancer patients attending outpatient clinics at a large Norwegian tertiary referral cancer hospital, and who reported either pain or analgesic use in a screening questionnaire. Overall, 21.4% of patients reported either pain or analgesic use, which is lower than would have been expected from the systematic review of van den Beuken-van Everdingen et al. (2007). On the basis of data from self-completed questionnaires, these patients' pain was categorized into three groups: pain due to cancer and/or cancer treatment (53%), pain due to non-cancer causes (25.3%), and pain due to both cancer and non-cancer causes (21.7%). Interestingly, these three groups were similar in terms of pain intensity and pain duration (the majority in each group reported pain of >6-months' duration). Both groups with cancer pain (alone or with non-cancer pain concurrently) had equal proportions of patients with metastatic disease. Compared to the cancer pain only group, the group with both cancer and non-cancer pain reported more pain sites and higher levels of interference with activities. In addition, the group with both cancer and non-cancer pain generally assigned higher severity scores to pain descriptors. Despite the poorer pain profile found in this group, it suffered the same degree of assessed analgesic under-treatment of pain as the other two groups.

This study provides some preliminary evidence that prior non-cancer pain matters in the subsequent expression of pain during cancer, and fits with evidence that multiple sites are prognostically significant in a range of pain conditions (Von Korff and Dunn, 2008; Mallen et al., 2007; Croft, 2009), most likely as an expression of central pain sensitization (Siddall and Cousins., 2004). The implication of this evidence is that effective pain assessment and interventions will still be needed in cancer populations, even if there is a shift to earlier diagnosis and longer survival.

Does chronic pain cause cancer?

This provocative question addresses another possible pathway by which chronic non-cancer pain and cancer-related pain may be related, if chronic non-cancer pain causes as well as precedes the onset of cancer. This is a topic that has only recently been studied in the context of research into the relationship between chronic pain and mortality. While there are some studies that have shown a small but statistically significant relationship between different forms of widespread pain and increased risk of cancer mortality (Macfarlane et al., 2001; McBeth et al., 2009), others have not (Macfarlane et al., 2007), and more scientific inquiry is needed to determine if a relationship exists, and to establish if it represents a causal relationship (candidate mechanisms including release of stress hormones, changes in immune function, and impairment of capacity to exercise or depression) or is the result of shared risk factors (such as obesity or smoking).

Conclusion

The global burden of cancer is increasing, and there have been gains in length of survival in many countries. These changes require us to reorient thinking about the causes and experience of pain in longer term cancer survivors, and to explore the interplay between pain due to cancer or its treatment, and pain from other causes. Ultimately, this will give us a clearer understanding of the public health burden of chronic pain which can be attributed to different causes, and clearer policies for tackling long-term pain in patients who have had cancer.[1]

References

Breivik H, Collett B, Ventafridda V, Cohen R, Gallacher D 2006: Survey of chronic pain in Europe: Prevalence, impact on daily life, and treatment. *Eur J Pain* **10**: 287–333.

Burton AW, Fanciullo GJ, Beasley RD, Fisch MJ 2007: Chronic pain in the cancer survivor: A new frontier. *Pain Med* **8**: 189–198.

Català E, Reig E, Artés M, Aliaga L, López JS, Segú JL 2002: Prevalence of pain in the Spanish population: telephone survey in 5000 homes. *Eur J Pain* **6**: 133–140.

Centres for Disease Control and Prevention (CDC). 2004: A National Action Plan for Cancer Survivorship: Advancing Public Health Strategies. Centres for Disease Control and Prevention and the Lance Armstrong Foundation.

Croft PR 2009: The question is not "have you got it?" but "how much of it have you got?" *Pain* **141**: 6–7.

Deandra S, Montanari M, Moja L, Apolone G 2008: Prevalence of undertreatment in cancer pain: A review of published literature. *Ann Oncol* **19**: 1985–1991.

Elliott AM, Smith BH, Penny KI, Smith WC, Chambers WA 1999: The epidemiology of chronic pain in the community. *Lancet* **354**: 1248–1252.

Ferrell BR, Rhiner M, Cohen M, Grant M 1991: Pain as a metaphor for illness Part I: Impact of cancer pain on family caregivers. *Oncol Nurs Forum* **18**: 1303–1309.

Ferrell BR and Winn R 2006: Medical and Nursing Education and training Opportunities to Improve Survivorship Care. *J Clin Oncol* **24**: 5142–5148.

Macfarlane GJ, McBeth J, Silman AJ 2001: Widespread body pain and mortality: a prospective population-based study. *BMJ* **323**: 1–5.

[1] Fiona Blyth's work was supported by a grant from the MBF Foundation. Frances Boyle's work was supported by the Friends of the Mater Foundation. We thank Madeleine King and Jung-Yoon Huh for feedback on earlier drafts of this chapter.

Macfarlane GJ, Jones GT, Kmekt A, Aromaa A, McBeth J, Mikkelsson M, et al. 2007: Is the report of widespread body pain associated with long-term increased mortality? Data from the Mini-Finland Health Survey. *Rheumatol* **46**: 805–807.

McBeth J, Symmons DP, Silman AJ, Allison T, Webb R, Brammah T, et al. 2009: Musculoskeletal pain is associated with a long-term increased risk of cancer and cardiovascular-related mortality. *Rheumatol* **48**: 74–77.

Mallen CD, Peat G, Thomas E, Dunn KM, Croft PR 2007: Prognostic factors for musculoskeletal pain in primary care: a systematic review. *Br J Gen Pract* **57**: 655–661.

Mullan F 1985: Seasons of survival: reflections of a physician with cancer. *New Engl J Med* **313**: 270–273.

Parkin DM 2001: Global cancer statistics in the year 2000. *Lancet Oncol* **2**: 533–543.

Portnoy RK, Miransky J, Thaler HT, Hornung J, Bianchi C, Cibas-Kong I, et al. 1992: Pain in ambulatory patients with lung or colon cancer. *Prevalence, characteristics and effect. Cancer* **70**: 1616–1624.

Reyes-Gibby CC, Aday LA, Anderson KO, Mendoza TR, Cleeland CS 2006: Pain, depression, and fatigue in community-dwelling adults with and without a history of cancer. *J Pain Symptom Manage* **32**: 118–128.

Siddall P and Cousins MJ 2004: Persistent pain as a disease entity: implications for clinical management. *Anesth Analg* **99**: 510–520.

Twycross R, Harcourt J, Bergl S 1996: A survey of pain in patients with advanced cancer. *J Pain Symptom Manage* **12**: 273–282.

Valeburg BT, Rustøen T, Bjordal K, Hanestad BR, Paul S, Miaskowski C 2008: Self-reported prevalence, etiology, and characteristics of pain in oncology outpatients. *Eur J Pain* **12**: 582–590.

Van den Beuken-van Everdingen MHJ, de Rijke JM, Kessels AG, Schouten HC, van Kleef M, Patijn J 2007: Prevalence of pain in patients with cancer: a systematic review of the past 40 years. *Ann Oncol* **18**: 1437–1439.

Von Korff M and Dunn KM 2008: Chronic pain reconsidered. *Pain* **38**: 267–276.

Zeppetella G, O'Doherty CA, Collins S 2000: Prevalence and characteristics of breakthrough pain in cancer patients admitted to a hospice. *J Pain Symptom Manage* **20**: 87–92.

Section 6

Public health and chronic pain

Chapter 22

Introduction to chronic pain as a public health problem

Fiona M. Blyth, Danielle van der Windt, and Peter Croft

We have argued in the introduction to this book, drawing on the writing of authors such as Siddall and Cousins (2004), that it is reasonable to view chronic pain as a condition in its own right. Does it then follow that it is reasonable to view this condition as a public health problem?

Defining chronic pain as a public health problem

'The starting point for identifying public health issues, problems and priorities, and for designing and implementing interventions, is the population as a whole, or population sub-groups'.

This statement from the Australian Public Health Partnership (Jorm et al., 2009) stresses the common-sense point that populations (the total number of people linked to a place or a setting) are the unit of interest for public health. Given that we can present population data on chronic pain and conclude that the problem is common and globally distributed, and also given that we can measure its societal impact in terms of aggregated distress, limitation of activity, health care consumption, reduced participation in work and social life, and economic consequences, it seems reasonable to summarize that chronic pain represents a pubic health problem.

However, 'public health' signifies an activity as well as a description. This is clearly encapsulated in the first part of the Australian Partnership's definition: '(Public health is . . .) the organised response by society to protect and promote health, and to prevent illness, injury and disability' (Jorm et al., 2009).

In this book we have pointed to evidence that chronic pain is not simply or only a consequence of an identifiable disease or injury, although prevention of triggering causes such as road traffic accidents is clearly one way of reducing population pain levels. Once again it seems more helpful to consider chronic pain as a condition in itself, which is worthwhile preventing. In treating or preventing this condition, population levels of disability may also be reduced or prevented, activity promoted, and participation in social and domestic life enhanced.

So far, this may amount to nothing more than stating that chronic pain is common and that treatment of pain should be widely available. To the extent that effective treatment of individuals may prevent long-term pain and its disabling consequences, this model implies that widespread availability of effective care is one way of dealing with chronic pain at the population level.

The traditional public health perspective however attempts much more than this – it seeks to identify population causes of occurrence, which might be amenable to population-level approaches to prevention. Some population causes of pain occurrence may be uniquely properties of populations, whereas others may be active in both populations and the individuals who live in them. Most examples of potential primary prevention targets that societies and populations could work towards as part of a policy for reducing chronic pain are of the latter sort (e.g. low education levels, low physical activity, overweight, or stress in the workplace), with a variable emphasis on interventions in systems (e.g. changes to the architectural and urban planning environment to encourage activity) or individuals (e.g. providing more opportunities for higher education).

The public health challenge with respect to chronic pain is to balance two perspectives:

◆ Pain is an inevitable part of life and cannot be completely prevented. Treatment is therefore going to be needed. Given the sheer number of people with pain who might self-care or seek treatment from health care professionals, this can be translated into one population-level approach, namely ensuring that effective treatments are universally available. However, this adds up to a lot of people worldwide getting treatments for an uncertain length of time. If these treatments carry risks, however small, this may result in large numbers of people experiencing side effects. It is not clear that using a treatment such as long-term opioids as a means of reducing the burden of chronic pain (compared with using it as a humane and necessary intervention for individuals) is either safe or effective (Von Korff and Deyo, 2004).

◆ The classic public health perspective is prevention – identify determinants of chronic pain that are preventable and can be targeted and addressed at the population level, either primary pathological triggers of pain, or the markers and mediators of risk and propensity for chronic pain, and intervene to reduce or remove them.

Chapters 23 and 24 provide examples of these two perspectives: Chapter 23, of the potential effectiveness of pharmacological treatment of osteoarthritis pain and, Chapter 24, of the relationship between work and pain. Characteristics which health care professionals address in order to reduce the likelihood of an individual developing chronic pain or the disability associated with chronic pain, or to improve social participation in people with chronic pain, might also provide the targets for public health interventions. The latter, however, must be deliverable at a population level to achieve an overall shift in risk of chronic pain or its consequences. In Chapter 25 Buchbinder discusses one example of a population-level intervention which worked in this way (i.e. community education about back pain). Other examples include obesity reduction, improved levels of physical activity through school programmes, environmental change to promote activity, improved levels of education in a society, and reduction of social inequalities to reduce psychological distress. For all of these factors, there is epidemiological evidence of associations with chronic pain occurrence, although little direct evidence (except in Buchbinder's study) of actual population change that has led to population reductions in chronic pain or its consequences.

There is stronger evidence of effectiveness for individual-level interventions directed at the same factors (e.g. weight reduction leading to reduced chronic knee pain (Zhang et al., 2008); physical activity reducing the pain of fibromyalgia (Jones et al., 2006); and depression treatment reducing pain and improving activity in persons with painful osteoarthritis (Lin et al., 2003)).

Neil Pearce (1996) calls such individual-level interventions the 'bottom-up approach' to improving public health, which

> . . . focuses on understanding the individual components of a process at the lowest possible level and using this information as the building block to gain knowledge about higher levels of organisation . . . The bottom-up approach lacks distinctive theory regarding the occurrence of diseases at population level (modern epidemiologic studies are conducted in populations, but the implicit etiologic theory is usually based at the individual-biologic level) . . . .(p.681)

There are ways, variable both in their short-term success and in the extent of their proven long-term effectiveness, to treat individuals with pain, reduce their risk of future chronicity, or promote their participation in social and domestic life despite pain. There is little evidence that this bottom-up approach is happening on a wide-enough scale to achieve population shifts in chronic pain, compared with improvements in small groups of treated individuals.

However, even if such population changes were achieved by this individual-level, bottom-up approach, long-term public health still requires population-level approaches, called by Pearce 'top-down public health' (Pearce, 1996).

The two approaches (individual- and population-level) are not incompatible and in the case of pain – particularly because it is a universal feature of life – the individual approach to pain relief will always be a crucial component of society's humane response to this symptom. However, it may not solve the population-level problem, and indeed may exacerbate it, directly (e.g. analgesic-induced headaches) or indirectly (e.g. through promoting the medicalization of pain and the search for a cure, rather than identifying stronger coping and adaptive strategies). Further, it seems even more important now, as chronic symptomatic diseases become increasingly common in the context of rising life expectancy, that population approaches to reducing the risks and consequences of chronic pain are a vital part of public health globally.

Despite this, population-level approaches can seem to ignore at times the stark reality of individuals in severe pain. This is because such approaches have a different purpose, theory, and target, compared with interventions for individuals. Reduction of chronic pain burden is the shared endeavour, but reduction in population risk is the primary target of top-down, population-level public health interventions as compared to the treatment of individuals in pain which is the objective of clinical care and of the bottom-up approach to improving public health. Geoffrey Rose characterized this as the difference between treating sick individuals and managing sick populations (Rose, 1985). But Rose was a clinician as well as an epidemiologist, who understood the paramount need to find strategies which combine both approaches, so that neither populations nor the individuals within them are neglected in health policy.

Pearce re-emphasizes the point when he considers the distinctive contribution of epidemiology to the public health endeavour:

> Epidemiologic techniques can be used in other settings . . . and for other purposes (e.g. studies of disease progression and prognosis) . . . but the key contribution of epidemiology to public health is its population focus.
>
> . . . Of course, epidemiologic studies in populations involve individuals who have specific exposures, but the important distinction is whether or not the etiologic framework is conceptualized at the population level and whether or not these exposures are placed in their social and historical context. (p.681)

Figure 22.1 demonstrates the two approaches. On the right side of the figure is a population with high levels of chronic pain and disability. The bottom-up risk-reduction effort within that population would be exemplified by focusing on identifying and intervening in individuals at high risk of adverse chronic pain outcomes (the approach which happens most commonly in practice) in order to lower that individual risk. As risk itself is not a static phenomenon, there will always be reservoirs of individuals moving between low- and high-risk states. On the left side of the figure is a population with lower levels of chronic pain and disability, where the entire population is at lower risk of adverse chronic pain outcomes. The classic hallmark of public health interventions is that they focus on shifting population risk from right to left.

Conceptualizing the aetiological framework at the population level

Summarizing earlier parts of the book, it seems that, unlike the case with many cancers or cardiovascular disease, the experience of chronic pain is remarkably consistent across different regions of the world. The likely explanations for this are:-

1. the universality of musculoskeletal conditions as the dominant cause of chronic pain at the population level, and

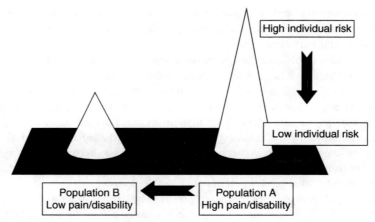

Fig. 22.1 'High risk' and 'low risk' population strategies

2. the universal presence across populations of characteristic subgroups of people with an under-lying propensity or increased risk for chronic pain, in the context of a wide range of different precipitating or underlying diseases and injuries.

Chapter 17 reviewed the potential contribution of underlying disease and injury to the patterns and occurrence of chronic pain. However, more important is the finding that groups within populations differ clearly in their occurrence of chronic pain or, more specifically, their risk of developing chronic pain and their likelihood of future activity and participation restrictions – and that these same subgroups and the same contrasting risks of chronic pain are found in very differ-ent geographic populations. The population construct of aetiology focuses on the causes of these differences or variations between population subgroups. To the extent that these might be pre-ventable, this will represent a public health perspective on chronic pain.

Drawing on the chapters and concepts developed, reviewed, or presented by contributors to this book, the prevention framework can be summarized as follows:

1. There is an extensive global burden of chronic pain across all populations.

2. Changing patterns of mortality and morbidity are resulting in an expanding number of long-term pain sufferers.

3. Although some of this rise is occurring in the context of changes in mortality patterns of spe-cific diseases, such as human immunodeficiency virus (HIV)/acquired immune deficiency syndrome (AIDS), the proportion of population chronic pain directly attributable to such underlying disease is unclear.

4. Musculoskeletal conditions dominate population chronic pain prevalence.

5. Psychological distress is a consistent accompaniment of chronic pain, both as a precursor and a consequence.

6. There is evidence for population-level influences on chronic pain development – physical, psychological, social, and cultural.

7. Genetic predisposition explains some individual variance in pain perception and diseases underlying pain. However, as the arguments and evidence presented by Macgregor in Chapter 8 make clear, this does not negate the potential and capacity for environmental change to shift

the population means of pain, although genetics would contribute to explaining continuing individual variation around the new population means.

8. We need to identify and research population approaches to reducing population risks for chronic pain, whilst at the same time identifying and ensuring continuing effective treatment for individuals with chronic pain or at risk of developing it.

Why does it matter if chronic pain is a public health problem or not?

We have considered some reasons for considering chronic pain as a public health problem above. If we accept that it can be conceptualized as such, then the reasons why this matters include:

♦ A traditional high-risk, individual-level approach to chronic pain will not succeed in substantially reducing the problem at the population level.

♦ Important intervention targets will be overlooked if unique population-level risk factors are not identified.

♦ Some individual-level risk factors that may appear unimportant because of their low relative risk – and which may be displaced from multivariable models by aetiologically stronger risk factors – may need to be reconsidered, if the population distribution of risk factors is taken into account and shows that these low-level risks are common across populations.

♦ Intervention strategies are not being optimized.

If chronic pain is accepted as a public health problem, and the reasons why it matters are also accepted, we finally need to consider the public health framework in which to place, not just this conceptualization and its epidemiology, but also public health action. What are the essential public health considerations to apply to thinking about chronic pain? The Australian National Public Health Partnership have proposed one multi-dimensional public health framework with six overarching classes (Jorm et al., 2009):

♦ Public health functions (i.e. the purpose of public health interventions, actions, activities, and programmes)

♦ Health issues

♦ Determinants of health

♦ Settings

♦ Methods of intervention

♦ Resources and infrastructure

Remaining questions include (following Jorm et al., 2009):

Are preventive services provided on a one-to-one basis part of the public health approach?

We do not see it as important to spend time worrying about what to classify where, but rather to debate and gain evidence about the pros and cons of individual prevention (e.g. pharmacological treatment for patients presenting with osteoarthritis pain) being an agent for population change. As the example in Chapter 23 illustrates clearly, individual approaches provide much evidence about efficacy and mechanisms of change in symptoms, but there is little evidence that they will deliver the public health outcome of population change. In addition, the evidence emerging from studies of analgesic medications for example is that, however good and important they are at an individual level, regarding them as population-level interventions may be attractive for pharmaceutical companies but may prove bad news for population health. Strong analgesics need highly individualized delivery to be safe as well as optimally effective, and we need more empirical evidence of how to target, choose, and monitor individual therapies for chronic long-term pain in the community.

Are prevention and management approaches, directed at risk factors for chronic pain, such as lifestyle or perceptions, and provided on a one-to-one or small group basis, part of the public health approach?

Just as the safety problem is less contentious here – it seems intuitively more difficult to do harm with widespread use of such interventions than with pharmaceutical agent – the argument about individual treatments forming part of the public health approach is rather more salient. Indeed the small positive effect sizes seen in many trials of pain treatment (see, e.g. Keller et al.'s review of non-surgical treatment effects in chronic low-back pain (Keller et al., 2007)), so often dispiriting reading for health care professionals trying to deliver evidence-based interventions in clinical practice, can be translated to much more positive statements of potential population effects. Given that pain is so common, and so commonly seen in primary care, such small effects may provide large shifts in the population's health. This is possible, even though evidence for such effects in practice is not generally available at present. One explanation for the evidence gap is that there is simply too little proper application of evidence-based treatment in practice. However, it seems unlikely that this approach will get beyond short-term effects, important as those might be for individuals. Achieving large, long-term shifts in population levels of pain demands more than this.

How much should the target be chronic pain itself rather than the consequences or context of the problem?

Approaches to the problem of chronic pain have embraced the idea of helping people to live with pain, e.g. to return to work despite pain and to focus on participation as an outcome (see, e.g. Chapter 24). Waddell's eloquent accounts of the potential for removing social influences on pain behaviour, such as changes in disability or sickness absence laws, provide one example of a population-level approach to address the consequences of chronic pain (Waddell, 1998). However, although this may be part of the picture of how society deals with the problem of the universality of the pain experience, it is not going to provide the whole picture of the public health approach to chronic pain.

How far to embrace a high-risk, individual-level strategy, i.e. a bottom-up approach to prevention?

This might take the form of screening for pre-morbid risk – equivalent to screening programmes for hypertension or high cholesterol. In the case of chronic pain, this is more likely to be comparable to the early case-finding concept of cancer screening – e.g. any significant episode of pain is a risk marker for future pain, the severity of current pain is part of Dunn and von Korff's prognostic model (Chapter 4), and the number of pain sites the key to Natvig and colleague's view (Chapter 7). This seems unlikely to produce a public health population approach – even though it may be a sensible extension of managing individuals with pain within a framework designed to reduce risk of future continuing chronic pain. Population-screening programmes to identify people at high risk of chronic pain seem rather less plausible. The frequency of high-risk people seeking health care is high anyway. On the other hand, many studies highlight the significant proportion of persons with severely disabling pain who are not accessing health care (e.g. Jinks et al., (2004), who noted that one-third of older adults with severe disabling knee pain had not used health care services in the course of a year) or who may not disclose significant pain in consultations about other health matters (e.g. Bedson et al., 2007). Such individuals might benefit from opportunistic screening or systematic case-finding. However, the evidence that this would result in overall population benefits has not been gathered or researched.

How to monitor and survey pain in populations? This provides a particular set of challenges for the public health approach to chronic pain. Routine health statistics are awkward as a basis for identifying chronic pain – witness the discussion about primary care data in some of the chapters in this book. There is a need for systems of measurement and surveillance of pain at a population level using an agreed set of definitions, such as the approach outlined and developed by Dionne in Chapter 5, and linked to dedicated condition codes in the 10th chapter of the International Classification of Diseases, for example. These could then be used for ongoing population health surveillance and in routinely collected episodes of care datasets.

Conclusion

An inclusive approach means that decisions about the boundaries between what is a population-level and what an individual-level strategy are made on a case-by-case basis (Jorm et al., 2009). These authors point out that notions of boundaries between public health and clinical practice may evolve with new knowledge about preventive interventions. Statin consumption by large numbers of persons in their middle years may eventually be categorized as a population intervention; brief behavioural therapy for everyone with more than three areas of chronic pain may perhaps also come to be regarded in the same way.

In terms of primary prevention of chronic pain, one approach, which could have a significant impact in some countries, is via primary prevention of underlying disease. Although, as we have argued, this is an incomplete view of chronic pain prevention, and there is surprisingly little evidence about the population attributable risk of these diseases in relation to pain, it still looks convincing that, were road traffic accidents, for example, to be curtailed in frequency, one outcome would be a reduction in chronic pain and its consequences. Primary prevention of accidents becomes one route to primary prevention of some chronic pain at least.

However, the most clear-cut traditional public health approach is to think, for example, about Natvig's distribution of number of pain sites as the marker of established risk, and ask if that can be 'shifted to the left'. This is equivalent to Rose's big idea that if blood pressure levels were to shift downwards as a whole in a population (i.e. the population mean reduces even if the variation around the mean is still the same pattern), this would produce major reductions in the population-level complications of blood pressure. The challenge is to identify underlying changeable population-level factors whose mean could be shifted downward to achieve the shift in numbers of pain sites. This would be the equivalent of mean population salt intake being shifted downwards to reduce population mean blood pressure, in Rose's example. The study described by Buchbinder in Chapter 25 attempted to achieve this for an important consequence of back pain (sickness absence from the workplace) by using a population-based approach to shift one specific risk factor: unhelpful beliefs regarding pain and exercise, and how they might interfere with keeping active when an episode of back pain starts. Physical activity, reduction of obesity, changes in the workplace, improving happiness levels in society – all may reduce the likelihood of pain episodes developing into chronic pain or reduce the consequences of the pain. This is real primary prevention in public health – delivered at a population level, with population benefits.

It is a plausible model that deserves to be tested. In 1990, Deyo and Bass (1989) identified this argument in relation to low-back pain, noting the implausibility of screening programmes achieving major population effects and observing that the major risk targets for primary prevention of back pain are shared with the risk targets for coronary heart disease, diabetes, mental health, and other chronic diseases.

Summary of prevention strategies

Primary

- Target group: The whole population.
- Objective:
  - Prevention of the underlying disease trigger for chronic pain, and/or prevention or reduction of the underlying propensity or risk of chronic pain – i.e. improving risk profile of a population.

Secondary

- Target group: Individuals presenting with episodes of pain or with disease carrying a risk of chronic pain.
- Objectives:
  - Better early treatment of trigger conditions.
  - Screening and tackling propensity for chronic pain.
  - Intervening on prognostic characteristics in people who present in clinical practice.

Tertiary

- Target group: Individuals with established chronic pain, defined prognostically.
- Objective:
  - To shift individual trajectories from their chronic persistent disabling course.

This takes us back to where the book started, and to the way in which the public health approach maps to the idea of the 2004 paper by Siddall and Cousins identifying chronic pain as a 'condition-in-itself'.

There are other considerations that will be familiar to anyone who has tried to advocate more resources and policy attention for chronic pain as a national health priority. Chronic pain faces hurdles that other common but better recognized and better-funded conditions such as obesity have already cleared. These include the need for recognition as a condition in its own right (the symptom vs. condition debate), underpinned by an agreed set of definitions and dedicated coding within routinely collected data sources and disease registries. With this will come routine population and health system surveillance of chronic pain and, crucially, visibility.

Another set of tasks is to make explicit the extent to which chronic pain links to existing, commonly acknowledged health priority areas such as cancer, injury, obesity, and healthy ageing. These would contribute to advocacy of chronic pain (see Figure 22.2) within initiatives such as national pain summits in the USA and Australia. This is all part of giving chronic pain a 'shape' and a 'voice' in the public arena.

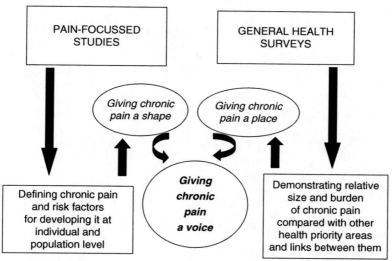

Fig. 22.2 A public health model

References

Bedson J, Mottram S, Thomas E, Peat G. 2007: Knee pain and osterarthritis in the general population: what influences patients to consult? *Fam Pract* **24**, 443–53.

Deyo RA and Bass JE. 1989: Lifestyle and low-back pain. The influence of smoking and obesity. *Spine* **14**, 501–6.

Jinks C, Jordan K, Ong BN, Croft P. 2004: A brief screening tool for knee pain in primary care (KNEST). 2. Results from a survey in the general population aged 50 and over. *Rheumatology* **43**, 55–61.

Jones KD, Adams D, Winters-Stone K, Burckhardt CS. 2006: A comprehensive review of 46 exercise treatment studies in fibromyalgia (1988-2005). *Health Qual Life Outcomes* **4**, 67.

Jorm LR, Gruszin S, Churches TR. 2009: A multidimensional classification of public health activity in Australia. *Australia and New Zealand Health Policy* **6**, 9.

Keller A, Hayden J, Bombardier C, van Tulder M. 2007: Effect sizes of non-surgical treatments of non-specific low-back pain. *Eur Spine J* **16**, 1776–88.

Lin EH, Katon W, Von Korff M, Tang L, Williams JW Jr, Kroenke K, et al., IMPACT Investigators. 2003: Effect of improving depression care on pain and functional outcomes among older adults with arthritis: a randomized controlled trial. *JAMA* **290**, 2428–9.

Pearce N. 1996: Traditional epidemiology, modern epidemiology and public health. *Am J Pub Health* **86**, 678–83.

Rose G 1985: Sick individuals and sick populations. *Int J Epidemiol* **14**, 32–5.

Siddall PJ and Cousins MJ. 2004: Persistent pain as a disease entity: implications for clinical management. *Anaesth Analg* **99**, 510–20.

Von Korff M and Deyo RA. 2004: Potent opioids for chronic musculoskeletal pain: flying blind? *Pain* **109**, 207–9.

Waddell G. 1998: *The Back Pain Revolution*. Edinburgh: Churchill Livingstone.

Zhang W, Moskowitz RW, Nuki G, Abramson S, Altman RD, Arden N, et al. 2008: OARSI recommendations for the management of hip and knee osteoarthritis, Part II: OARSI evidence-based, expert consensus guidelines. *Osteoarthritis Cartilage* **16**, 137–62.

Chapter 23

Pharmacological treatments: the example of osteoarthritis

Weiya Zhang and Michael Doherty

Introduction

A number of drugs are available for the treatment of chronic pain. 'Minor' analgesics, such as paracetamol and non-steroidal anti-inflammatory drugs (NSAIDs), are commonly used for rapid-onset, short-acting relief of mild-to-moderate pain due to chronic musculoskeletal conditions. Stronger analgesics, such as opioids, other narcotics, and inhibitors of central and peripheral neurotransmitters, are often used for severe pain such as those caused by cancer and neuropathy. In inflammatory diseases, agents that inhibit specific aspects of inflammation, such as tumour necrosis factor alpha (TNF), interleukins, or leucocyte subpopulations, may have indirect, slow-onset analgesic effects. This class of drugs has been developed recently and clinical evidence to support their use has yet to be confirmed. Nutraceuticals and herbs are widely used to control chronic pain as adjuvant therapy but their mechanism of action is largely unknown. Clinical effectiveness observed from analgesics, even from strong analgesics, varies greatly from patient to patient, confirming the complexity of pain experience and supporting an important role for non-specific (meaning and contextual) effects. This raises the issue of minimum quality of care for chronic pain management that optimizes such contextual responses. In this chapter, we discuss common pharmacological and nutraceutical treatments in the management of chronic pain. We use a common musculoskeletal disease – osteoarthritis (OA) (Peat et al., 2001), as an example to discuss benefits and harms of each treatment and possible optimization of management.

Evidence-based medicine (EBM): principle and clinical application

EBM is defined as 'the conscientious, explicit and judicious use of current best evidence in making decisions about the care of individual patients' (Sackett et al., 1996). EBM aims to apply the best evidence into clinical practice. The best research evidence depends on the clinical question. For example, for therapeutic efficacy, randomized controlled trials (RCTs) are the usual gold standard and systematic reviews of RCTs offer the best evidence (Table 23.1) (Shekelle et al., 1999). For diagnosis, however, case-control studies are more appropriate and systematic reviews of case-control studies offer best evidence (Zhang et al., 2006). For causality and questions concerning prognosis and side effects, observational cohort studies are the ideal design and systematic reviews of cohort studies offer best evidence. Evidence for efficacy, together with the evidence for side effects and cost-effectiveness, form the basis of research evidence. However, this is just one of three essential components of evidence-based decision-making (Figure 23.1) (Hynes et al., 1996). Contrary to popular belief, research evidence, expert experience and opinion, and patient beliefs and acceptability are equally weighted, and it is only when all three concur that we approach current best practice.

Table 23.1 Evidence hierarchy (efficacy)

Ia – meta-analysis of randomized controlled trials
Ib – randomized controlled trial
IIa – controlled study without randomization
IIb – quasi-experimental study
III – non-experimental descriptive studies, such as comparative, correlation, and case-control studies
IV – expert committee reports or opinion or clinical experience of respected authorities, or both

EBM originated from the search for the gold standard to test the effect of a medical intervention. The idea can be traced back to ancient Greece, but it was not until the 20th century, at a time when effective drug treatments were being produced, that Professor Archie Cochrane, a Scottish epidemiologist, through his book *Effectiveness and Efficiency: Random Reflections on Health Services* (1972) and subsequent advocacy, caused increasing acceptance of the application of the RCT. Cochrane's contribution was honoured through the Cochrane Collaboration – an international organization to systematically review RCTs. The term 'evidence-based medicine' first appeared in the medical literature in 1992 in a paper by the Evidence-Based Medicine Working Group (1992).

Systematic review is the foundation of EBM. It aims to systematically review and critically appraise the research evidence before application. Quantitative analysis may be undertaken within a systematic review to form meta-analysis. Systematic review and meta-analysis aim to summarize information on study selection, characteristics (age, gender, etc), heterogeneity, and overall estimate of effect. The common measurements of effect of therapy include weighted mean difference (WMD), standardized mean difference (or effect size (ES)), relative risk (RR), odds ratio (OR), number needed to treat (NNT), or number needed to harm (NNH).

EBM has been used widely to guide clinical practice, drug regulation, guideline development, and health care policy. EBM is evolving, from a focus on RCTs to observational studies; from clinical effectiveness to cost-effectiveness; and from summarizing research evidence to integrating clinical opinions. The concept then broadens as both expert opinion and patient perspectives are incorporated.

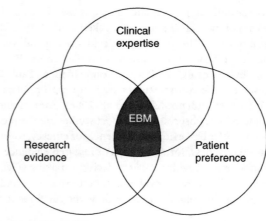

Fig. 23.1 Evidence based practice (EBM)

Pharmacological treatments for OA

Treatment objectives

OA is the most common type of arthritis and a major cause of chronic musculoskeletal pain and mobility disability in elderly populations worldwide (Peat et al., 2001). The objectives of management of OA are universally agreed (Zhang et al., 2008a; National Collaborating Centre for Chronic Conditions, 2008), including

- Educating patients about the nature of the disorder and its management.
- Reducing pain and stiffness.
- Maintaining and improving joint mobility and function.
- Reducing physical disability and handicap.
- Improving health-related quality of life.
- Limiting the progression of joint damage.

Treatment options and classification

Over 20 pharmacological and nutraceutical treatments are available for the treatment of OA (Zhang et al., 2007b). They can be classified according to the route of delivery (i.e. oral, topical, and intra-articular (IA); Table 23.2). In addition to common analgesics (e.g. paracetamol, non-steroidal anti-inflammatory drugs (NSAIDs), opioids), IA corticosteroid, IA hyaluronans, nutraceuticals (e.g. glucosamine sulphate, chondroitin sulphate, avocado soybean unsaponifiables (ASU), and vitamins), herbs (rosehip and S-adenosylmethionine (SAM-e)), the anti-interleukin agent diacerhein and antidepressants are also used to treat OA. They all claim to have symptomatic relief effects. Some of them (e.g. glucosamine sulphate, chondroitin sulphate, ASU, and diacerhein) may modify diseased structures in the joint, which previously warranted their inclusion in a class of 'symptomatic slow acting drugs for OA' (SYSADOA; Zhang and Doherty et al., 2006), more recently termed 'disease modification OA drugs' (DMOAD) (Qvist et al., 2008).

Table 23.2 Drugs and nutrients for osteoarthritis

Oral	Topical	Intra-articular
Paracetamol	Topical NSAIDs	Intra-articular corticosteroid
NSAIDs	Topical capsaicin	Intra-articular hyaluronic acid
NSAIDs + PPI	Topical rubefacients	
NSAIDs + misoprostol		
COX-2 inhibitors		
Opioids		
Glucosamine sulphate		
Chondroitin sulphate		
Avocado soybean unsaponifiables (ASU)		
Vitamins		
Rosehip		
S-adenosylmethionine (SAM-e)		
Diacerhein		
Antidepressants		
Oestrogen		
Bisphosphonates		

For simplicity and clinical convenience, we discuss these drugs according to the route of delivery, regardless of the mechanism of action. Table 23.3 summaries evidence for their efficacy.

Oral agents

Paracetamol

Paracetamol (acetaminophen) is recommended as a first-line pharmacological therapy for OA (Zhang et al., 2008a; National Collaborating Centre for Chronic Conditions, 2008; Jordan et al., 2003; Zhang et al., 2005). The Current Osteoarthritis Research Society International (OARSI) recommendations suggest that paracetamol (up to 4 g/day) can be an effective initial oral analgesic for treatment of mild-to-moderate pain in patients with knee or hip OA (Zhang et al., 2008a). In the absence of an adequate response, or in the presence of severe pain and/or inflammation, alternative pharmacological therapy should be considered based on relative efficacy and safety, as well as concomitant medications and co-morbidities.

Two systematic reviews have been undertaken to support the use of paracetamol (Towheed et al., 2006; Zhang et al., 2004). The earlier systematic review of 10 RCTs (2 vs. placebo, 6 vs. NSAIDs, 2 vs. both) in 2004 revealed a small but statistically significant effect size for pain relief compared to placebo (effect size (ES) = 0.21, 95% confidence interval (CI): 0.02–0.41; Zhang et al., 2004; Table 23.3). This ES, however, reduced to 0.13 (95% CI: 0.04–0.22) when more RCTs were added in the later Cochrane systematic review which included 15 RCTs (7 vs. placebo and 10 vs. NSAIDs; Towheed et al., 2006). Side effects of paracetamol at recommended doses are controversial (Table 23.4; Zhang et al., 2007). A case-control study showed that paracetamol was associated with increased risk of gastrointestinal (GI) perforation and bleeding (odds ratio (OR) = 3.60, 95%CI: 2.60–5.10; Garcia Rodriguez and Hernandez-Diaz, 2001), whereas a systematic review of RCTs and a meta-analysis of case-control studies using individual patient data did not show any increase in GI side effects from paracetamol compared to placebo or non-use (Lewis et al., 2002; Zhang et al., 2004). More recently, a population-based cohort study ($n = 644 \ 183$) found that the high dose (>3000 mg/day) of paracetamol was associated with greater risk of hospitalization due to GI perforation, ulceration, or bleeding (PUB) compared with the low dose (≤3000 mg/day; Rahme et al., 2008). The hazard ratio (HR) was 1.20 (95%CI: 1.03–1.40). In addition, the HR was 1.63 (95%CI: 1.44–1.85) for NSAIDs and 2.55 (95% CI: 1.98–3.28) for combined use of NSAIDs plus paracetamol. This graded risk suggests that paracetamol may indeed have modest potential to cause peptic ulceration complications. This side effect may become significant when full treatment doses (e.g. 3000–4000 mg/day) are used. The combination of paracetamol plus oral NSAID should not be encouraged as there is a potential risk of interaction between these drugs in terms of GI events. There may also be renal side effects when paracetamol is taken long term (Fored et al., 2001; Rexrode et al., 2001). In brief, paracetamol is effective for OA but its effect size is small and its long-term safety is increasingly being questioned. The benefit–risk ratio may change according to duration and regularity of treatment, the requirements for which necessitate monitoring as part of management of chronic pain.

NSAIDs, coxibs, and GI-protective agents

NSAIDs are widely used analgesics for chronic pain. A telephone survey of 1149 patients with OA in the UK in 2003 revealed that only 15% were taking paracetamol, while 32% were taking non-selective NSAIDs and 18% COX-2 selective drugs for analgesia (Arthritis Care, 2003).

A 2004 systematic review of 23 short-term, placebo-controlled RCTs of NSAIDs, including COX-2 selective agents in >10 000 patients with knee OA, showed that the ES for pain reduction was 0.32 (95%CI: 0.24–0.39; Table 23.3; Bjordal et al., 2004). Three other systematic reviews have

Table 23.3 Recent evidence for efficacy of pharmacological treatment of osteoarthritis

Modality	Joint	QoS*(%)	LoE	ES$_{pain}$ (95%CI)	ES$_{function}$ (95%CI)	ES$_{stiffness}$ (95%CI)	NNT (95%CI)
Paracetamol (Acetaminophen)	Any	100	Ia	0.13 (0.04–0.22)			2 (1–2)
NSAIDs	Any	100	Ia	0.32 (0.24–0.39)			
COX-2 inhibitors	Any	100	Ia	0.44 (0.33–0.55)			
Topical NSAIDs	Knee/hand	100	Ia	0.41 (0.22–0.59)	0.36 (0.24–0.48)	0.49 (0.17–0.80)	3 (2–4)
Topical capsaicin	Knee/hand	75	Ia				4 (3–5)
Opioids	Any	100	Ia	0.78 (0.59–0.98)	0.31 (0.24–0.39)		
IA Corticosteroid	Knee	100	Ia	0.72 (0.42–1.02)	0.06 (–0.17–0.30)		4 (2–11)
IA Hyaluronic acid	Knee	100	Ia	0.32 (0.17–0.47)	0.00 (–0.23–0.23)		
Glucosamine Sulphate	Knee/hip	100	Ia	0.35 (0.14–0.56)	0.07 (–0.08–0.21)	0.06 (–0.11–0.23)	5 (4–7)
Chondroitin Sulphate	Knee/hip	100	Ia	0.52 (0.37–0.67)			5 (4–7)
Diacerhein	Knee/hip	–	Ia	0.22 (0.01–0.42)			
ASU	Knee/hip	100	Ia	0.39 (0.01–0.76)			
Rosehip	Knee/hip	100	Ia	0.37 (0.13–0.60)			6 (4–13)
SAM-e	Knee	100	Ia	0.22 (–0.25–0.69)	0.31 (0.10–0.52)		

ES: effect size, ES = 0.2 is considered small, ES = 0.5 is moderate, and ES > 0.8 is large; NNT: number needed to treat for symptom relief, e.g. ≥50% pain relief, unless otherwise specified; CI: confidence interval; SR: systematic review; SAM-e: S-adenosylmethionine; ASU: avocado soybean unsaponifiables ¹ LoE (level of evidence): Ia: meta-analysis of RCTs; Ib: RCT; IIa: controlled study without randomization; IIb: quasi-experimental study (e.g. uncontrolled trial, one-arm dose-response trial, etc.); III: observational studies (e.g. case-control, cohort, and cross-sectional studies); IV: expert opinion.

* QoS **(Quality of study)** was assessed using validated scales, e.g. the Oxman and Guyatt Scale for systematic review and the Jadad scale for clinical trials. The percentage score was calculated for each study. The best available evidence was presented, i.e. systematic review with the highest quality, randomized controlled trial with highest quality followed by uncontrolled or quasi-experiment, cohort, and case-control studies.

Adapted from Zhang et al., 2007, with permission from Elsevier.

Adapted and updated from the OARSI treatment guidelines (Zhang et al., 2008a) with permission. Figures are derived from data in Towheed et al., 2006; Zhang et al., 2004; Bjordal et al., 2004; Lee et al., 2005; Lin et al., 2004; Zhang and Li Wan Po, 1994; Avouac et al., 2007; Bellamy et al., 2005b; Lo et al., 2003; Arrich et al., 2005; Vlad et al., 2007; Towheed et al., 2005; Richy et al., 2003; Zhang et al., 2007b; Christensen et al., 2008a and 2008b; Soeken et al., 2002.

Table 23.4 Side effects – relative risk (RR) or odds ratio (OR) and 95% confidence interval (CI)

Intervention*	Adverse events	RR/OR (95%CI)	Evidence
Paracetamol (Acetaminophen)	GI discomfort	0.80 (0.27–2.37)	RCTs
	GI perforation/bleed	3.60 (2.60–5.10)	CC
	GI bleeding	1.20 (0.80–1.70)	CCs
	Renal failure	0.83 (0.50–1.39)	CS
	Renal failure	2.50 (1.70–3.60)	CC
NSAIDs	GI perforation/ulcer/bleed	5.36 (1.79–16.10)	RCTs
	GI perforation/ulcer/bleed	2.70 (2.10–3.50)	CSs
	GI perforation/ulcer/bleed	3.00 (2.50–3.70)	CCs
	Myocardial infarction	1.09 (1.02–1.15)	CSs
Topical NSAIDs	GI events	0.81 (0.43–1.56)	RCTs
	GI bleed/perforation	1.45 (0.84–2.50)	CC
H2 blocker + NSAID vs. NSAID	Serious GI complications	0.33 (0.01–8.14)	RCTs
	Symptomatic ulcers	1.46 (0.06–35.53)	RCTs
	Serious CV or renal events	0.53 (0.08–3.46)	RCTs
PPI + NSAID vs. NSAID	Serious GI complications	0.46 (0.07–2.92)	RCTs
	Symptomatic ulcers	0.09 (0.02–0.47)	RCTs
	Serious CV or renal events	0.78 (0.10–6.26)	RCTs
Misoprostol + NSAID vs. NSAID	Serous GI complications	0.57 (0.36–0.91)	RCTs
	Symptomatic ulcers	0.36 (0.20–0.67)	RCTs
	Serious CV or renal events	1.78 (0.26–12.07)	RCTs
	Diarrhoea	1.81 (1.52–2.61)	RCTs
COX-2 inhibitors			
Coxibs vs. NSAIDs	Serious GI complications	0.55 (0.38, 0.80)	RCTs
	Symptomatic ulcers	0.49 (0.38, 0.62)	RCTs
	Serious CV or renal events	1.19 (0.80, 1.75)	RCTs
Celecoxib	Myocardial infarction	2.26 (1.00, 5.10)	RCTs
	Myocardial infarction	0.97 (0.86, 1.08)	CSs/CCs
Rofecoxib	Myocardial infarction	2.24 (1.24, 4.02)	RCTs
	Myocardial infarction	1.27 (1.12, 1.44)	CSs/CCs
Valdecoxib	CV events	2.30 (1.10, 4.70)	RCTs
Opioids	Any	1.40 (1.30, 1.60)	RCTs
	Constipation	3.60 (2.70, 4.70)	RCTs
Glucosamine sulphate	Any	0.97 (0.88, 1.08)	RCTs
Diacerhein	Diarrhoea	3.98 (2.90, 5.47)	RCTs
IA hyaluronic acid	Local transient pain	1.08 (1.01, 1.15)	RCTs

RCT: randomized controlled trial; CC: case-control study; CS: cohort study. Pooled RR/OR was provided if more than one study were included.

*Compared with placebo/non-exposure unless otherwise stated.

H_2-blockers: histamine type 2 receptor antagonists; PPIs: proton-pump inhibitors; GI: gastrointestinal; CV: cardiovascular.

Adapted from Zhang et al., 2007, with permission from Elsevier.

Adapted and updated from the OARSI treatment guidelines (Zhang et al., 2008a) with permission. Figures are derived from data in Zhang et al., 2004; Garcia Rodriguez and Hernandez-Diaz 2001; Lewis et al., 2002; Rexrode et al., 2001; Fored et al., 2001; Ofman et al., 2002; Hernandez-Diaz et al., 2006; Lin et al., 2004; Evans and Macdonald., 1996; Hooper et al., 2004; Capurso and Koch, 1991; Caldwell et al., 2006; Juni et al., 2004; Aldington et al., 2005; Kalso et al., 2004; Towheed et al., 2005; Dougados et al., 2001; Pham et al., 2004; Arrich et al., 2005.

confirmed this result in OA pain relief (Towheed et al., 2006; Bjordal et al., 2004; Bjordal et al., 2007; Zhang et al., 2004). Twenty-seven placebo-controlled RCTs ($n = 14 523$) have been undertaken so far. The pooled ES for pain relief was 0.29 (95%CI: 0.22–0.35; Figure 23.2), which is superior to the ES obtained for paracetamol (ES = 0.13, 95%CI: 0.04–0.22; Towheed et al., 2006).

Evidence that NSAIDs are superior to paracetamol for pain relief is directly supported by a systematic review of head-to-head comparisons between NSAIDs versus paracetamol (ES = 0.20, 95%CI: 0.10–0.30; Zhang et al., 2004). The clinical response rate was higher (relative risk (RR) = 1.24, 95%CI: 0.10–1.41) and the number of patients preferring NSAIDs to paracetamol was consistently greater (RR = 2.46, 95%CI: 1.50–4.12; Zhang et al., 2004).

However, there is abundant evidence that NSAIDs are associated with more frequent adverse effects than paracetamol. The 2004 meta-analysis (Zhang et al., 2004) showed that NSAIDs were associated with GI discomfort more frequently than paracetamol (RR = 1.35, 95% CI: 1.05–1.75) and this was confirmed in the more recent Cochrane systematic review of RCTs (RR = 1.47, 95%

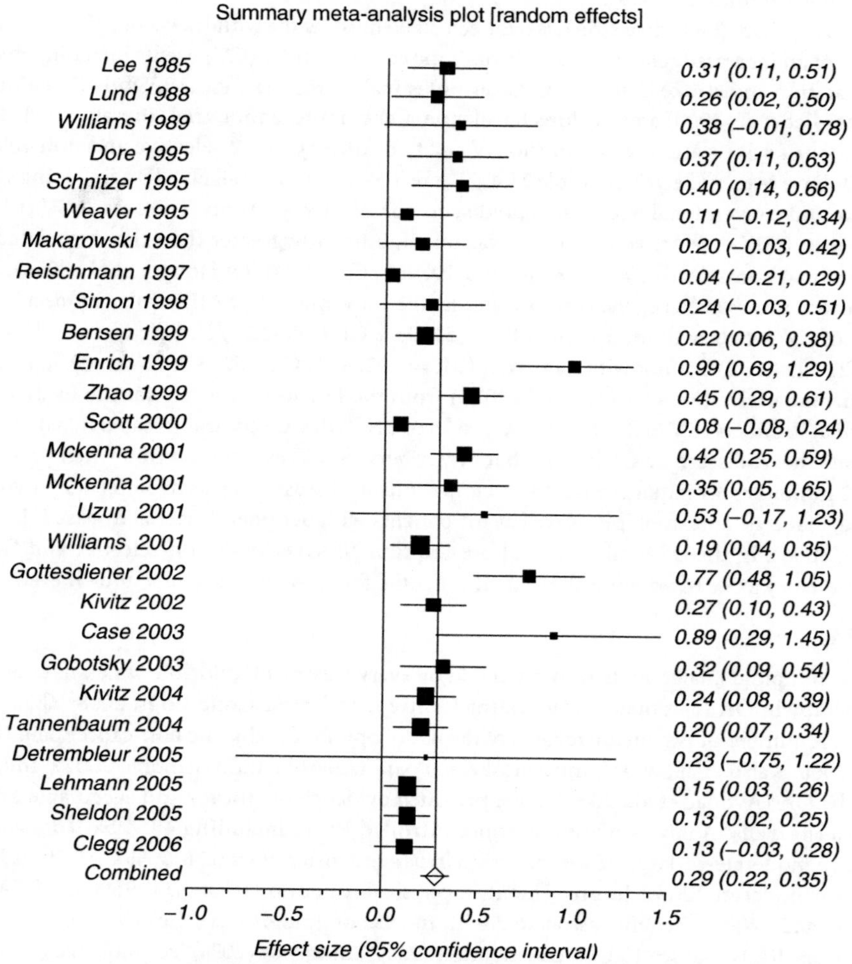

Summary meta-analysis plot [random effects]

Study	Effect size (95% CI)
Lee 1985	0.31 (0.11, 0.51)
Lund 1988	0.26 (0.02, 0.50)
Williams 1989	0.38 (−0.01, 0.78)
Dore 1995	0.37 (0.11, 0.63)
Schnitzer 1995	0.40 (0.14, 0.66)
Weaver 1995	0.11 (−0.12, 0.34)
Makarowski 1996	0.20 (−0.03, 0.42)
Reischmann 1997	0.04 (−0.21, 0.29)
Simon 1998	0.24 (−0.03, 0.51)
Bensen 1999	0.22 (0.06, 0.38)
Enrich 1999	0.99 (0.69, 1.29)
Zhao 1999	0.45 (0.29, 0.61)
Scott 2000	0.08 (−0.08, 0.24)
Mckenna 2001	0.42 (0.25, 0.59)
Mckenna 2001	0.35 (0.05, 0.65)
Uzun 2001	0.53 (−0.17, 1.23)
Williams 2001	0.19 (0.04, 0.35)
Gottesdiener 2002	0.77 (0.48, 1.05)
Kivitz 2002	0.27 (0.10, 0.43)
Case 2003	0.89 (0.29, 1.45)
Gobotsky 2003	0.32 (0.09, 0.54)
Kivitz 2004	0.24 (0.08, 0.39)
Tannenbaum 2004	0.20 (0.07, 0.34)
Detrembleur 2005	0.23 (−0.75, 1.22)
Lehmann 2005	0.15 (0.03, 0.26)
Sheldon 2005	0.13 (0.02, 0.25)
Clegg 2006	0.13 (−0.03, 0.28)
Combined	0.29 (0.22, 0.35)

Effect size (95% confidence interval)

Fig. 23.2 Effect size of NSAIDs for pain relief. Figure calculated and constructed using data and references drawn from the systematic review of Bjordal et al., 2007 and the randomized controlled trial of Clegg et al., 2006. Data adapted from Zhang et al., 2007.

CI: 1.08–2.00; Towheed et al., 2006). More importantly, NSAIDs can cause serious GI complications such as PUBs, and this risk increases with age, concurrent use of other medications, and probably with the duration of therapy (Tramer et al., 2000). A meta-analysis of severe upper GI complications of NSAIDs showed relative risks of 5.36 (95% CI: 1.79–16.1) in 16 NSAID versus placebo trials with 4431 patients, 2.7 (95% CI: 2.1–3.5) in nine cohort studies with >750 000 person-years of drug exposure, and 3 (95% CI: 2.5–3.7) in 23 case-control studies with 25 732 patients (Ofman et al., 2002). The recommendation that, in patients with increased GI risk, either a COX-2 selective agent or a non-selective NSAID with co-prescription of a proton-pump inhibitor (PPI) or misoprostol for gastroprotection should be considered is supported by evidence from a systematic review of 112 RCTs which included ~75 000 patients (Hooper et al., 2004). The relative risks for symptomatic ulcers and serious GI complications with these different strategies are shown in Table 23.4. Recently, NICE (National Institute for Clinical Excellence), in the UK, has recommended addition of gastroprotection (PPI) to both traditional NSAIDs and COX-2 selective agents, irrespective of estimated individual patient risk (National Collaborating Centre for Chronic Conditions, 2008).

The use of COX-2 selective NSAIDs has been challenged by the withdrawal of rofecoxib in 2004 because of an increased relative risk of thrombotic cardiovascular (CV) events including myocardial infarction and stroke in the Vioxx Gastrointestinal Outcomes Research Study (VIGOR) trial (Bombardier et al., 2000) and a colorectal adenoma-chemoprevention trial (Bresalier et al., 2005). A number of systematic reviews of the CV safety of other COX-2 selective and non-selective NSAIDs have been undertaken (Table 23.4). There is a tendency for all NSAIDs, including COX-2 selective and conventional NSAIDs, to predispose to CV adverse events. The overall CV risk associated with COX-2 selective inhibitors was not significantly greater than that associated with conventional non-selective NSAIDs (RR = 1.19, 95% CI: 0.80–1.75; Hooper et al., 2004). There was, however, some heterogeneity in risk among the conventional NSAIDs with a modest increase in risk of CV events with ibuprofen (RR = 1.51, 95% CI: 0.96–2.37) and diclofenac (RR = 1.63, 95% CI: 1.12–2.37) but not with naproxen (RR = 0.92, 95% CI: 0.67–1.26; Kearney et al., 2006). The current advice (Heim and Broich, 2006) from the European Agency for the Evaluation of Medicinal Products (EMEA) is that COX-2-selective NSAIDs are contraindicated in patients with ischaemic heart disease or stroke and that prescribers should exercise caution when prescribing COX-2 inhibitors for patients with risk factors for heart disease, such as hypertension, hyperlipidaemia, diabetes, and smoking, as well as for patients with peripheral arterial disease (Heim and Broich, 2006). In the USA, all marketed prescription NSAIDs, both non-selective and COX-2-selective, carry a boxed warning about their potential for causing serious CV and GI events.

Opioids

The use of opioid analgesics is recommended by every treatment guideline which has addressed this therapy in OA (National Collaborating Centre for Chronic Conditions, 2008; Zhang et al., 2007b). A number of systematic reviews of the use of opioids for chronic non-cancer pain (Furlan et al., 2006; Kalso et al., 2004), musculoskeletal pain (Abasolo and Carmona, 2007), and, more recently, OA (Avouac et al., 2007), have provided evidence of efficacy and acceptable safety in short-term trials. Analysis of 18 placebo-controlled RCTs including 4856 patients with OA showed a moderate-to-large ES for reduction in pain intensity (ES = 0.78, 95% CI: 0.59–0.98) and small-to-moderate ES for improvement in physical function (ES = 0.31, 95% CI: 0.24–0.39; Avouac et al., 2007). Benefits associated with the use of opioids were, however, limited by frequent side effects; nausea (30%), constipation (23%), dizziness (20%), somnolence (18%), and vomiting (13%) (Avouac et al., 2007). Overall, 25% of patients treated with opioids withdrew from studies compared with 7% of placebo-treated patients with a NNH of 5. The withdrawal rate for strong opioids (e.g. oxymorphone, oxycodone, oxytrex, fentanyl, and morphine sulphate) was 31% (NNH: 4) compared with a withdrawal rate of 19% (NNH: 9) for the weaker opioids (e.g. tramadol, tramadol/paracetamol, codeine, and propoxyphene; Avouac et al., 2007). Combination use of opioid and minor analgesics, such as paracetamol, is suggested. A systematic review conducted a decade earlier, however, confirmed that paracetamol–codeine combinations did provide a small (~5%) but statistically significant analgesic benefit when compared with paracetamol alone, but adverse effects were more frequent (RR = 2.5, 95% CI: 1.5–4.2; De Craen et al., 1996). In addition, the risks of dependence or addiction to opiates have to be considered (Von Korff and Deyo, 2004). Irrespective of recommendation, as much as 25% of general practitioners in the UK have never prescribed opioids for patients with persistent non-cancer-related pain (Hutchinson et al., 2007).

Nutraceuticals

The claim of symptomatic benefit (e.g. pain relief) of glucosamine products is not fully supported by research evidence. The latest systematic review of 15 RCTs in 2007 demonstrated an ES for pain relief of 0.35 (95%CI: 0.14–0.56) but there was a considerable variation in outcomes between studies (I^2 = 0.80; Vlad et al., 2007). It was suggested that allocation concealment may affect the results (Vlad et al., 2007). The most striking differences, however, seemed to be related to the glucosamine preparations. The ES for trials which used glucosamine sulphate was 0.44 (95% CI: 0.18–0.70) compared with 0.06 (95% CI: −0.08–0.20) for those that used glucosamine hydrochloride. The ES for trials utilizing the Rottapharm preparation of glucosamine sulphate was 0.55 (95% CI: 0.29–0.82) compared with an ES of 0.11 (95% CI: −0.16–0.38) for trials with other products. Three large-scale well-designed RCTs have been published recently (2006–08): two for glucosamine sulphate 1500 mg/day (Herrero et al., 2007; Rozendaal et al., 2008) and one for glucosamine hydrochloride 1500 mg/day (Clegg et al., 2006). The results are predominantly negative. Only one showed that glucosamine sulphate 1500 mg daily was significantly better than placebo in improving the Lequesne score but not the Western Ontario and McMaster Osteoarthritis Index (WOMAC) score in knee OA (Herrero et al., 2007). The other two showed that neither glucosamine sulphate 1500 mg/day in hip OA (Rozendaal et al., 2008) nor glucosamine hydrochloride 1500 mg/day in knee OA (Clegg et al., 2006) were better than placebo for pain relief.

Evidence for structure-modifying effect of glucosamine products is controversial. Three RCTs have been undertaken for this outcome, two for knee OA (Pavelka et al., 2002; Reginster et al., 2001), and one for hip OA (Rozendaal et al., 2008). Although one demonstrated a significant effect of glucosamine sulphate in reducing loss of joint space width, two did not. The overall ES of these three RCTs is 0.20 (95%CI: 0.04–0.35) (Figure 23.3). More recently, a follow-up observational study examined the risk of total knee replacement in participants involved in the two RCTs in knee OA. The results showed that the 5-year incidence rate of total knee replacement in people who took glucosamine sulphate 1500 mg/day across 12 months (14.5%) was 2 times lower than those who took placebo (6.3%; p = 0.0024; Bruyere et al., 2008b).

Evidence to support the symptomatic benefit of chondroitin sulphate in OA is also controversial. Five meta-analyses have been undertaken so far (Bjordal et al., 2007; Leeb et al., 2000; McAlindon et al., 2000; Reichenbach et al., 2007; Richy et al., 2003). Analysis of eight RCTs involving 755 patients in 2003 showed a moderate ES for pain reduction (ES = 0.52, 95% CI: 0.37–0.67) with an NNT of 5 (Michaels, 2001; Good, 1994) and no evidence of serious side effects (Richy et al., 2003). However, in a meta-analysis of 20 trials involving 3846 patients in 2007 (Reichenbach et al., 2007), the ES for pain relief was large (ES = 0.75, 95% CI: 0.50–0.99) but there was very marked heterogeneity of outcomes between trials (I^2 = 92%). Small trials with poor-quality features, such as uncertain allocation concealment and a failure to analyse results on

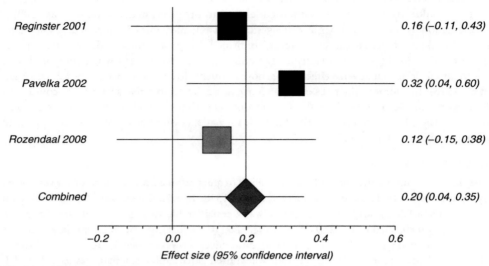

Fig. 23.3 Effect size of glucosamine sulphate for joint space width

an intention-to-treat basis, showed larger effects in favour of chondroitin sulphate. When the analysis was restricted to three recent trials with large sample sizes and an intention-to-treat analysis, the ES for pain reduction was only 0.03 (95% CI: −0.07–0.13) with an I^2 of 0% (Reichenbach et al., 2007). The pooled RR for adverse events was 0.99 (95% CI: 0.76–1.21; Reichenbach et al., 2007). A critical appraisal has been undertaken of the published meta-analyses of the symptomatic benefits of chondroitin sulphate (Monfort et al., 2008). In addition to the heterogeneity of the trials, this critical appraisal noted that the effect of chondroitin sulphate increases between weeks 4 and 12, whilst pain relief from NSAIDs decreases over this period. Whether the long-term symptomatic benefit from chondoitin sulphate is different from that of standard analgesics requires further research.

The structure-modification effect of chondroitin sulphate has been systematically reviewed (Hochberg et al., 2008). Five RCTs were included in this review where no heterogeneity was found across the trials. Pooled results demonstrated a small but significant effect of chondroitin sulphate over placebo on the reduction in rate of decline of minimum joint-space width (JSW) in people with knee OA (ES = 0.26, 95%CI: 0.14–0.38, $p < 0.0001$). The result was reinforced by the recent RCT published in 2009 (Kahn et al., 2009), where the minimum JSW loss over 2 years of observation was significantly lower in the treatment (JSW: −0.07, standard error of mean (SEM): 0.03) than in the placebo group (JSW: 0.031, SEM: 0.04; p<0.0001).

Evidence for symptomatic efficacy of ASU in patients with OA came from a systematic review of four RCTs ($n = 664$) for either hip (41%) or knee (59%) OA (Christensen et al., 2008b). Alhough based on heterogeneous results ($I^2 = 83.5\%$), the ES for pain reduction was 0.39 (95%CI: 0.01–0.76). Applying the Lequesne Index also favoured ASU ($I^2 = 61.0\%$, ES = 0.45, 95% CI: 0.21–0.70). Secondarily, the number of responders taking ASU compared to those taking placebo (OR = 2.19, $p = 0.007$) resulted in an NNT of 6 (95%CI: 4–21) patients.

Six RCTs were systematically reviewed for vitamin E in OA, including four placebo and two active (i.e. diclofenac) controlled trials (Canter et al., 2007). The studies are generally of poor quality and results are controversial. Whilst two short-term placebo-controlled trials found that vitamin E was superior to placebo, the other two long-term trials showed no benefit from vitamin E over placebo. Two subsequent active-control trials, however, suggested that vitamin E was equivalent to diclofenac for OA. Further high-quality trials are needed.

In summary, many nutraceuticals have been used to treat OA and appear generally safe. Although the mechanism of action remains substantially unknown, RCTs demonstrate small but heterogeneous effects over placebo. Largely because of the heterogeneity of trials in glucosamine and chondroitin sulphate, and their cost, recent NICE recommendations are to not prescribe these agents for patients with OA in the UK (National Collaborating Centre for Chronic Conditions, 2008). They also receive only weak support from European (Jordan et al., 2003; Zhang et al., 2005; Zhang et al., 2007a) and the Osteoarthritis Research Society International (OARSI) guidelines (Zhang et al., 2008a).

Herbs (e.g. rosehip, SAM-e, etc.)

Herbal medicines recently have gained popularity as treatments for OA. A meta-analysis of three RCTs demonstrated a small ES of 0.37 (95%CI: 0.13–0.60) of rosehip over placebo to relieve pain due to hip and knee OA, corresponding to an NNT of 6 (95%CI: 4–13; Christensen et al., 2008b).

SAM-e is a popular dietary product in the USA available as a treatment for OA. A systematic review of 11 RCTs found that SAM-e was effective in reducing functional limitation from OA (ES: 0.31; 95% CI: 0.10–0.52), but not in reducing pain (ES: 0.22; 95% CI: −0.25–0.69). This result, however, is based on only two studies. SAM-e seems to be comparable with NSAIDs (pain, ES: 0.12; 95% CI: −0.029–0.273; functional limitation, ES: 0.03; 95% CI: −0.13–0.18). However, those treated with SAM-e were less likely to report adverse effects than those receiving NSAIDs (Soeken et al., 2002).

Other herbal remedies which are used to treat OA include *Harpagophytum* preparations, ginger, seed powder, *Boswellia serrata* gum resin, and willow bark extract. However, the evidence for all of these is sparse (Chrubasik et al., 2007).

Other oral agents (e.g. diacerhein, antidepressants, etc)

Diacerhein has been developed as the first anti-interleukin-1 therapy for OA (Solignac, 2004). However, its clinical effectiveness has yet to be confirmed. The pooled efficacy of four RCTs for pain reduction is small and marginal (ES = 0.22, 95%CI: 0.01–0.42) but the side effects are clinically significant – about fourfold greater than placebo (RR for diarrhoea: 3.98, 95%CI: 2.90–5.47; Zhang et al., 2007b). More RCTs have been undertaken in the past 2 years, especially for possible long-term structure modification, but evidence for this has yet to be reviewed.

The use of antidepressants (e.g. low-dose amitriptyline) for relieving pain from OA, especially for patients with non-restorative sleep, is predominantly supported by clinical expertise, and there is no RCT evidence to support this effect. However, depression is a common co-morbidity in older patients with OA (Sale et al., 2008), and there is limited evidence that successful treatment of coexisting depression can improve OA outcomes (Lin et al., 2003).

Topical agents
Topical NSAIDs

Topical NSAIDs are widely used as adjunctive or alternative therapy by patients with hand or knee OA. The ES pooled from patients with OA was 0.41 (95%CI: 0.16–0.59) for pain relief, 0.36 (95% CI: 0.24–0.48) for function, and 0.49 (95% CI: 0.17–0.80) for stiffness, corresponding to an NNT of 3 (95% CI: 2–4) i.e. one-third patients would have symptomatic improvement after using topical NSAIDs (Lin et al., 2004). However, the effect of topical NSAIDs may reduce with time due to the large placebo effect (Zhang et al., 2008). Some topical NSAIDs are as effective, but safer, than oral NSAIDs (Tugwell et al., 2004; Underwood et al., 2008; Evans et al., 1995). A number of new RCTs have been undertaken in the past 5 years (Tugwell et al., 2004; Underwood et al., 2008; Baer et al., 2005; Bookman et al., 2004; Roth and Stainhouse, 2004) and the efficacy and safety of topical NSAIDs in OA has been reinforced. Topical NSAIDs have been recommended by both NICE and OARSI guidelines as either a single or adjuvant therapy for OA (Zhang et al., 2008a; National Collaborating Centre for Chronic Conditions, 2008). However, whether topical NSAIDs are cost effective remains controversial, especially for long-term therapy (Roth and Stainhouse, 2004).

Topical capsaicin

Capsaicin is a lipophilic alkaloid extracted from chilli peppers which activates and sensitizes peripheral c-nociceptor fibres by binding and activating the vanilloid transient receptor potential vanilloid 1 (TRPV1) cation channel. Paradoxically, although the application of topical capsaicin to the skin may cause initial burning discomfort at the site of application, continued regular application results in progressive analgesia that is maximal after 10–14 days. Evidence for the efficacy of topical capsaicin (0.025% cream × 3–4 times daily) in patients with knee or hand OA is supported by a meta-analysis of RCTs of topical capsaicin in the treatment of chronic painful conditions (Zhang and Li Wan Po, 1994). This included a single placebo-controlled trial in 70 patients with knee OA as well as two RCTs in patients with hand OA. The mean reduction in pain was 33% with an NNT of 4 (95% CI: 3–5) after 4 weeks of therapy but adequate blinding is not possible in trials with this agent. Treatment with topical capsaicin is safe but up to 40% of patients may be troubled initially by local burning, stinging, or erythema.

IA injections

IA hyaluronic acid (hyaluronan)

Hyaluronic acid (HA) is a large-molecular-weight glycosaminoglycan which is a constituent of many connective tissues including joint synovial fluid. IA injection of HA (IAHA) is widely used for patients with knee OA, and occasionally other joint sites, and is variably registered as a medical device ('viscosupplement') or as a pharmaceutical (Zhang et al., 2007b). It has limited support from many existing guidelines as a therapeutic modality for knee OA despite considerable ongoing controversy with regard to its efficacy, cost-effectiveness, and benefit–risk ratio.

Seventeen systematic reviews and meta-analyses have been undertaken to assess the therapeutic effects of IAHA in OA – the majority of them being for knee OA (Aggarwal and Sempowski, 2004; Arrich et al., 2005; Bellamy et al., 2005; Bellamy et al., 2006; Bruyere et al., 2008a; Divine et al., 2007; Espallargues and Pons, 2003; Fenandez Lopez and Ruano-Ravina, 2006; Lo et al., 2003; Maheu et al., 2002; Modawal et al., 2005; Pagnano and Westrich, 2005; Reichenbach et al., 2007; Strand et al., 2006; Van den Bekerom et al., 2008; Wang et al., 2004). The results of these systematic reviews are controversial because of the different HA preparations, different search strategies and selection criteria, differences in the outcome measures and time points selected for outcome; and different statistical methods for data synthesis (Campbell et al., 2007). More than 70 RCTs have been undertaken so far for IAHA in the treatment of knee OA, either compared with placebo or active control, or against different preparations of HA. The pooled ES for pain reduction at 2–3 months following at least three IA injections at weekly intervals in 22 placebo-controlled RCTs in 2003 was 0.32 (95%CI: 0.17–0.47; Lo et al., 2003). There was, however, significant heterogeneity among studies. An asymmetric funnel plot and a positive

Egger test also suggested the possibility of publication bias; and the identification of two unpublished trials with a pooled effect size of 0.07 (95% CI: -0.15–0.28) further suggested that the overall ES might have been overestimated. In 10 trials comparing IAHA injections with IA corticosteroids, there were no significant differences 4 weeks after injection but IAHA was shown to be more effective 5–13 weeks post injection (Bellamy et al., 2006). No major safety issues were detected, apart from local adverse events such as temporary pain and swelling at the injection site (RR = 1.08, 95% CI: 1.01–1.15; Arrich et al., 2005). A recent meta-analysis of 13 RCTs comparing high-molecular-weight HA with standard HA showed that the former was no better (ES = 0.27, 95%CI: -0.01–0.55) but more harmful in terms of triggering acute flares of pain and swelling (RR = 2.04, 95%CI: 1.18–3.53; Reichenbach et al., 2007).

Evidence to support the use of IAHA in patients with hip OA are sparse. Two systematic reviews (Fernandez Lopez and Ruano-Ravina, 2006; van den Bekerom et al., 2008) have been undertaken, where only two RCTs were identified (Tikiz et al., 2005; Qvistgaard et al., 2006): one comparing a higher with a low-molecular-weight HA in 43 patients with hip OA (Tikiz et al., 2005), the other being a double-blind, three-armed RCT in 101 patients with hip OA in which IA injections of a low-molecular-weight HA preparation were compared with IA saline and IA corticosteroid injections (Qvistgaard et al., 2006). In the randomized comparison of three injections of high- and low-molecular-weight HA given at weekly intervals under fluoroscopic control, there were significant improvements of ~40% in visual analogue scale (VAS), WOMAC, and Lequesne Index scores at 1, 3, and 6 months after treatment, but there were no significant differences at any of the time points between the two groups (Tikiz et al., 2005). In the placebo-controlled trial in which three injections of HA, corticosteroid or saline were given with ultrasound guidance at two-weekly intervals, there were no significant differences among the HA-, corticosteroid-, or saline-treated groups in pain on walking, WOMAC, or Lequesne indices at 14, 28, or 90 days after the course of injections (Qvistgaard et al., 2006). Using OARSI response criteria, responses at 14 days were 53% in patients treated with HA, 56% in those receiving corticosteroid, and 33% in those receiving placebo. At 28 days, 53% responded to HA, 66% to corticosteroids, and 44% to placebo (Qvistgaard et al., 2006).

In summary, the symptomatic effects of IAHA in OA require further confirmation because of the heterogeneity and controversial results between studies. A systematic review of systematic reviews will not solve the problem, whereas a systematic review of all placebo-controlled RCTs with adequate examination of quality of trials, publication bias, heterogeneity, cumulative meta-analysis, and sensitivity analysis may be helpful. However, it does seem clear that high-molecular-weight HA is no better than normal HA and is more likely to trigger local reactions. Because of trial heterogeneity, high cost, and logistical issues related to a course of weekly joint injections, NICE does not recommend the use of IAHA in OA (National Collaborating Centre for Chronic Conditions, 2008).

IA corticosteroid

IA injections of corticosteroids have been widely used as adjunctive therapy in the treatment of patients with knee OA for >50 years (Miller et al., 1958), and are recommended as a treatment option in 11/13 existing treatment guidelines where this modality of therapy was considered (Zhang et al., 2007b). The efficacy of IA corticosteroid injections in patients with knee OA is well supported by evidence from a Cochrane systematic review (Bellamy et al., 2006), which examined data from 13 placebo-controlled RCTs. The ES for relief of pain was in the moderate range (ES = 0.72, CI: 0.42–1.02) with an NNT of 4 (95% CI: 2–11) at 2 and 3 weeks after injection, although function was not significantly improved (ES = 0.06, 95% CI: -0.17–0.30) and evidence for relief of pain 4 and 24 weeks post injection was lacking.

One RCT has demonstrated better outcome in patients with knee effusion (Gaffney et al., 1995), but others have not found that clinical signs of inflammation or the presence of a joint effusion (Dieppe et al., 1980; Jones and Doherty, 1996) are predictors of a good clinical response, supporting the recommendation in NICE that IA steroid injections should not be restricted to patients with physical signs of inflammation and/or joint effusion.

By contrast, the evidence to support the recommendation for IA steroid injection in patients with OA hip is mainly limited to two RCTs (Flanagan et al., 1988; Kullenberg et al., 2004). In one RCT an IA injection combining bupivacaine and triamcinolone gave no better pain relief than IA injection of saline after 1 month (RR = 1.18; 95% CI: 0.68–2.15) or after 3 months (RR = 0.61, CI: 0.23–1.60); and the combination containing IA steroid was no better than IA injection of local anaesthetic alone in patients with OA awaiting hip-joint replacement (Flanagan et al., 1988). A second RCT in 80 patients with severe symptomatic hip OA compared the effects of fluoroscopically controlled IA injection of 80 mg triamcinolone hexacetonide or 1% mepivacaine and demonstrated significant reduction in pain and improved mobility after 3 weeks and 3 months in the steroid-treated patients but not in those treated with IA injection of local anaesthetic (Kullenberg et al., 2004).

No serious adverse events were reported as a consequence of IA steroid injections in 1973 patients in 28 controlled trials in patients with knee OA (Bellamy et al., 2006). Possible side effects include local post-injection flares of pain and systemic corticosteroid effects such as temporary facial flushing (up to 72 h), fluid retention, or aggravation of hypertension or diabetes mellitus. Although introduction of sepsis is a theoretical concern, this seems negligible provided simple aseptic precautions are observed. Cartilage and other joint-tissue atrophy from repeated injections is another concern, but there are limited data at present to indicate how frequently it is safe to administer IA steroid injections to patients with knee or hip OA. Most experts recommend caution regarding too-frequent use, although repeat injections up to 3–4 times per year into the same large joint are generally considered safe.

Non-specific treatment

Placebo has been used as a standard therapy for decades. It literally means 'I will please' and was a term that was first used for the presumed inactive compounds (e.g. bread pills, saline injections, coloured water, etc.) that doctors gave to patients with the assurance that they would help them and allow them to better cope with chronic disease (Shapiro, 1968). At a time when there were few effective treatments, such deception was considered benevolent and ethical. However, since the 1950s, when many new and effective treatments were being developed, placebo became a standard comparator in RCTs to determine the efficacy and side effects of a treatment (Kaptchuk, 1998). Placebo is still a common therapy in clinical practice for many conditions, irrespective of its ethical problems (Hrobjartsson and Norup, 2003). However, the placebo effect is often substantial, whether it is obtained from an inert pill, cream, injection, inactive electrodes, sham acupuncture, or sham surgery (Kaptchuk et al., 2006; Mercado et al., 2006; Moseley et al., 2002). It is also clear that, even without the 'ritual' of receiving a specific item of treatment, positive aspects of the practitioner–patient encounter can result in improved patient outcomes (Thomas, 1987). This resulted in the change of the concept of placebo from an item of treatment to broader non-specific elements of treatment which now are more commonly called 'contextual' or 'meaning' responses.[1] This concept is especially relevant to chronic conditions, such as OA, for which there are no very effective treatments, where optimization of the non-specific aspects of treatment can improve patient-centred outcomes (Doherty and Dieppe, 2009).

A recent meta-analysis of 198 RCTs demonstrated that placebo was effective at relieving pain (ES: 0.51, 95% CI: 0.46–0.55 for the placebo group and 0.03, 95% CI: −0.13–0.18 for untreated control; Zhang et al., 2008b). Placebo was also effective at improving function and stiffness. The pain-relieving effect increased when the active-treatment effect, baseline pain, and sample size increased, and when placebo was given by needles/injection. This meta-analysis confirmed that the effect size of non-specific therapy in OA cannot be ignored since it is usually larger than the ES obtained from the specific effects of any OA treatment. Factors that modify the size of this effect include patient and practitioner expectation of improvement, relief of anxiety, positive patient–practitioner interaction, and meaning response and 'contextual healing' (Doherty and Dieppe, 2009).

Treatment optimization

Benefit and harm

Clinical decision-making is based on the trade-off between benefits and harms, especially with respect to drug therapy and surgery. For example, although conventional NSAIDs are effective, they also cause GI bleeding and perforation, and therefore should not be used in patients at high risk of GI events. The combination of paracetamol and codeine may be more effective than either alone, but codeine should be used with caution in the elderly since it can cause marked constipation and other central nervous system (CNS) side effects. COX-2 inhibitors may be safer than traditional NSAIDs for the gut but are more risky for the CV system. Whilst diacerhein is as effective as NSAIDs in relieving pain, it has a high incidence of diarrhoea. Nutraceuticals such as glucosamine sulphate, chondroitin sulphate, ASU, and vitamins are generally harmless but their clinical benefits are marginal and even questionable.

Cost-effectiveness

The cost and logistics of any treatment is an important consideration given the shortage of resource. Although COX-2 inhibitors cause fewer GI complications, they are far more expensive than a conventional NSAID. The cost per quality-adjusted life-year (QALY) gained by COX-2 inhibitors is £33 889, in addition to the cost incurred by NSAIDs (Table 23.5; Zhang et al., 2007b). This exceeds the NICE cost-effective threshold of £20 000–30 000/QALY (Appleby et al., 2007). NSAID plus PPI (£36 923/QALY) is also not cost-effective therapy for OA from the perspective of the UK National Health Services (Zhang et al., 2007b). In contrast, NSAID plus misoprostol (£8889/QALY) is cost effective according to this threshold. This makes the clinical decision even more difficult. Direct use of the incremental cost-effectiveness ratio (ICER) for all patients may not be adequate, as it may vary from individual to individual according to the disease severity, risk exposures, co-morbidities, affordability, and personal preference.

Treatment algorithm and toolbox

NICE has recommended a stepwise treatment for OA (Figure 23.4), although emphasizing that every management plan needs to be tailored to the individual, taking into account the severity of OA, co-morbidity, and patient needs and preferences. Non-pharmacological therapy (such as education and information access, exercise, weight reduction if overweight, and reduction of other adverse mechanical factors) should be the core therapy that is considered for every patient with OA. If, in addition, pharmacological treatment for pain relief is required, oral paracetamol and/or topical NSAIDs are the recommended first-line agents to consider. If required, there are then a wide variety of additional treatments (including both pharmacological and non-pharmacological interventions) from which to select. These may be used alternatively or as adjuncts, for patients in whom sufficient symptomatic control cannot be achieved (National Collaborating Centre for

Table 23.5 Cost per QALY

Intervention	Comparator	Perspective*	Time horizon	Discounting	Year published	Country	Cost/QUALY Original	Cost/QUALY Converted ($)#
Water-based exercise	Usual care	Societal	1 year	No	2005	UK	£5738	10 483
Acupuncture	Sham acupuncture	Societal	3 months	No	2005	Germany	17 845 euros	22 297
NSAID + PPI	NSAIDs	NHS	6 months	No	2005	UK	£33 889	61 915
NSAID + misoprostol	NSAIDs	NHS	6 months	No	2005	UK	£8889	16 240
COX-2 specifics	NSAIDs	NHS	6 months	No	2005	UK	£36 923	74 298
COX-2 selectives	NSAIDs	NHS	6 months	No	2005	UK	£30 000	60 367
Intra-articular hyaluronic acid	Standard care	Societal	1 year	No	2002	Canada	$10 000	10 453
Total hip replacement	Conventional therapy	Societal	Life	5%	1996	US	$4754	8131
Total knee replacement	Pre-operation	Institutional	2 years	No	1997	US	$5856	10 325

*Perspective = perspective for economic evaluation (Societal = costs and benefits to whole society; NHS = costs and benefits to UK National Health Service; Institutional = costs and benefits to other payers, e.g. insurance company)

The original cost/quality-adjusted life year (QALY) was converted into US$ with a discount rate of 5% p.a. from the date of the publication to the current value on 10 March 2006.

Adapted from Zhang et al., 2007, with permission from Elsevier.

Adapted from the OARSI treatment guidelines (Zhang et al., 2008a) with permission. Figures are derived from data in Cochrane et al., 2005; Witt et al., 2005; Elliott et al., 2005; Torrance et al., 2002; Chang et al., 1996; Lavernia et al., 1997.

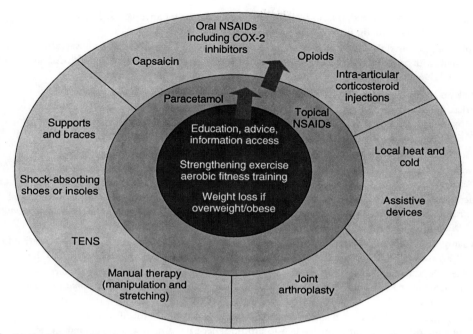

Fig. 23.4 NICE algorithm. Adapted from: National Collaborating Centre for Chronic Conditions. *Osteoarthritis: national clinical guideline for care and management in adults.* London: Royal College of Physicians, 2008. Copyright © 2008 Royal College of Physicians. Adapted by permission.

Chronic Conditions, 2008). EULAR (Jordan et al., 2003; Zhang et al., 2005; Zhang et al., 2007a) and OARSI (Zhang et al., 2008a), however, used a 'toolbox' system to recommend treatments. Each recommendation is examined for the best available research evidence, and the strength of recommendation and confidence of the recommendation from experts is provided, without any specific guide to follow. Such recommendations may be more adaptable to different countries, whereas NICE recommendations are developed specifically for the UK National Health Service and are therefore explicit in what to do, including what not to prescribe for OA.

Concluding remarks

Management of patients with chronic pain needs to be individualized, but usually requires a combination of non-pharmacological and pharmacological treatments. More than 20 groups of drugs and nutraceuticals are available for OA, including oral, topical, and IA agents. They may reduce symptoms, have structure-modification effects, or do both. However, most of the agents for OA have only mild-to-moderate ES. Furthermore, their side effects may be significant (and even life-threatening from NSAIDS and COX-2 selective drugs), especially with long-term therapy. The use of these agents is based on the balance between benefits and harms, as well as the cost incurred in the treatment of OA and the costs of any adverse events. Pharmacological agents should be considered as adjuncts to non-pharmacological core therapy and given within a holistic context of care that optimizes the non-specific effects of treatment and takes into account individual patient features and preference.

References

Abasolo, L. and Carmona, L. 2007: Systematic review: are major opioids effective in the treatment of musculoskeletal pain? *Medicina Clinica* **128**, 291–301.

Aggarwal, A. and Sempowski, I.P. 2004: Hyaluronic acid injections for knee osteoarthritis. Systematic review of the literature. *Canadian Family Physician* **50**, 249–56.

Aldington, S., Shirtcliffe, P., Weatherall, M. and Beasley, R. 2005: Increased risk of cardiovascular events with parecoxib/valdecoxib: A systematic review and meta-analysis. *New Zealand Medical Journal* **118**, U1755.

Appleby, J., Devlin, N. and Parkin, D. 2007: NICE's cost effectiveness threshold. *BMJ* **335**, 358–9.

Arrich, J., Piribauer, F., Mad, P., Schmid, D., Klaushofer, K. and Mullner, M. 2005: Intra-articular hyaluronic acid for the treatment of osteoarthritis of the knee: systematic review and meta-analysis. *CMAJ Canadian Medical Association Journal* **172**, 1039–43.

Arthritis Care. 2003: OA Nation Report. *TNS/arthritis care survey* www.arthritiscare.org.uk.

Avouac, J., Gossec, L. and Dougados, M. 2007: Efficacy and safety of opioids for osteoarthritis: a meta-analysis of randomized controlled trials. *Osteoarthritis and Cartilage* **15**, 957–65.

Baer, P.A., Thomas, L.M. and Shainhouse, Z. 2005: Treatment of osteoarthritis of the knee with a topical diclofenac solution: a randomised controlled, 6-week trial [ISRCTN53366886]. *BMC Musculoskeletal Disorders* **6**, 44.

Bellamy, N., Campbell, J., Robinson, V., Gee, T., Bourne, R. and Wells, G. 2005: Viscosupplementation for the treatment of osteoarthritis of the knee. *Cochrane Database of Systematic Reviews* CD005321.

Bellamy, N., Campbell, J., Robinson, V., Gee, T., Bourne, R. and Wells, G. 2006: Intraarticular corticosteroid for treatment of osteoarthritis of the knee. *Cochrane Database of Systematic Reviews* CD005328.

Bjordal, J.M., Klovning, A., Ljunggren, A.E. and Slordal, L. 2007: Short-term efficacy of pharmacotherapeutic interventions in osteoarthritic knee pain: A meta-analysis of randomised placebo-controlled trials. *European Journal of Pain* **11**, 125–38.

Bjordal, J.M., Ljunggren, A.E., Klovning, A. and Slordal, L. 2004: Non-steroidal anti-inflammatory drugs, including cyclo-oxygenase-2 inhibitors, in osteoarthritic knee pain: Meta-analysis of randomised placebo controlled trials. *British Medical Journal* **329**, 1317–20.

Bombardier, C., Laine, L., Reicin, A., Shapiro, D., Burgos-Vargas, R., Davis, B., et al. 2000: Comparison of upper gastrointestinal toxicity of rofecoxib and naproxen in patients with rheumatoid arthritis. VIGOR Study Group.[see comment]. *New England Journal of Medicine* **343**, 1520–8.

Bookman, A.A., Williams, K.S. and Shainhouse, J.Z. 2004: Effect of a topical diclofenac solution for relieving symptoms of primary osteoarthritis of the knee: a randomized controlled trial. *CMAJ Canadian Medical Association Journal* **171**, 333–8.

Bresalier, R.S., Sandler, R.S., Quan, H., Bolognese, J.A., Oxenius, B., Horgan, K., et al. 2005: Cardiovascular Events Associated with Rofecoxib in a Colorectal Adenoma Chemoprevention Trial. *N Engl J Med* **352**, 1092–102.

Bruyere, O., Burlet, N., Delmas, P.D., Rizzoli, R., Cooper, C. and Reginster, J-Y. 2008a: Evaluation of symptomatic slow-acting drugs in osteoarthritis using the GRADE system. *BMC Musculoskeletal Disorders*. **9**, Article Number: 165

Bruyere, O., Pavelka, K., Rovati, L.C., Gatterova, J., Giacovelli, G., Olejarova, M., et al. 2008b: Total joint replacement after glucosamine sulphate treatment in knee osteoarthritis: results of a mean 8-year observation of patients from two previous 3-year, randomised, placebo-controlled trials. *Osteoarthritis and Cartilage* **16**, 254–60.

Caldwell, B., Aldington, S., Weatherall, M., Shirtcliffe, P. and Beasley, R. 2006: Risk of cardiovascular events and celecoxib: A systematic review and meta-analysis. *Journal of the Royal Society of Medicine* **99**, 132–40.

Campbell, J., Bellamy, N. and Gee, T. 2007: Differences between systematic reviews/meta-analyses of hyaluronic acid/hyaluronan/hylan in osteoarthritis of the knee. *Osteoarthritis and Cartilage* **15**, 1424–36.

Canter, P.H., Wider, B. and Ernst, E. 2007: The antioxidant vitamins A, C, E and selenium in the treatment of arthritis: a systematic review of randomized clinical trials. *Rheumatology* **46**, 1223–33.

Capurso, L. and Koch, M. 1991: Prevention of NSAID-induced gastric lesions: H2 antagonists or misoprostol? A meta-analysis of controlled clinical studies. *Clinica Terapeutica* **139**, 179–89.

Castelnuovo, E., Cross, P., Mt-Isa, S., Spencer, A., Underwood, M. and TOIB study team. 2008: Cost-effectiveness of advising the use of topical or oral ibuprofen for knee pain; the TOIB study. *Rheumatology* **47**, 1077–81.

Chang, R.W., Pellissier, J.M. and Hazen, G.B. 1996: A cost-effectiveness analysis of total hip arthroplasty for osteoarthritis of the hip (Structured abstract). *JAMA* **275**, 858–65.

Christensen, R., Bartels, E.M., Altman, R.D., Astrup, A. and Bliddal, H. 2008a: Does the hip powder of Rosa canina (rosehip) reduce pain in osteoarthritis patients? - a meta-analysis of randomized controlled trials. *Osteoarthritis and Cartilage* **16**, 965–72.

Christensen, R., Bartels, E.M., Astrup, A. and Bliddal, H. 2008b: Symptomatic efficacy of avocado-soybean unsaponifiables (ASU) in osteoarthritis (OA) patients: a meta-analysis of randomized controlled trials. *Osteoarthritis and Cartilage* **16**, 399–408.

Chrubasik, J.E., Roufogalis, B.D. and Chrabasik, S. 2007: Evidence of effectiveness of herbal antiinflammatory drugs in the treatment of painful osteoarthritis and chronic low back pain. *Phytotherapy Research* **21**, 675–83.

Clegg, D.O., Reda, D.J., Harris, C.L., Klein, M.A., O'Dell, J.R., Hooper, M.M., et al. 2006: Glucosamine, chondroitin sulfate, and the two in combination for painful knee osteoarthritis. *New England Journal of Medicine* **354**, 795–808.

Cochrane, T., Davey, R.C. and Matthes Edwards, S.M. 2005: Randomised controlled trial of the cost-effectiveness of water-based therapy for lower limb osteoarthritis. *Health Technology Assessment (Winchester, England)* **9**, iii–iiv.

de Craen, A.J., Di Giulio, G., Lampe-Schoenmaeckers, J.E., Kessels, A.G. and Kleijnen, J. 1996: Analgesic efficacy and safety of paracetamol-codeine combinations versus paracetamol alone: a systematic review. *Britis Medical Journal* **313**, 321–5.

Dieppe, P.A., Sathapatayavongs, B. and Jones, H.E. 1980: Intra-articular steroids in osteoarthritis. *Rheumatology and Rehabilitation* **19**, 212–17.

Divine, J.G., Zazulak, B.T. and Hewett, T.E. 2007: Viscosupplementation for knee osteoarthritis: a systematic review. *Clinical Orthopaedics and Related Research* **455**, 113–22.

Doherty, M. and Dieppe, P.A. 2009: The "placebo" response in osteoarthritis and its relevance to clinical practice. *Osteoarthritis and Cartilage* **17**, 1255–62.

Dougados, M., Nguyen, M., Berdah, L., Mazieres, B., Vignon, E., Lequesne, M., et al. 2001: Evaluation of the structure-modifying effects of diacerein in hip osteoarthritis: ECHODIAH, a three-year, placebo-controlled trial. Evaluation of the Chondromodulating Effect of Diacerein in OA of the Hip. *Arthritis and Rheumatism* **44**, 2539–47.

Elliott, R.A., Hooper, L., Payne, K., Brown, T.J., Roberts, C. and Symmons, D. 2006: Preventing non-steroidal anti-inflammatory drug-induced gastrointestinal toxicity: are older strategies more cost-effective in the general population? *Rheumatology* **45**, 606–13.

Espallargues, M. and Pons, J.M. 2003: Efficacy and safety of viscosupplementation with Hylan G-F 20 for the treatment of knee osteoarthritis: a systematic review. *International Journal of Technology Assessment in Health Care* **19**, 41–56.

Evans, J.M. and MacDonald, T.M. 1996: Tolerability of topical NSAIDs in the elderly: do they really convey a safety advantage? *Drugs and Aging* **9**, 101–8.

Evans, J.M.M., McMahon, A.D., McGilchrist, M.M., White, G., Murray, F.E., McDevitt, D.G., et al. 1995: Topical non-steroidal anti-inflammatory drugs and admission to hospital for upper gastrointestinal bleeding and perforation: a record linkage case-control study. *British Medical Journal* **311**, 22–6.

Evidence-Based Medicine Working Group. 1992: Evidence-based Medicine. A new approach to teaching the practice of medicine. *JAMA* **268**, 2420–5.

Fernandez Lopez, J.C. and Ruano-Ravina, A. 2006: Efficacy and safety of intraarticular hyaluronic acid in the treatment of hip osteoarthritis: a systematic review. *Osteoarthritis and Cartilage* **14**, 1306–11.

Flanagan, J., Casale, F.F., Thomas, T.L. and Desai, K.B. 1988: Intra-articular injection for pain relief in patients awaiting hip replacement. *Annals of the Royal College of Surgeons of England* 70, 156–7.

Fored, C.M., Ejerblad, E., Lindblad, P., Fryzek, J.P., Dickman, P.W., Signorello, L.B., et al. 2001: Acetaminophen, aspirin, and chronic renal failure. *New England Journal of Medicine* 345, 1801–8.

Furlan, A.D., Sandoval, J.A., Mailis-Gagnon, A. and Tunks, E. 2006: Opioids for chronic noncancer pain: a meta-analysis of effectiveness and side effects. *CMAJ Canadian Medical Association Journal* 174, 1589–94.

Gaffney, K., Ledingham, J. and Perry, J.D. 1995: Intra-articular triamcinolone hexacetonide in knee osteoarthritis: Factors influencing the clinical response. *Annals of the Rheumatic Diseases* 54, 379–381.

Garcia Rodriguez, L.A. and Hernandez-Diaz, S. 2001: Relative risk of upper gastrointestinal complications among users of acetaminophen and nonsteroidal anti-inflammatory drugs. *Epidemiology* 12, 570–6.

Heim, H.K. and Broich, K. 2006: Selective COX-2 inhibitors and the risk of thromboembolic events – regulatory aspects. *Thromb Haemost* 96, 423–32.

Hernandez-Diaz, S., Varas-Lorenzo, C. and Garcia Rodriguez, L.A. 2006: Non-steroidal antiinflammatory drugs and the risk of acute myocardial infarction. *Basic and Clinical Pharmacology and Toxicology* 98, 266–74.

Herrero, B.G., Ivorra, J.A., Del Carmen, T.M., Blanco, F.J., Benito, P., Martín, M.E., et al. 2007: Glucosamine sulfate in the treatment of knee osteoarthritis symptoms: a randomized, double-blind, placebo-controlled study using acetaminophen as a side comparator. *Arthritis and Rheumatism* 56, 555–67.

Hochberg, M.C., Zhan, M. and Langenberg, P. 2008: The rate of decline of joint space width in patients with osteoarthritis of the knee: a systematic review and meta-analysis of randomized placebo-controlled trials of chondroitin sulfate: *Curr. Med Res* 24, 3029–35.

Hooper, L., Brown, T.J., Elliott, R., Payne, K., Roberts, C. and Symmons, D. 2004: The effectiveness of five strategies for the prevention of gastrointestinal toxicity induced by non-steroidal anti-inflammatory drugs: systematic review. *British Medical Journal* 329, 948–52.

Hrobjartsson, A. and Norup, M. 2003: The use of placebo interventions in medical practice–a national questionnaire survey of Danish clinicians. *Eval Health Prof* 26, 153–65.

Hutchinson, K., Moreland, A.M., de C Williams, A., Weinman, J. and Horne, R. 2007: Exploring beliefs and practice of opioid prescribing for persistent non-cancer pain by general practitioners. *European Journal of Pain* 11, 93–8.

Hynes, R.B., Sacket, D.L., Gray, J.M.A., Cook, D.J. and Guyatt, G.H. 1996: Transferring evidence from research into practice: 1. The role of clinical care research evidence in clinical decisions. *Evidence*-Based *Medicine* 1, 196–7.

Jones, A. and Doherty, M. 1996: Intra-articular corticosteroids are effective in osteoarthritis but there are no clinical predictors of response. *Annals of the Rheumatic Diseases* 55, 829–32.

Jordan, K.M., Arden, N.K., Doherty, M., Bannwarth, B., Bijlsma, J.W., Dieppe, P., et al. 2003: EULAR Recommendations 2003: an evidence based approach to the management of knee osteoarthritis: Report of a Task Force of the Standing Committee for International Clinical Studies Including Therapeutic Trials (ESCISIT). *Annals of the Rheumatic Diseases* 62, 1145–55.

Juni, P., Nartey, L., Reichenbach, S., Sterchi, R., Dieppe, P.A. and Egger, M. 2004: Risk of cardiovascular events and rofecoxib: cumulative meta- analysis. *Lancet* 364, 2021–9.

Kahan, A., Uebelhart, D., De Vathaire, F., Delmas, P.D. and Reginster, J.Y. 2009: Long-term effects of chondroitins 4 and 6 sulfate on knee osteoarthritis: The study on osteoarthritis progression prevention, a two-year, randomized, double-blind, placebo-controlled trial. *Arthritis Rheum* 60, 524–33.

Kalso, E., Edwards, J.E., Moore, R.A. and McQuay, H.J. 2004: Opioids in chronic non-cancer pain: systematic review of efficacy and safety. *Pain* 112, 372–80.

Kaptchuk, T.J. 1998: Powerful placebo: the dark side of the randomised controlled trial. *Lancet* 351, 1722–5.

Kaptchuk, T.J., Stason, W.B., Davis, R.B., Legedza, A.R., Schnyer, R.N., Kerr, C.E., et al. 2006: Sham device v inert pill: randomised controlled trial of two placebo treatments. *British Medical Journal* **332**, 391–7.

Kearney, P.M., Baigent, C., Godwin, J., Halls, H., Emberson, J.R. and Patrono, C. 2006: Do selective cyclo-oxygenase-2 inhibitors and traditional non-steroidal anti-inflammatory drugs increase the risk of atherothrombosis? Meta-analysis of randomised trials. *British Medical Journal* **332**, 1302–8.

Kullenberg, B., Runesson, R., Tuvhag, R., Olsson, C. and Resch, S. 2004: Intraarticular corticosteroid injection: Pain relief in osteoarthritis of the hip? *Journal of Rheumatology* **31**, 2265–8.

Lavernia, C.J., Guzman, J.F. and Gachupin, G.A. 1997: Cost effectiveness and quality of life in knee arthroplasty. *Clinical Orthopaedics and Related Research* 134–9.

Lee, C., Hunsche, E., Balshaw, R., Kong, S.X. and Schnitzer, T.J. 2005: Need for common internal controls when assessing the relative efficacy of pharmacologic agents using a meta-analytic approach: Case study of cyclooxygenase 2-selective inhibitors for the treatment of osteoarthritis. *Arthritis Care and Research* **53**, 510–18.

Leeb, B.F., Schweitzer, H., Montag, K. and Smolen, J.S. 2000: A metaanalysis of chondroitin sulfate in the treatment of osteoarthritis. *Journal of Rheumatology* **27**, 205–11.

Lewis, S.C., Langman, M.J.S., Laporte, J-R., Matthres, N.S., Rawlins, M.D. and Wiholm, B-E. 2002: Dose-response relationships between individual nonaspirin nonsteroidal anti-inflammatory drugs (NSAIDs) and serious upper gastrointestinal bleeding: a meta-analysis based on individual patient data. *British Journal of Clinical Pharmacology* **54**, 320–6.

Lin, E.H.B., Katon, W., Von Korff, M., Tang, L., Williams, J.W., Jr., Kroenke, K., et al. 2003: Effect of Improving Depression Care on Pain and Functional Outcomes Among Older Adults With Arthritis: A Randomized Controlled Trial. *JAMA* **290**, 2428–9.

Lin, J., Zhang, W., Jones, A. and Doherty, M. 2004: Efficacy of topical non-steroidal anti-inflammatory drugs in the treatment of osteoarthritis: meta-analysis of randomised controlled trials. *British Medical Journal* **329**, 324.

Lo, G.H., LaValley, M., McAlindon, T. and Felson, D.T. 2003: Intra-articular hyaluronic acid in treatment of knee osteoarthritis: a meta-analysis. *JAMA* **290**, 3115–21.

Maheu, E., Ayral, X. and Dougados, M. 2002: A hyaluronan preparation (500-730 kDa) in the treatment of osteoarthritis: a review of clinical trials with Hyalgan. *International Journal of Clinical Practice* **56**, 804–13.

McAlindon, T.E., LaValley, M.P., Gulin, J.P. and Felson, D.T. 2000: Glucosamine and chondroitin for treatment of osteoarthritis: a systematic quality assessment and meta-analysis. *JAMA* **283**, 1469–75.

Mercado, R., Constantoyannis, C., Mandat, T., Kumar, A., Schulzer, M., Stoessl, A.J., et al. 2006: Expectation and the placebo effect in Parkinson's disease patients with subthalamic nucleus deep brain stimulation. *Movement Disorders* **21**, 1457–61.

Miller, J.H., White, J. and Norton, T.H. 1958: The value if intra-articular injections in osteoarthritis of the knee. *British Journal of Bone and Joint Surgery* **40**, 636–43.

Modawal, A., Ferrer, M., Choi, H.K. and Castle, J.A. 2005: Hyaluronic acid injections relieve knee pain. *Journal of Family Practice* **54**, 758–67.

Monfort, J., Martel-Pelletier, J. and Pelletier, J.P. 2008: Chondroitin sulphate for symptomatic osteoarthritis: critical appraisal of meta-analyses. *Current Medical Research Opinion* **24**, 1303–8.

Moseley, J.B., O'Malley, K., Petersen, N.J., Menke, T.J., Brody, B.A., Kuykendall, D.H., et al. 2002: A controlled trial of arthroscopic surgery for osteoarthritis of the knee. *New England Journal of Medicine* **347**, 81–8.

National Collaborating Centre for Chronic Conditions. 2008: *Osteoarthritis: national clinical guideline for care and management in adults.* London: Royal College of Physicians.

Ofman, J.J., MacLean, C.H., Straus, W.L., Morton, S.C., Berger, M.L., Roth, E.A., et al. 2002: A meta-analysis of severe upper gastrointestinal complications of nonsteroidal antiinflammatory drugs. *Journal of Rheumatology* **29**, 804–12.

Pagnano, M. and Westrich, G. 2005: Successful nonoperative management of chronic osteoarthritis pain of the knee: safety and efficacy of retreatment with intra-articular hyaluronans. *Osteoarthritis and Cartilage* **13**, 751–61.

Pavelka, K., Gatterova, J., Olejarova, M., Machacek, S., Giacovelli, G. and Rovati, L.C. 2002: Glucosamine sulfate use and delay of progression of knee osteoarthritis: a 3-year, randomized, placebo-controlled, double-blind study. *Archives of Internal Medicine* **162**, 2113–23.

Peat, G., McCarney, R. and Croft, P. 2001: Knee pain and osteoarthritis in older adults: a review of community burden and current use of primary health care. *Annals of Rheumtic Diseases* **60**, 91–7.

Pham, T., Le Henanff, A., Ravoud, P., Dieppe, P., Paolozzi, L. and Dougados, M. 2004: Evaluation of the symptomatic and structural efficacy of a new hyaluronic acid compound, NRD101, in comparison with diacerein and placebo in a 1 year randomised controlled study in symptomatic knee osteoarthritis. *Annals of Rheumatic Diseases* **63**, 1611–17.

Qvist, P., Bay-Jensen, A-C., Christiansen, C., Dam, E.B., Pastoureau, P. and Karsdal, M.A. 2008: The disease modifying osteoarthritis drug (DMOAD): Is it in the horizon? *Pharmacological Research* **58**, 1–7.

Qvistgaard, E., Christensen, R., Torp-Pedersen, S. and Bliddal, H. 2006: Intra-articular treatment of hip osteoarthritis: a randomized trial of hyaluronic acid, corticosteroid, and isotonic saline. *Osteoarthritis and Cartilage* **14**, 163–70.

Rahme, E., Barkun, A., Nedjar, H., Gaugris, S. and Watson, D. 2008: Hospitalizations for upper and lower GI events associated with traditional NSAIDs and acetaminophen among the elderly in Quebec, Canada. *American Journal of Gastroenterology* **103**, 872–82.

Reichenbach, S., Blank, S., Rutjes, A.W., Shang, A., King, E.A., Dieppe, P.A., et al. 2007: Hylan versus hyaluronic acid for osteoarthritis of the knee: a systematic review and meta-analysis. *Arthritis and Rheumatism* **57**, 1410–18.

Reginster, J.Y., Deroisy, R., Rovati, L.C., Lee, R.L., Lejeune, E., Bruyere, O., et al. 2001: Long-term effects of glucosamine sulphate on osteoarthritis progression: a randomised, placebo-controlled clinical trial. *Lancet* **357**, 251–6.

Reichenbach, S., Sterchi, R., Scherer, M., Trelle, S., Burgi, E., Burgi, U., et al. 2007: Meta-analysis: chondroitin for osteoarthritis of the knee or hip. *Annals of Internal Medicine* **146**, 580–90.

Rexrode, K.M., Buring, J.E., Glynn, R.J., Stampfer, M.J., Youngman, L.D. and Gaziano, J.M. 2001: Analgesic use and renal function in men. *JAMA* **286**, 315–21.

Richy, F., Bruyere, O., Ethgen, O., Cucherat, M., Henrotin, Y. and Reginster, J-Y. 2003: Structural and symptomatic efficacy of glucosamine and chondroitin in knee osteoarthritis: A comprehensive meta-analysis. *Archives of Internal Medicine* **163**, 1514–22.

Roth, S.H. and Shainhouse, J.Z. 2004: Efficacy and safety of a topical diclofenac solution (Pennsaid) in the treatment of primary osteoarthritis of the knee: A randomized, double-blind, vehicle-controlled clinical trial. *Archives of Internal Medicine* **164**, 2017–23.

Rozendaal, R.M., Koes, B.W., van Osch, G.J.V.M., Uitterlinden, E.J., Garling, E.H., Willemsen, S.P., et al. 2008: Effect of Glucosamine Sulfate on Hip Osteoarthritis: A Randomized Trial. *Annals of Internal Medicine* **148**, 268–77.

Sackett, D.L., Rosenberg, W.M., Gray, J.A., Haynes, R.B. and Richardson, W.S. Evidence based medicine: what it is and what it isn't. *BMJ* 1996;**312**:71–2.

Sale, J.E., Gignac, M. and Hawker, G. 2008: The relationship between disease symptoms, life events, coping and treatment, and depression among older adults with osteoarthritis. *Journal of Rheumatology* **35**, 335–42.

Shapiro, A.K. 1968: Semantics of the placebo. *Psychiatr Q* **42**, 653–95.

Shekelle, P.G., Woolf, S.H., Eccles, M. and Grimshaw, J. 1999: Clinical guidelines: developing guidelines. *BMJ* **318**, 593–6.

Soeken, K.L., Lee, W.L., Bausell, R.B., Agelli, M. and Berman, B.M. 2002: Safety and efficacy of S-adenosylmethionine (SAMe) for osteoarthritis. *Journal of Family Practice* **51**, 425–30.

Solignac, M. 2004: Mechanisms of action of diacerein, the first inhibitor of interleukin-1 in osteoarthritis. *Presse Medicale* **33**, t-2.

Strand, V., Conaghan, P.G., Lohmander, L.S., Koutsoukos, A.D., Hurley, F.L., Bird, H., et al. 2006: An integrated analysis of five double-blind, randomized controlled trials evaluating the safety and efficacy of a hyaluronan product for intra-articular injection in osteoarthritis of the knee. *Osteoarthritis and Cartilage* **14**, 859–66.

Thomas, K.B. 1987: General practice consultations: is there any point in being positive? *British Medical Journal (Clin Res Ed)* **294**, 1200–2.

Tikiz, C., Unlu, Z., Sener, A., Efe, M. and Tuzun, C. 2005: Comparison of the efficacy of lower and higher molecular weight viscosupplementation in the treatment of hip osteoarthritis. *Clinical Rheumatology* **24**, 244–50.

Torrance, G.W., Raynauld, J.P., Walker, V., Goldsmith, C.H., Bellamy, N., Band, P.A., et al. 2002: A prospective, randomized, pragmatic, health outcomes trial evaluating the incorporation of hylan G-F 20 into the treatment paradigm for patients with knee osteoarthritis (Part 2 of 2): economic results. *Osteoarthritis and Cartilage* **10**, 518–27.

Towheed, T.E., Maxwell, L., Anastassiades, T.P., Shea, B., Houpt, J., Robinson, V., et al. 2005: Glucosamine therapy for treating osteoarthritis. *The Cochrane Library.(Oxford)* CD002946.

Towheed, T.E., Maxwell, L., Judd, M.G., Catton, M., Hochberg, M.C. and Wells, G. 2006: Acetaminophen for osteoarthritis. *Cochrane Database of Systematic Reviews* CD004257.

Tramer, M.R., Moore, R.A., Reynolds, D.J.M. and McQuay, H.J. 2000: Quantitative estimation of rare adverse events which follow a biological progression: A new model applied to chronic NSAID use. *Pain* **85**, 169–82.

Tugwell, P.S., Wells, G.A. and Shainhouse, J.Z. 2004: Equivalence study of a topical diclofenac solution (Pennsaid) compared with oral diclofenac in symptomatic treatment of osteoarthritis of the knee: A randomized controlled trial. *Journal of Rheumatology* **2004**, 2002–12.

Underwood, M., Ashby, D., Cross, P., Hennessy, E., Letley, L., Martin, J., et al. 2008: Advice to use topical or oral ibuprofen for chronic knee pain in older people: randomised controlled trial and patient preference study. *British Medical Journal* **336**, 138–42.

van den Bekerom, M.P., Lamme, B., Sermon, A. and Mulier, M. 2008: What is the evidence for viscosupplementation in the treatment of patients with hip osteoarthritis? Systematic review of the literature. *Archives of Orthopaedic and Trauma Surgery* **128**, 815–23.

Vlad, S.C., LaValley, M.P., McAlindon, T.E. and Felson, D.T. 2007: Glucosamine for pain in osteoarthritis: Why do trial results differ? *Arthritis and Rheumatism* **56**, 2267–77.

Von Korff, M. and Deyo, R.A. 2004: Potent opioids for chronic musculoskeletal pain: flying blind. *Pain* **109**, 207–9.

Wang, C.T., Lin, J., Chang, C.J., Lin, Y.T. and Hou, S.M. 2004: Therapeutic effects of hyaluronic acid on osteoarthritis of the knee. A meta-analysis of randomized controlled trials. *Journal of Bone and Joint Surgery - American* **86-A**, 538–45.

Witt, C., Selim, D., Reinhold, T., Jena, S., Brinkhaus, B., Liecker, B. et al. 2005: Cost-effectiveness of acupuncture in patients with headache, low back pain and osteoarthritis of the hip and the knee. 12th Annual Symposium on Complementary Health Care. *Focus on Alternative and Complementary Therapies* **10**, 57–8.

Zhang, W. and Doherty, M. 2006: EULAR recommendations for knee and hip osteoarthritis: a critique of the methodology. *British Journal of Sports Medicine* **40**, 664–9.

Zhang, W., Jones, A. and Doherty, M. 2004: Does paracetamol (acetaminophen) reduce the pain of osteoarthritis?: a meta-analysis of randomised controlled trials. *Annals of Rheumatic Diseases* **63**, 901–7.

Zhang, W., Doherty, M., Arden, N., Bannwarth, B., Bijlsma, J., Gunther, K.P., et al. 2005: EULAR evidence based recommendations for the management of hip osteoarthritis: report of a task force of the EULAR Standing Committee for International Clinical Studies Including Therapeutics (ESCISIT). *Annals of Rheumatic Diseases* **64**, 669–81.

Zhang, W., Doherty, M., Leeb, B.F., Alekseeva, L., Arden, N.K., Bijlsma, J.W., et al. 2007a: EULAR evidence based recommendations for the management of hand osteoarthritis: Report of a Task Force of the EULAR Standing Committee for International Clinical Studies Including Therapeutics (ESCISIT). *Annals of Rheumatic Diseases* **66**, 377–88.

Zhang, W., Doherty, M., Pascual, E., Bardin, T., Barskova, V., Conaghan, P., et al. 2006: EULAR evidence based recommendations for gout. Part I: Diagnosis. Report of a task force of the standing committee for international clinical studies including therapeutics (ESCISIT). *Annals of Rheumatic Diseases* **65**, 1301–11.

Zhang, W.Y. and Li Wan Po, P.A. 1994: The effectiveness of topically applied capsaicin. A meta-analysis. *European Journal of Clinical Pharmacology* **46**, 517–22.

Zhang, W., Moskowitz, R.W., Nuki, G., Abramson, S., Altman, R.D., Arden, N., et al. 2007b: OARSI recommendations for the management of hip and knee osteoarthritis, Part I: Critical appraisal of existing treatment guidelines and systematic review of current research evidence. *Osteoarthritis and Cartilage* **15**, 981–1000.

Zhang, W., Moskowitz, R.W., Nuki, G., Abramson, S., Altman, R.D., Arden, N. et al. 2008a: OARSI recommendations for the management of hip and knee osteoarthritis, Part II: OARSI evidence-based, expert consensus guidelines. *Osteoarthritis and Cartilage* **16**, 137–62.

Zhang, W., Robertson, J., Jones, A.C., Dieppe, P.A. and Doherty, M. 2008b: The placebo effect and its determinants in osteoarthritis: meta-analysis of randomised controlled trials. *Annals of Rheumatic Diseases* **67**, 1716–23.

Chapter 24

The potential for prevention: occupation

Gwenllian Wynne-Jones and Chris J. Main

Overview

Work is a common exposure. For example, almost three-quarters of the UK population of working age are in employment (73.8%) (Office for National Statistics, 2009): in the 3 months to February 2009, a total of 21.7 million individuals were working full time, 13.9 million men and 7.8 million women, average weekly hours of 31.7. The number of employees in the UK is greatest in the private sector where 23.6 million individuals are employed compared to the public sector where 5.7 million individuals are employed (Office for National Statistics, 2009).

Most people reporting pain are of working age (Natvig and Picavet, 2002). Pain is a common phenomenon for many people and may extend from an acute phase to a chronic condition. Chronic pain can significantly affect quality of life (Clark, 2002; Blyth et al., 2001; Verhaak et al., 1998; Crook et al., 1984, Elliott et al., 2002; Woolf and Pfleger, 2003). Chronic pain of moderate-to-severe intensity is estimated to occur in 19% of adult Europeans, seriously affecting their daily activities and social and working lives (Blyth et al., 2001).

Work is an important component of the public health perspective on chronic pain. This chapter considers work and the working environment as causes of pain; the consequences of chronic pain for work and working life; and the public health perspective on work and chronic pain.

Background concepts

The World Health Organization's International Classification of Function (ICF)

The conceptual framework for thinking about occupation and chronic pain in this chapter is provided by the World Health Organization's International Classification of Function (ICF), which has been summarized by Raspe in Chapter 6 (see Figure 6.2). In this framework:

◆ pain (an impairment) can restrict the capacity to do specific occupational activities and, more broadly, can lead to restricted participation in work,

◆ work can also be the cause of the impairment (pain), and pre-existing individual factors (the 'propensity' for chronic pain) may predispose a person to developing chronic pain in the context of occupational triggers for pain, and

◆ both the work environment and the wider cultural and social environment may influence whether the person in pain (whatever the cause of the pain) can or cannot participate fully in work.

Traditional approaches to health and safety use a model of work as being hazardous to health. This is based on an injury model whereby individuals with injuries are advised to rest, take time away from the workplace, and avoid activity. Patients expect that a period of work absence is necessary (Verbeck et al., 2004).

By contrast, the vocational rehabilitation model advocates helping individuals with health problems to stay at, return to, or remain in work (Waddell et al., 2008). This fits with the ICF model – work, from this perspective, is seen as a means to reduce some of the broader biopsychosocial risks for chronic pain and to promote musculoskeletal health, as distinct from being seen exclusively as an inappropriate place or source of risk for persons with ill-health.

This rehabilitation concept also forms the basis for public health strategies to minimize the effects of injuries and reinforce positive messages about remaining active (Buchbinder et al., 2001; Waddell et al., 2007). The benefits of remaining active despite pain have been well documented, e.g. in workers with back pain, leading to less sick leave, less time on modified duties, and a reduction in pain recurrence (Buchbinder et al., 2001; Waddell et al., 1997; McGuirk and Bogduk, 2007; Waddell and Burton, 2006).

The importance of work

Waddell has highlighted that welfare systems rewarding sickness absence may promote the problem of disability. The belief that work is generally harmful or prevents recovery, and lack of health care professional training, understanding, time, and motivation can all affect judgements about the complex issue of fitness for work (Waddell and Aylward, 2005). Long-term worklessness poses a serious risk to physical, mental, and social well-being, while return to work can improve recovery for people with common health problems (Waddell and Burton, 2006). Sick certification can reinforce the 'sick role' and adaptation to invalidity, which can potentially have 'catastrophic social consequences for the patient, including loss of employment and long-term incapacity' (Waddell and Aylward, 2005). The beliefs that people hold about illness determine their coping strategies and actions (Leventhal, 1998).

In the light of these observations and ideas, it can be argued that society needs to move from a systems-level approach in which all stakeholders (e.g. patients, employers, health professionals, and government departments/policy-makers) are working as individuals, towards one more aligned with public health, in which all stakeholders are working together to provide appropriate preventive messages to the wider population. Promotion of work as good for health may result in less long-term disabling pain.

The importance of demography

Populations are ageing. In the UK, for example, there has been a 1% increase in the percentage of the population aged >65 over the past 25 years (from 15% to 16%), an increase of 1.5 million individuals in real terms (Office for National Statistics, 2009). Although many people are living with better health, this increase in the proportion of older adults will inevitably bring with it an increase in the proportion of people working with pain conditions. Furthermore, the proposed increases in state pension age in the UK and other countries will mean that more people are having to work longer (DirectGov, 2009), so that more people will be working with painful conditions. However, in order to maintain health and function in old age, the social, economic, and environmental aspects of ageing must be taken into account (Andrews, 2001). Given the projected increase in the state pension age, appropriate messages about working with musculoskeletal conditions need to reach this older population.

The effect of work on pain

The contribution of work to the onset of pain symptoms has played a large part in understanding the aetiology of chronic pain. Historically, there has been much debate in the medical and legal literature about the contribution of physical injury at work to the development of chronic pain symptoms, but the arguments for injury being a precursor to pain symptoms are limited in their scope and rarely address the psychosocial factors which are known to be important in the onset and maintenance of pain. One important question is whether occupational factors, physical or psychosocial, cause chronic pain, or do such factors precipitate the onset of chronic pain in vulnerable individuals? Not all workers exposed to overuse, injury, or an adverse psychosocial environment at work go on to develop chronic pain syndromes. The two historical accounts below provide examples of where it seems as if psychologically and socially vulnerable individuals were influenced by industrial, political, physical, and iatrogenic effects (Awerbuch, 2004).

Two historical examples
Railway spine

With the advent of the railway system in the UK during the 18th century, the precursor to some of the chronic pain symptoms seen currently was known as 'railway spine'. Railway spine was considered to be the development of chronic pain and other symptoms as a result of involvement in a railway accident. Railway spine fast became a contentious issue, with injured passengers and staff making claims for compensation from the railway companies through the courts. In 1867, Dr Erichsen, an eminent London doctor, published a book containing a case series of patients who had developed chronic pain and other chronic symptoms following involvement in railway accidents (Erichsen, 1867). This book was used by the courts who found that 'railway spine' was a reasonable basis on which to argue for compensation for passengers and employees injured in railway accidents (Ferrari and Shorter, 2003). The onset of symptoms was generally some time after the accident and, interestingly, was considered by Erichsen (a surgeon) to originate in the psychological and emotional reaction to the accident. It was such cases that contributed to the medical and legal debates about railway spine; all parties had their own interests with doctors striving to uphold the credibility of the medical profession and railway companies trying to avoid expensive claims, whilst the courts and public sought to ensure that, if railway companies had been negligent, they were to be sufficiently punished (Harrington, 2003). Railway spine, however, has not been alone in its ability to generate fierce medical and legal debate resulting from non-specific symptoms due to injury.

Repetitive strain injury

Repetitive strain injury (RSI) provided a particularly dramatic story in Australia, where it was first observed in electrical process workers in the 1970s (Ferguson, 1971), with the concept of RSI becoming accepted amongst the medical, research, and governmental bodies during the 1980s. The symptoms of RSI are non-specific pain, usually in the forearm, which may or may not be associated with neck pain. There are generally no objective clinical signs and symptoms (Awerbuch, 2004). RSI was strongly considered to be an injury caused by work and this assumption was strengthened by guidelines issued by the National Health and Medical Research Council of Australia advocating approved occupational health management of the condition (National Health and Medical Research Council, 1982). Epidemiological studies have demonstrated that psychosocial workplace factors, such as low decision latitude, monotonous work, and poor relationships within the workplace, are associated with the onset of RSI (Walker-Bone and Cooper, 2005). However, there is little evidence for effective treatment of the condition (van Tulder et al., 2007). Within the community setting, arm pain is reported to be transient and not severe, whereas in the workplace these same arm-pain symptoms are often described as chronic or disabling (Awerbuch, 2004). In the UK there were strong debates in the courts about the existence of RSI, with many judges commenting that the condition was not proved to exist (Dyer, 1994).

Physical occupational risk factors for chronic pain

A range of physical factors in the workplace can cause or contribute to pain, such as working posture, suitability of work stations, or occupational injuries (Harkness et al., 2003). Pain symptoms are generally more common in blue collar workers, who are more likely to consult their general practitioner (GP) with a new occurrence of pain (Aggarwal et al., 2003; Papageorgiou et al., 1997; Andersson et al., 1993). The risk of pain in these groups remains even after taking into account the influence of individual psychosocial factors (Papageorgiou et al., 1997).

There is evidence that mechanical risk factors are important predictors of the onset and site of regional musculoskeletal pains. In a public health context, this means that preventing occupational injury or overuse might be an important strategy for primary prevention of chronic pain, regardless of the causes of persistence of such symptoms. The degree to which chronic pain might be reduced by removing a particular risk factor among those persons exposed to that factor is estimated by the attributable or aetiological fraction: the proportion of all chronic pain among such persons attributable to that factor. It has been estimated that physical work-environment exposures explain between 10% and 30% of long-term sickness absence in the exposed groups. For example, in men the aetiological fraction for long-term sickness absence associated with working in mainly a standing or squatting position and lifting or carrying loads was estimated to be 23% and 28%, respectively (Bang et al., 2007). In women, 27% of long-term sickness absence was attributable to bending or twisting of the neck or back. The potential for reducing sickness absence in groups with specific physical exposures by addressing these work-environment factors appears substantial (Bang et al., 2007), but must be interpreted in the context of the many other factors that might be influencing sickness absence in these persons.

Psychosocial occupational risk factors for chronic pain

Other chapters in this book have emphasized that, whilst mechanical factors can explain the onset and the site of pain, other factors, such as psychological distress or cultural beliefs, are involved in whether the pain becomes chronic and in the wider consequences of the pain.

Individuals reporting chronic musculoskeletal pain also report a range of co-morbid psychological conditions, such as anxiety and depression, and such individual psychological factors might be either cause or consequence of chronic pain (Macfarlane et al., 2000; Harkness et al., 2003; Nahit et al., 2003; Linto et al., 1989; Bongers et al., 1993). What is the evidence that phenomena related to the psychological, social, and organizational environments ('psychosocial factors') influence the onset or persistence of pain.

The study of work-related psychosocial risk factors stems from the work of Karasek who developed the 'demand–control–support' model (Karasek, 1979), and Siegrist who developed the 'effort–reward imbalance' model (Siegrist, 1996). The demand–control–support model assumes that the combination of high psychological demands and low decision-making autonomy leads to a negative state or 'job strain'. Job strain increases the risk of psychophysiological stress reactions and subsequent ill-health. The effort–reward imbalance model is based on the concept of high effort with low rewards and work-related over-commitment. However, both these models are limited in their scope and may not include all important aspects of the psychosocial work environment (Saastamoinen et al., 2009). More recently, the concept of the psychosocial work environment has been expanded to include organizational justice, including the relationships between employees and supervisors (Elovainio et al., 2002), and work–life balance (Winter et al., 2006).

There are a number of systematic reviews that have attempted to summarize the range of work-related psychosocial factors that may cause or contribute to pain in the working-age population.

These systematic reviews have identified strong evidence for the effect of job satisfaction, monotonous tasks, relationships with colleagues and supervisors (also described as social support in the workplace), and self-reported work stress and job demands, with moderate evidence for a range of other factors (Macfarlane et al., 2009; Hoogendoorn et al., 2000; Linton, 2001; Ariens et al., 2001). Although these reviews focus on pain in specific locations, the similar findings from each of them would suggest that these factors have an impact on pain regardless of location.

As before, the potential impact of removing psychosocial risks from the workplace can be estimated by identifying the proportion of pain cases among those exposed to a particular factor, which could be prevented if the exposure were removed. Linton (2001) conducted a systematic review and calculated the attributable fraction for back pain associated with a range of psychosocial factors in the workplace. He reported that the attributable fraction associated with job satisfaction ranged from 41% to 69% across four studies, for job stress was 17% in one study, work pace 48% in one study, and lack of variation in work was 23% (Linton, 2001). In addition, Linton considered studies that looked at the attributable fraction associated with work absence linked to back pain rather than back pain alone. One study reported job satisfaction to have an attributable risk of 17% for sick leave related to back pain, whilst another study estimated that it had different effects in men and women – job satisfaction had an attributable risk of 49% in men and 25% in women for <7 days absence, and having >7 days absence had an attributable risk of 33% in men and 20% in women.

The consequences of pain for work: sickness absence and work incapacity

The size of the problem

The economic costs of poor health to the workforce and the resulting reduction in work capacity are very high globally (Office for National Statistics, 2009). In the UK in 2007 the Confederation of British Industry (CBI) estimated that poor health in the workplace accounted for 175 million days lost at a cost of £13.4 billion (CBI, 2007). Chronic pain contributes substantially to this. It has been estimated that the odds of quitting one's job as a result of pain is 7 times higher than for those without pain (Jonsson, 2000). Pain and musculoskeletal complaints account for ~20% of claims for long-term state incapacity benefit in the UK (Blyth et al., 2003). Approximately 75% of these health problems are classed as being mild to moderate rather than severe in the medical sense, as there is limited or inconsistent evidence of pathology despite the potential for considerable functional impairment (Blyth et al., 2003).

The costs of reduced work capacity due to pain greatly outweigh its direct medical costs (Phillips et al., 2008). There is evidence that remaining in work, or returning to work as soon as possible, is potentially beneficial to persons with health problems, and reduces the risk of experiencing the negative social, psychological, and physical effects of long-term sickness absence (Waddell et al., 2008; Waddell and Burton, 2006).

The sociological perspective

From a sociological viewpoint, people who are ill may adopt the 'sick role', in which they become exempt from normal social roles and responsibilities and are entitled to special care (Glenton, 2003). This sick role may be perpetuated by the medical profession who often 'prescribe' sick leave as a treatment for chronic pain (Glenton, 2003). There are some medical professionals who view work as harmful to their patients, but the opposite is often true and lack of work can have negative consequences in terms of social exclusion, financial security, and physical and mental health (Waddell and Burton, 2006). Furthermore, the longer someone is out of work, the more distant they become from the workforce and the more difficult it is for them to return (Waddell and Burton, 2006).

Risk factors for sickness absence and work incapacity

We have considered above the role of physical factors and injury, including studies which used long-term incapacity as an outcome measure. However, in this section, we concentrate on the potential additional or independent influence of psychosocial factors on this outcome.

Psychosocial risk factors which influence how pain impacts on work can be subdivided into two factors (Sullivan et al., 2005): type I factors *within* the individual (e.g. beliefs and fears), and Type II factors *outside* the individual (e.g. the workplace and insurance systems; Sullivan et al., 2005). The socioeconomic situation of the individual, cultural factors, labour market forces, and regional deprivation can all affect the impact of an injury on an individual's work (Waddell and Aylward, 2005).

The list of psychosocial risk factors for long-term disability and incapacity for work as a result of pain conditions is extensive. Psychosocial risk factors include psychological distress, fear/avoidance, catastrophizing, pain behaviour and beliefs, job dissatisfaction, and social support in the workplace, in addition to a range of working conditions, e.g. repetitive or boring work (Shaw et al., 2001; Crook et al., 2002; Kendall et al., 2009; Larsson et al., 2007; Niedhammer et al., 2008; Bartys et al., 2005; Griffiths et al., 2006; Schultz et al., 2004). Many of these risk factors are modifiable and may be used to identify and support individuals who are at risk of reduced work capacity as a result of their pain symptoms (Kendall et al., 2009).

There is also some evidence to suggest that work-related psychosocial factors are associated with recurrence of sickness absence in employees with musculoskeletal pain. Again, relationships within the workplace and high job strain or demands were strongly related to repeated absences (Ijzelenberg and Burdorf, 2005).

Taken in conjunction with the earlier discussion, individual psychosocial factors and the psychosocial and cultural environment in the workplace and wider society appear to be important contributors both to the propensity of pain to become chronic and to the consequences of pain for sickness absence and incapacity for work.

The consequences of pain for work: performance at work

Poor health not only affects work absence but also affects productivity whilst at work (Burton et al., 1999). Some individuals, who suffer an occupational injury, which causes chronic pain in other workers, either do not develop chronic pain symptoms or more specifically do not become incapacitated from work as a result. Evidence suggests that a substantial number of people maintain work whilst being in pain (Wynne-Jones et al., 2008; Blyth et al., 2003) and that the culture of presenteeism (defined as being at work in spite of illness) as the norm does appear to partly account for this (Barnes et al., 2008). This may be related to higher levels of vulnerability in those who do develop chronic ill-health and work incapacity, or it may be that those who remain at work may be more resilient or desire to be viewed as a valued member of society and a 'good worker', in the context of a culture of presenteeism in their workplace (Barnes et al., 2008). Additionally, establishing the legitimacy of 'unseen' complaints such as pain, as compared, say, to a broken bone visible as a plaster splint on a limb, can be problematic and lead to stigmatization of these complaints (Barnes et al., 2008).

Certain occupations or companies may have lower rates of chronic pain and sickness absence. In addition to a presenteeism culture in those workplaces, healthy worker effects may also be in operation. The healthy worker effect relates to the observation that people in particular occupations may have lower-than-expected mortality and morbidity compared with age- and sex-matched general population figures. The suggested explanation is a selection effect generated by employers, where individuals who are fit for the job are more likely to be employed than those who are not (Osmotherly and Attia, 2006). This effect may also be apparent in pre-employment screening checks, where the aim is to match workers to their job demands. Vulnerable persons may be selectively excluded.

The size and costs of the problem

The large public health impact of chronic pain may extend to the consequences of being at work in pain. Measurement of presenteeism depends to a greater or lesser extent on the type of employment an individual undertakes, e.g. Burton et al. (2002) found that presenteeism accounted for higher productivity losses in telephone operatives with migraine. Productivity was measured here as handle time per call and time unavailable for calls. Productivity therefore defines the degree to which an individual is or is not performing in their job. The degree to which pain is impacting on an individual's functional ability is likely to have an impact on an individual's performance in their workplace.

Overall, it has been estimated that 25% of absentees experienced a loss of productivity during their presence at work prior to sickness absence and 20% after return (Brouwer et al., 1999). Musculoskeletal conditions in the workplace, principally back and neck pain, make up approximately half the total reported ill-health at work, accounting for 9.5 million days of work absence in the UK (Health and Safety Executive, 2007). Presenteeism is estimated to account for 1.5 times more productive working time lost than absenteeism, and costs are higher because it is more common among higher-paid staff (Stewart et al., 2003). It has been demonstrated that productivity losses may occur without absence from the workplace and that, on an average day, ~7% of employees work with health problems, suggesting that loss of productivity without absence is common (Brouwer et al., 1999).

It has also been estimated that reduced productivity is prevalent for ~60% of employees after return-to-work from a period of sickness absence (Lotters et al., 2005). This would suggest that there are cycles of risk with poor health reducing performance until a period of absence is taken, followed by a period of reduced performance when an employee re-enters the workplace. This reduced performance does not only occur before and after a period of absence but at any time during an episode of pain, it has been reported that men have a higher number of reduced effectiveness work-days when compared to women and that the 35–44- and 45–54-year age groups are the most affected for men and women, respectively (van Leeuwen et al., 2006).

Including the costs of lost productive time as a result of chronic pain increased the estimates of costs of chronic pain in one Australian study by fivefold to $5.1 billion Australian dollars (van Leeuwen et al., 2006). Lost productive time associated with back pain in workers in the age range of 40–65 years costs US employers an estimated $7.4 billion/year, those with back-pain exacerbations accounting for 72% of this cost (Ricci et al., 2006). Average annual productivity losses in 1996 per worker due to chronic back pain have been calculated at $1230 per male worker and $773 per female worker. These figures translate into aggregate annual productivity losses from chronic back pain of ~$28 billion in the USA (Rizzo et al., 1998).

The picture in the UK workforce is similar with an estimated cost of £9090 million in lost productivity due to both absence and reduced performance as a result of back pain (Maniadakis and Gray, 2000). Neck pain is also very common in the workplace with a reported 12-month prevalence of 56% (Ijzelenberg and Burdorf, 2005). With a similar prevalence to back pain, the costs associated with lost productivity and absence attributable to neck pain are likely to be close to those reported in the back-pain literature. However, if the costs of lost productive time as a result of *any* musculoskeletal pain are included, then the economic costs are likely to be higher.

The sociological view

It is useful to look in more detail at the reasons why people either take absence from work or maintain work despite their pain. A small number of qualitative studies have attempted to explain how people make decisions about sickness absence and attendance, and how these decisions are related to the psychosocial work environment. The illness-flexibility model suggests that 'attendance requirements', the negative consequences of absence for the employee (e.g. impact on work tasks or colleagues), and 'adjustment latitude', the opportunities to work despite illness (e.g. modifications to work), act as 'push and pull' factors in determining sickness absence and attendance behaviour (Johansson and Lundberg, 2004). Work-related demands for presence may also influence the decision to remain in work or to take a period of sickness absence (Aronsson and Gustafsson, 2005). These work-related demands include 'replaceability' (work left undone), sufficient resources, conflicting demands at work, control, pace of work, and time pressure. They also encompass personally orientated demands for presence, such as 'boundarylessness' (difficulty in resisting the demands or expectations of others) and private financial demands.

Psychosocial influences on pain and work are also bound by social and cultural norms, which can be strong influences on attitudes and behaviour. In a community-based qualitative study, attitudes towards working with common health problems were found to have a strong moral dimension, with a culture of presenteeism being the norm (Barnes et al., 2008). The moral dimension to health has been noted in the medical sociological literature (Blaxter, 2004; Nettleton, 2006; Pinder, 1995; Williams, 1993). The moral dimensions of health compounded by the moral dimension of work (and being seen to work), may lead to a desire to prove one's self-'worth' to others by not taking time off (Barnes et al., 2008). These social and cultural norms need further exploration and their interactions with specific work-related psychosocial factors should be examined to assess the impact of each.

Moving towards a public health approach

With the estimated prevalence of chronic pain in the UK at 10%, representing 2150 million chronic pain days per year, the public health challenge of pain is clear (Phillips et al., 2008). From the overview above of occupational risk factors for pain and risk factors for sickness absence and lowered productivity at work, we can draw the tentative conclusion that addressing these exposures, both physical and psychosocial, could reduce both the incidence and prevalence of pain and the personal, social, and economic consequences for the workforce which follow from chronic pain, work absence, and performance difficulties at work (Labriola et al., 2006). When assessing the overall impact of work on sickness absence, the aetiological fraction attributable to differences in work-environment exposures has been calculated to be 40% (Labriola et al., 2006). The literature provides very variable figures on which to base an estimate of how much of the burden of chronic pain in populations as a whole might be related to occupational factors (population attributable fraction). However, with a lower limit of chronic pain associated with work at almost a quarter of those employed, it is likely to be substantial.

Tackling barriers to recovery

Barriers to recovery from chronic pain in the work and wider psychosocial environment are potential population targets for a public health strategy to prevent sickness absence and incapacity for work because of chronic pain.

The bio-psychosocial model highlights the multi-factorial nature of the influences on an individual's experiences of pain, and the impacts of this pain on the individual's daily life, with physical factors and symptoms being included with the psychosocial aspects (Wade and Halligan, 2004). The bio-psychosocial model has been useful in clarifying the relationship between pain complaints and work, and setting the individual in the context of health care services, their immediate work environment, the organization, and the socioeconomic environment (Buck et al., 2009). In relation to managing pain, each aspect of the bio-psychosocial model can provide triggers for treatment, but can also highlight barriers to recovery or management of pain.

Recently, these barriers to recovery and pain management have been synthesized into the concept known as the 'Flags' system. This focuses on the identification of various types of modifiable risk factors (or 'flags' for intervention targets) and highlights the multi-factorial nature of disability and incapacity (Kendall et al., 2009). Originating with clinical Red Flags indicating serious pathology (Kendall, 1999), the system developed to include Yellow Flags, encompassing psychological and social/environmental risk factors (Kendall et al., 1997), whilst Orange Flags are indicators of psychopathology (Kendall et al., 2009). In occupational contexts, barriers to recovery can be divided into Blue Flags and Black Flags. The former refer to 'perceptions' of work (e.g. relationships with managers, control over workload), and the latter to more 'objective' features (e.g. contract type, sickness absence policies), which are more 'contextual in nature'. Identification of these barriers or risk factors can help to identify both targets for treatment and barriers to managing pain in the workplace. The flags framework has recently been integrated into a set of management guidelines for the clinic and the workplace. (Kendall et al., 2009)

The example of RSI demonstrated the influence that external agencies can have on the occurrence and course of pain symptoms. It would seem reasonable, therefore, to presume that interventions designed to elicit a social or cultural change, such as changes in government policy or public health campaigns, could also have an impact on pain symptoms. Australia and Scotland have both run public information campaigns aimed at changing health professionals' and the public's attitudes towards managing back pain through keeping active (Buchbinder et al., 2001; Waddell et al., 2007). Government policies influence a number of areas relevant to working with pain, including the social welfare system, access to health care services, provision of education, and labour market/economic factors (Buck et al., 2009). Avoiding work loss through changing perceptions of work and health, the wider provision of pain services and the right support from health professionals and employers, are potentially important components in recovery for individuals and for reducing the economic impact of pain (Phillips et al., 2008).

Several factors beyond the control of the individual can act as barriers to working with health problems, particularly in the context of long-term incapacity for work, including age, poor work history, low skills, and employer discrimination (Waddell and Aylward, 2005). These problems can be compounded in socioeconomically deprived communities where people face multiple disadvantages, such as dependency on benefits extending across subsequent generations, shifting social norms, poor health, low levels of education and skills, and limited availability of jobs that command a high-enough wage to make work pay (Phillips et al., 2006). Capacity for work is a complex and morally charged issue and contextual factors need to be considered in developing and implementing interventions and policies relating to health and work.

Promoting return-to-work

There is a strong case to be made – on moral, political, and economic grounds (Buchbinder et al., 2001) – that, if employees are injured as a consequence of work, they should receive appropriate support to return to, or maintain, work (Waddell et al., 2007; Buchbinder et al., 2001). There is clear evidence that the concept of vocational rehabilitation is a good business strategy, providing cost–benefits for many health conditions including musculoskeletal pain (Waddell et al., 2008). There is a consensus, in the UK at least, for moving the emphasis away from putting a financial value on the injury or the harm done to the individual, and towards minimizing the effects of injuries (Waddell et al., 2007).

Appropriately managing return to work after a period of absence is very important; Shaw et al. (2002) aimed to identify how individual perceptions of personal and environmental issues influence return to work. The authors found that one of the key aspects of returning to work was the individuals' expectations – if opportunities in their current workplace were limited, other options were explored such as retraining or other employment opportunities. It has been suggested that some of this expectation of returning to work, and also presenteeism which impacts upon performance, can be related to a 'duty to work'. This may have a positive impact on an individual in maintaining, or returning to, work, or may be detrimental to an individual's health and performance (Ostlund et al., 2002). Shaw et al (2009) have recommended a specific focus on seven key workplace factors as a precursor to a stepped approach to workplace interventions. A systematic review of the qualitative literature on return to work after a musculoskeletal injury identified that goodwill and trust between all stakeholders are central to successful return to work. The authors also reported that there are often social and communication barriers to return-to-work, and intermediaries have a key role in facilitating the return-to-work process (Maceachen et al., 2006).

Not only does the culture of the workplace impact upon return to work, but there is also some evidence to suggest that it is associated with recurrence of sickness absence in those employees with musculoskeletal pain. Ijzelenberg and Burdorf (2005) reported that poor social support and high job strain in the workplace were associated with the recurrence of sickness absence. The involvement of all stakeholders in the return to work process is paramount in developing a successful return -to -work plan for employees. However, this return -to -work goal needs to be articulated and operationalized clearly, and set within the context of the competing goals and environments in which the stakeholders are located (Ijzelenberg and Burdorf, 2005).

Primary prevention

Attitudes and beliefs about back pain have consistently been important predictors in identifying persons who are likely to develop long-term and disabling pain, and recent guidelines run contrary to current opinions of many health care practitioners and the public (Gross et al., 2006). These guidelines advocate remaining active, whereas traditional advice advocates rest, whilst work in particular has been identified as good for health and wellbeing (Waddell and Burton, 2006; Hagen et al., 2002). It is clear then that, to mediate the effect that pain has on an individual, the attitudes and beliefs of the public and health care providers need to be changed to ensure that evidence-based health care is in place. Media campaigns have been used to deliver health messages for many years with greater or lesser success (Grilli et al., 2001). As mentioned above, there have been two recent public health campaigns aimed at changing both health professionals and the public's attitudes towards managing back pain (Buchbinder et al., 2001; Buchbinder and Jolley, 2004; Buchbinder and Jolley, 2005; Waddell et al., 2007), and the first of these (from Australia) is reviewed in detail in the next chapter. Improvements in knowledge, attitudes, and beliefs remained after 3 years (Buchbinder and Jolley, 2005), although these effects did begin to reduce over the years, suggesting that reminders or other strategies may be useful to continue promoting positive messages about back pain (Buchbinder and Jolley, 2004).

Similar results were found in Scotland, where a media campaign was undertaken with a specific emphasis on improving work outcomes (Waddell et al., 2007). Again there was a significant change in beliefs about pain, with more people reporting the stay active message after the campaign, and again this change in beliefs was maintained 3 years subsequent to the campaign. However, there was no change in the advice provided by professionals about work and consequently no change in work absence or new benefit awards (Waddell et al., 2007).

It has been hypothesized that providing information about remaining active despite pain is not sufficient to change patient's actions in terms of work absence, and the Working Backs Scotland study would certainly support this view. A systematic review looking at the effectiveness of information provided in primary care has identified that if information is provided it should be based on the biopsychosocial model, but that provision of information is not sufficient to prevent work absence or reduce health care costs (Henrotin et al., 2006). Work is very individual to each person and it may be that any information provided needs to be more specific to patients rather than general to the population as whole (Henrotin et al., 2006; Lorig et al., 2002). However, improving the baseline understanding of the general population would undoubtedly enhance any further information and advice provided by health care professionals (Lorig et al., 2002).

Focusing on improving the advice provided by primary health care professionals may be one way to address pain and work as a public health issue. Health care provider training and expertise has been demonstrated to impact on the duration of sickness absence from back pain (Webster et al., 2005). It seems that, although GPs are aware of the guidelines and recommendations surrounding work, they are not always successful in implementing these in practice (Bishop et al., 2008). A key reason for this is that patients often have an expectation that they will receive a sickness certificate when they consult their GP with an episode of pain (Verbeek et al., 2004), and avoiding conflict in the doctor–patient relationship accounts for much of the problem of implementing evidence relating to the management of back pain in general practice (Breen et al., 2007). Public health campaigns, such as those conducted in Australia and Scotland, may go some way to altering this expectation of patients that they should receive a sickness certificate and therefore take time away from the workplace.

Coupling national campaigns with improved training of health care providers may address the issue of pain and work in a more comprehensive manner. The aim of any such approach should be to reduce the impact of work on chronic pain and the impact of chronic pain on work, and to improve the working lives of persons with pain conditions. Given the frequency of both work and pain, such approaches are likely to benefit populations as well as individuals.

References

Aggarwal VR, Macfarlane TV, Macfarlane GJ. 2003: Why is pain more common amongst people living in areas of low socio-economic status? A population-based cross-sectional study. *Br Dent J* **194**, 383–7.

Andersson HI, Ejlertsson G, Leden I, Rosenberg C. 1993: 2001: Chronic pain in a geographically defined general population: studies of differences in age, gender, social class, and pain localization. *Clin J Pain* **9**, 174–82.

Andrews GR. Promoting health and function in an ageing population. *BMJ* **322**, 728–9.

Ariens GA, van MW, Bongers PM, Bouter LM, van der WG. 2001: Psychosocial risk factors for neck pain: a systematic review. *Am J Ind Med* **39**, 180–93.

Aronsson G, Gustafsson K. 2005: Sickness presenteeism: prevalence, attendance-pressure factors, and an outline of a model for research. *J Occup Environ Med* **47**, 958–66.

Awerbuch M. 2004: Repetitive strain injuries: has the Australian epidemic burnt out? *Intern Med J* **34**, 416–19.

Bang CK, Lund T, Labriola M, Villadsen E, Bultmann U. 2007: The fraction of long-term sickness absence attributable to work environmental factors: prospective results from the Danish Work Environment Cohort Study. *Occup Environ Med* **64**, 487–9.

Barnes MC, Buck R, Williams G, Webb K, Aylward M. 2008: Beliefs about common health problems and work: a qualitative study. *Soc Sci Med* **67**, 657–65.

Bartys S, Burton K, Main C. 2005: A prospective study of psychosocial risk factors and absence due to musculoskeletal disorders-implications for occupational screening. *Occup Med* **55**, 375–9.

Bishop A, Foster NE, Thomas E, Hay EM. 2008: How does the self-reported clinical management of patients with low back pain relate to the attitudes and beliefs of health care practitioners? A survey of UK general practitioners and physiotherapists. *Pain* **135**, 187–95.

Blaxter M. 2004: *Health*. Cambridge: Policy Press.

Blyth FM, March LM, Brnabic AJ, Jorm LR, Williamson M, Cousins MJ. 2001: Chronic pain in Australia: a prevalence study. *Pain* **89**, 127–34.

Blyth FM, March LM, Nicholas, MK and Cousins, MJ. 2003: Chronic pain, work performance and litigation. *Pain* **103**, 41–47.

Bongers PM, de Winter CR, Kompier MA, Hildebrandt VH. 1993: Psychosocial factors at work and musculoskeletal disease. *Scand J Work Environ Health* **19**, 297–312.

Breen A, Austin H, Campion-Smith C, Carr E, Mann E. 2007: "You feel so hopeless": A qualitative study of GP management of acute back pain. *Eur J Pain* **11**, 21–9.

Brouwer WB, Koopmanschap MA, Rutten FF. 1999: Productivity losses without absence: measurement validation and empirical evidence. *Health Policy* **48**, 13–27.

Buchbinder R, Jolley D, Wyatt M. 2001: Population based intervention to change back pain beliefs and disability: three part evaluation. *BMJ* **322**, 1516–20.

Buchbinder R, Jolley D. 2004: Population based intervention to change back pain beliefs: three year follow up population survey. *BMJ* **328**, 321.

Buchbinder R, Jolley D. 2005: Effects of a media campaign on back beliefs is sustained 3 years after its cessation. *Spine* **30**,1323–30.

Buck R, Wynne-Jones G, Varnava A, Main CJ, Phillips CJ. 2009: Working with musculoskeletal pain. *Reviews in Pain* **3**, 6–10.

Burton WN, Conti DJ, Chen CY, Schultz AB, Edington DW. 1999: The role of health risk factors and disease on worker productivity. *J Occup Environ Med* **41**, 863–77.

Burton WN, Conti DJ, Chen CY, Schultz AB, Edington DW. 2002: The economic burden of lost productivity due to migraine headache: a specific worksite analysis. *J Occup Environ Med* **44**, 523–9.

CBI, AXA. 2007: Workplace absence rises amid concerns over long-term sickness - BI/AXA survey. *CBI News Release*.

Clark JD. 2002: Chronic pain prevalence and analgesic prescribing in a general medical population. *J Pain Symptom Manage* **23**, 131–7.

Crook J, Rideout E, Browne G. 1984: The prevalence of pain complaints in a general population. *Pain* **18**, 299–314.

Crook J, Milner R, Schultz IZ, Stringer B. 2002: Determinants of occupational disability following a low back injury: a critical review of the literature. *J Occup Rehabil* **12**, 277–95.

DirectGov. Changes to the state pension age. http://www direct gov uk/en/Pensionsandretirementplanning/StatePension/DG_4017919 2009

Dyer C. 1994: Court awards record settlement for worker with RSI. *BMJ* **308**, 293.

Elliott AM, Smith BH, Hannaford PC, Smith WC, Chambers WA. 2002: The course of chronic pain in the community: results of a 4-year follow-up study. *Pain* **99**, 299–307.

Elovainio M, Kivimaki M, Vahtera J. 2002: Organizational justice: evidence of a new psychosocial predictor of health. *Am J Public Health* **92**, 105–8.

Erichsen J. 1867: *On railway and other injuries of the nervous system*. Philadelphia: Lea.

Ferguson D. 1971: Repetition injuries in process workers. *Medical Journal of Australia* **2**, 408–12.

Ferrari R, Shorter E. 2003: From railway spine to whiplash--the recycling of nervous irritation. *Medical Science Monitor* **9**, HY27–HY37.

Glenton C. 2003: Chronic back pain sufferers—striving for the sick role. *Soc Sci Med* **57**, 2243–52.

Griffiths A, Cox T, Karanika M, Khan S, Tomás JM. 2006: Work design and management in the manufacturing sector: development and validation of the Work Organisation Assessment Questionnaire. *Occup Environ Med* **63**, 669–75.

Grilli R, Freemantle N, Minozzi S, Domenighetti G, Finer D. 2001: Mass media interventions: effects on health service utilisation. *Cochrane Database Syst Rev* CD000389.

Gross DP, Ferrari R, Russell AS, Battie MC, Schopflocher D, Hu RW, et al. 2006: A population-based survey of back pain beliefs in Canada. *Spine* **31**, 2142–5.

Hagen KB, Hilde G, Jamtvedt G, Winnem MF. 2002: The Cochrane review of advice to stay active as a single treatment for low back pain and sciatica. *Spine* **27**, 1736–41.

Harkness EF, Macfarlane GJ, Nahit ES, Silman AJ, McBeth J. 2003: Mechanical and psychosocial factors predict new onset shoulder pain: a prospective cohort study of newly employed workers. *Occup Environ Med* **60**, 850–7.

Harrington R. 2003: On the tracks of trauma: railway spine reconsidered. *Social History of Medicine* **16**, 209–23.

Health and Safety Executive. 2007: Self-reported work-related illness and workplace injuries in 2005/06: Results from the Labour Force Survey. UK: National Statistics;

Henrotin YE, Cedraschi C, Duplan B, Bazin T, Duquesnoy B. 2006: Information and low back pain management: a systematic review. *Spine* **31**, E326–E334.

Hoogendoorn WE, van Poppel MN, Bongers PM, Koes BW, Bouter LM. 2000: Systematic review of psychosocial factors at work and private life as risk factors for back pain. *Spine* **25**, 2114–25.

Ijzelenberg W, Burdorf A. 2005: Risk factors for musculoskeletal symptoms and ensuing health care use and sick leave. *Spine* **30**, 1550–6.

Johansson G, Lundberg I. 2004: Adjustment latitude and attendance requirements as determinants of sickness absence or attendance. *Empirical tests of the illness flexibility model. Soc Sci Med* **58**, 1857–68.

Jonsson E. 2000: Back pain, Neck pain. Swedish Council on Techonology Assessment in Health Care Report. Stockholm; Report No. 145.

Karasek RA. 1979: Job demands, job decision latitude and mental strain: Implications for job redesign. *Adm Sci Q* **24**, 285–311.

Kendall N, Linton SL, Main CJ. 1997: Guide to assessing psychosocial yellow flags in acute low back pain: Risk factors for long term disability and work loss. Wellington, New Zealand: Accident Rehabilitation and Compensation Insurance Compensation of New Zealand and the National Health Committee;

Kendall NA. 1999: Psychosocial approaches to the prevention of chronic pain: the low back paradigm. *Baillieres Best Pract Res Clin Rheumatol* 13:545–54.

Kendall N.A.S., Burton A.K., Main C.J., Watson P.J. 2009: *Tackling musculosketal problems. The Psychosocial Flags Framework: a guide for clinic and workplace.* London: The Stationary Office.

Labriola M, Lund T, Burr H. 2006: Prospective study of physical and psychosocial risk factors for sickness absence. *Occup Med* **56**, 469–74.

Larsson B, Sogaard K, Rosendal L. 2007: Work related neck-shoulder pain: a review on magnitude, risk factors, biochemical characteristics, clinical picture and preventive interventions. *Best Pract Res Clin Rheumatol* **21**, 447–63.

Leventhal HEA. 1998: Self-regulation, health, and behaviour: A perceptual-cognitive approach. *Psychology and Health* **13**, 717–33.

Linton SJ, Kamwendo K. 1989: Risk factors in the psychosocial work environment for neck and shoulder pain in secretaries. *J Occup Med* **31**, 609–13.

Linton SJ. 2001: Occupational psychological factors increase the risk for back pain: a systematic review. *J Occup Rehabil* **11**, 53–66.

Lorig KR, Laurent DD, Deyo RA, Marnell ME, Minor MA, Ritter PL. 2002: Can a Back Pain E-mail Discussion Group improve health status and lower health care costs?: A randomized study. *Arch Intern Med* **162**, 792–6.

Lötters F, Meerding W, Burdorf A. 2005: Reduced productivity after sickness absence due to musculoskeletal disorders and its relation to health outcomes. *Scandinavian Journal of Work, Environment and Health* **31**, 367–74.

Maceachen E, Clarke J, Franche RL, Irvin E. 2006: Systematic review of the qualitative literature on return to work after injury. *Scand J Work Environ Health* **32**, 257–69.

Macfarlane GJ, Hunt IM, Silman AJ. 2000: Role of mechanical and psychosocial factors in the onset of forearm pain: prospective population based study. *BMJ* **321**, 676–9.

Macfarlane GJ, Pallewatte N, Paudyal P, Blyth FM, Coggon D, Crombez G, et al. 2009: Evaluation of work-related psychosocial factors and regional musculoskeletal pain: results from a EULAR Task Force. *Ann Rheum Dis* **68**, 885–91.

Maniadakis N, Gray A. 2000: The economic burden of back pain in the UK. *Pain* **84**, 95–103.

McGuirk B, Bogduk N. 2007: Evidence-based care for low back pain in workers eligible for compensation. *Occup Med* **57**, 36–42.

Nahit ES, Hunt IM, Lunt M, Dunn G, Silman AJ, Macfarlane GJ. 2003: Effects of psychosocial and individual psychological factors on the onset of musculoskeletal pain: common and site-specific effects. *Ann Rheum Dis* **62**, 755–60.

National Health and Medical Research Council. 1982: Approved Occupational Health Guide – Repetition Strain Injuires. Canberra: Commonwealth Department of Health.

Natvig B, Picavet HS. 2002: The epidemiology of soft tissue rheumatism. *Best Pract Res Clin Rheumatol* **16**, 777–93.

Nettleton S. 2006: 'I just want permission to be ill': towards a sociology of medically unexplained symptoms. *Soc Sci Med* **62**, 1167–78.

Niedhammer I, Chastang JF, David S. 2008: Importance of psychosocial work factors on general health outcomes in the national French SUMER survey. *Occup Med* **58**, 15–24.

Office for National Statistics. Ageing: Fastest increase in the "oldest old". http://www statistics gov uk/cci/nugget asp?ID=949 2009 August.

Office for National Statistics. 2009: Labour Market Statistics April 2009. London: Office for National Statistics.

Osmotherly P, Attia J. The healthy worker survivor effect in a study of neck muscle performance measures in call-centre operators2006: . *Work* **26**, 399–406.

Östlund G, Cedersund E, Alexanderson K, Hensing G. 2002: Developing a typology of the "duty to work", as experienced by lay persons with musculoskeletal pain. *Intl J Soc Welfare* **11**, 150–8.

Papageorgiou AC, Macfarlane GJ, Thomas E, Croft PR, Jayson MI, Silman AJ. 1997: Psychosocial factors in the workplace—do they predict new episodes of low back pain? Evidence from the South Manchester Back Pain Study. *Spine* **22**, 1137–42.

Phillips C, Main CJ, Buck R, Button L, Farr A, Havard L, et al. 2006: Profiling the community in Merthyr Tydfil: Problems, challenges and opportunities. http://www.wellbeinginwork.org/.

Phillips C, Main C, Buck R, Aylward M, Wynne-Jones G, Farr A. Prioritising pain in policy making: The need for a whole systems perspective2008: . *Health Policy* **88**, 166–75.

Pinder R. 1995: Bringing back the body without the blame? The experience of ill and disabled people at work. *Sociol Health & Illness* **17**, 605–31.

Ricci JA, Stewart WF, Chee E, Leotta C, Foley K, Hochberg MC. 2006: Back pain exacerbations and lost productive time costs in United States workers. *Spine* **31**, 3052–60.

Rizzo JA, Abbott TA, III, Berger ML. 1998: The labour productivity effects of chronic backache in the United States. *Med Care* **36**, 1471–88.

Saastamoinen P, Laaksonen M, Leino-Arjas P, Lahelma E. 2009: Psychosocial risk factors of pain among employees. *Eur J Pain* **13**, 102–8.

Schultz IZ, Crook J, Meloche GR, Berkowitz J, Milner R, Zuberbier OA, et al. 2004: Psychosocial factors predictive of occupational low back disability: towards development of a return-to-work model. *Pain* **107**, 77–85.

Shaw W.S., van der Windt., Main C.J., Loisel P and Linton S.J. "Now tell me about your work: the feasibility of early screening and intervention to address occupational factors ("Blue Flags") in back disability". *J Occup Rehab* **19**, 64–80.

WS, Pransky G, Fitzgerald TE. 2001: Early prognosis for low back disability: intervention strategies for health care providers. *Disabil Rehabil* **23**, 815–28.

Shaw L, Segal R, Polatajko H, Harburn K. 2002: Understanding return to work behaviours: promoting the importance of individual perceptions in the study of return to work. *Disabil Rehabil* **24**, 185–95.

Siegrist J. 1996: Adverse health effects of high-effort/low-reward conditions. *J Occup Health Psychol* **1**, 27–41.

Stewart WF, Ricci JA, Chee E, Morganstein D. 2003: Lost productive work time costs from health conditions in the United States: results from the American Productivity Audit. *J Occup Environ Med* **45**, 1234–46.

Sullivan MJ, Feuerstein M, Gatchel R, Linton SJ, Pransky G. 2005: Integrating psychosocial and behavioral interventions to achieve optimal rehabilitation outcomes. *J Occup Rehabil* **15**, 475–89.

van Leeuwen MT, Blyth FM, March LM, Nicholas MK, Cousins MJ. 2006: Chronic pain and reduced work effectiveness: The hidden cost to Australian employers. *Eur J Pain* **10**, 161–6.

van Tulder MW, Malmivaara A, Koes B. 2007: Repetitive Strain Injury. *The Lancet* **369**, 1815.

Verbeek J, Sengers MJ, Riemens L, Haafkens J. 2004: Patient expectations of treatment for back pain: a systematic review of qualitative and quantitative studies. *Spine* **29**, 2309–18.

Verhaak PF, Kerssens JJ, Dekker J, Sorbi MJ, Bensing JM. 1998: Prevalence of chronic benign pain disorder among adults: a review of the literature. *Pain* **77**, 231–9.

Waddell G, Feder G, Lewis M. 1997: Systematic reviews of bed rest and advice to stay active for acute low back pain. *Br J Gen Pract* **47**, 647–52.

Waddell G, Aylward M. 2005: *The scientific and conceptual basis of incapacity benefits.* London: The Stationary Office.

Waddell G, Burton AK. *Is work good for your health and wellbeing?* 2006: London: TSO.

Waddell G, O'Connor M, Boorman S, Torsney B. 2007: Working Backs Scotland: a public and professional health education campaign for back pain. *Spine* **32**, 2139–43.

Waddell G, Burton AK, Kendall N. 2008: *Vocational rehabilitation: What works, for whom, and when?* London: The Stationary Office.

Wade DT, Halligan PW. 2004: Do biomedical models of illness make for good healthcare systems? *BMJ* **329**, 1398–401.

Walker-Bone K, Cooper C. 2005: Hard work never hurt anyone—or did it? A review of occupational associations with soft tissue musculoskeletal disorders of the neck and upper limb. *Ann Rheum Dis* **64**, 1112–17.

Webster BS, Courtney TK, Huang YH, Matz S, Christiani DC. 2005: Physicians' initial management of acute low back pain versus evidence-based guidelines. Influence of sciatica. *J Gen Intern Med* **20**, 1132–5.

Williams GH. 1993: Chronic illness and the pursuits of virtue in everyday life. In: Radley A, ed. *Worlds of illness: biographical and cultural perspectives of health and disease.* London: Routledge;

Winter T, Roos E, Rahkonen O, Martikainen P, Lahelma E. 2006: Work-family conflicts and self-rated health among middle-aged municipal employees in Finland. *Int J Behav Med* **13**, 276–85.

Woolf AD, Pfleger B. 2003: Burden of major musculoskeletal conditions. *Bull World Health Organ* **81**, 646–56.

Wynne-Jones G, Dunn KM, Main CJ. 2008: The impact of back pain on work: A study amongst primary care consulters. *Eur J Pain* **12**, 180–8.

Chapter 25

Can we change a population's perspective on pain?

Rachelle Buchbinder

Introduction

Social marketing (also known as public health interventions/campaigns, public education campaigns, and mass media campaigns) involves the systematic application of marketing along with other concepts and techniques to achieve specific behavioural goals for the social good (Weinreich, 1999; Andreasen, 2006; Kotler et al., 2002). It is an approach that is being increasingly used to prevent and manage various health conditions, based on the premise that targeting the health or well-being of the population as a whole has the advantage of potentially modifying the knowledge or attitudes of a large proportion of the community simultaneously, thereby providing social support for behavioural change (Redman et al., 1990). For example, the mass media has been used to influence population attitudes and beliefs to change risky health behaviours such as smoking, excessive sun exposure, unprotected sex, and driving under the influence of alcohol or without a seatbelt. Mass media has also been used to promote healthy behaviours, such as cancer screening and increasing physical activity, and to promote effective and efficient use of health services such as cancer and human immunodeficinecy virus (HIV) screening, immunization programmes, and emergency services for suspected myocardial infarction.

Social marketing public health strategies appear to be effective in combating major health issues which are strongly influenced by societal views. Back pain is an archetypal example of an important public health problem that is negatively influenced by societal ideas. Unfortunately, many people, including patients, health professionals, and the general public, still have mistaken beliefs about its nature and likely outcome. These cover a range of issues such as erroneous beliefs about the cause of the problem including the role of work, overly pessimistic beliefs about the future consequences of back trouble and long-term damage, and unfounded beliefs about the most appropriate management.

The significant rise in back-pain disability and workers' compensation costs for back-pain claims that occurred in developed countries in the mid-1990s is hypothesized to have been driven by erroneous beliefs contributing to a complex interaction of individual, health care, workplace, and societal factors (Loisel et al., 2005). This may be analogous to the workplace epidemic of repetitive strain injuries seen in Australia in the 1980s, also believed to have arisen as a result of mistaken beliefs and resulting in over-medicalization of the phenomenon, coincident with other industrial, political, and social causes. (Ireland, 1998). This conjecture is supported by the recent observation that the low prevalence of back pain and related disability seen in East Germany early after reunification had risen to rates comparable to West Germany by 2003 (Raspe et al., 2008). The authors postulated back pain to be a 'communicable disease' transmitted by the sharing or exchanging of information.

Taken together, these data suggest that a social marketing approach may be a highly appropriate strategy to simultaneously shift the attitudes and beliefs of the whole population to be in line with the best available evidence-based care for back pain. If this results in a more behaviourally appropriate appreciation of back pain and its management, it has the potential to achieve a significant reduction in the overall burden of back pain in the community.

This chapter describes just such a social marketing campaign – a mass media intervention that took place in the Victorian state of Australia from 1997 to 1999.

This 3-year campaign entitled *Back Pain: Don't Take It Lying Down*, came about in response to a significant rise in workers' compensation costs for back-pain claims which had tripled over the previous decade (Victorian WorkCover Authority, 1995–96), a trend that had also been observed in other developed countries (Waddell, 1996). The campaign was initiated by the Victorian WorkCover Authority, the manager of the Australian state of Victoria's workers' compensation system, and was the first time, anywhere in the world, that a population-based strategy had been used to influence a population's perspective on back pain. At the time, the traditional biomedical approach to back-pain management had been accepted to have been playing an important role in the development of disability, and contributing to the escalating costs. It had also been recognized that targeting health care providers alone had had limited impact upon changing clinical practice.

In addition to presenting a detailed examination of the Australian campaign, the results of similar interventions for back pain that have now been undertaken in other settings are also described. The strong rationale for using a social marketing approach to shift population beliefs about back pain is explored, together with a discussion of the advantages of changing a population's perspective on pain compared with more targeted interventions. Finally, the chapter concludes with some considerations that may be helpful in planning and evaluating future social marketing campaigns targeting population perceptions about pain.

What do we know about acute simple (non-specific) low back pain?

Simple acute back pain is a common complaint with a lifetime prevalence as high as 80% in adults (Nachemson et al., 2000) and 84% in adolescents (Jeffries et al., 2007). A systematic review of prognostic studies performed in 2003 found that the typical clinical course of acute non-specific low back pain (LBP) is of rapid recovery within the first month, with further improvements apparent until ~3 months (Pengel et al., 2003). Despite the fact that symptoms often persist or recur, with many people still having symptoms at 12 months, most people are able to either maintain or quickly resume normal function, including work, whether the pain has fully resolved or not, while only a few will not improve much at all despite treatment (Pengel et al., 2003).

A recent study has now suggested that nearly one-third of individuals do not achieve a full recovery and return to work 12 months after initial onset of pain (Henschke et al., 2008). In the workplace, back pain is an enormous contributor to lost productivity, second only to mental health. Back pain and intervertebral disc disorders were identified as by far the most significant work-related problems in the period 2004–05 Australian National Health Survey (Australian Bureau of Statistics, 2007), associated with significant workforce absenteeism and presenteeism.

Back pain also imposes a significant personal and societal burden. An investigation of the burden of all diseases in Australia in 2003 found back pain to be among the top 20 burden-imposing diseases in terms of disability-adjusted life-years (Australian Institute of Health and Welfare, 2006). Although the greatest burden of back pain occurs during middle age, important from a societal work-productivity perspective, it is *not* trivial in youth or old age. While prevalence of back pain is reportedly low in children (1–6%), this rises sharply during adolescence (18–50%) to approach adult rates (Leboeuf-Yde and Kyvik, 1998; Taimela et al., 1997). Back pain experienced by children and adolescents is associated with disability in up to 94% of cases (Watson et al., 2002), and of imminent concern is the increasing prevalence of back pain in adolescents, suggesting a growing burden into adulthood (Hakala et al, 2002) accompanied by a threat to future workforce productivity. At the other end of the age spectrum, while it is commonly believed that the prevalence of back pain decreases around the middle of the sixth decade, recent epidemiological evidence now suggests that this may only be true for benign back pain, with severe back pain increasing into old age (Dionne et al., 2006; Hartvigsen and Christensen, 2008).

While the vast majority of acute presentations are considered to be due to non-specific mechanical factors, it is not possible to give a precise patho-anatomical diagnosis in most cases. Since the mid-1990s, it has been known that individual clinical treatments have had limited impact upon long-term outcomes for back pain (van der Weide et al., 1997; Deyo, 1996a). There is only modest evidence that treatment significantly helps symptoms (van Tulder et al., 1997), and a substantial amount of evidence about the adverse effects of rest, surgery, medication, and focusing on the problem itself (Deyo, 1996b; Malmivaara et al., 1995; Indahl et al., 1995).

On the other hand there is mounting evidence that fear-avoidance beliefs, pain-coping strategies, and illness behaviours are more influential than biomedical or biomechanical factors in determining outcome from back pain (Symonds et al., 1996; Burton et al., 1995). Interventions that have been designed to promote a more positive approach to managing back pain, with an emphasis on addressing fear-avoidance beliefs and poor coping strategies, have been demonstrated to improve outcomes in both primary care and occupational settings (Symonds et al., 1995; Burton et al., 1999) and their benefits may far outweigh those derived from specific traditional treatments (Indahl et al., 1995). Educational interventions specifically intended to modify patient expectations have also been shown to reduce inappropriate imaging and costs, without compromising symptom resolution, functional improvement, satisfaction, or detection of serious pathology (Deyo et al., 1987).

Lack of significant shifts in clinicians' management of back pain towards more evidence-based care over the past 10 years

Numerous evidence-based clinical practice guidelines, advocating a biopsychosocial approach to treating back pain, have been developed in recent years in an effort to shift doctors' and other health professionals' management of back pain towards more evidence-based care (Australian Acute Musculoskeletal Pain Guidelines Group, 2003; AHCPR, 1994; van Tulder et al., 2004; Staal et al., 2003; Borkan et al., 1995). In general, they stress that back pain is a benign, self-limiting condition requiring minimal medical intervention; they counsel clinicians to provide reassurance and positive advice to stay active and continue or resume ordinary activities, because it is more effective than rest (Waddell et al., 1997); and advise that early investigation and specialist referral are unwarranted in the majority of cases (Deyo and Phillips, 1996).

Nevertheless, physician surveys have continued to demonstrate only partial adherence to their recommendations (Bishop and Wing, 2003; Di Iorio et al., 2000; Little et al., 1996; Frankel et al., 1999; Fullen et al., 2007; Gonzalez-Urzelai et al., 2003; Schers et al., 2001; Turner et al., 1998; Schroth et al., 1992; Jackson and Browning, 2005; Espeland et al., 1999; Werner et al., 2005; Rozenberg et al., 2004; Poiraudeau et al., 2006). For example, while there is sound evidence that imaging is unnecessary for acute back pain in most patients (Deyo and Phillips, 1996), and may be harmful (Orchard et al., 2005), LBP remains the most common reason for imaging requests in primary care (Britt et al., 2007). An Australian study found that 28.7 per 100 new back-pain presentations to general practice lead to an imaging request (Britt et al., 2001), while up to 48% of those who present to primary care in the USA and Europe may undergo X-ray imaging (Di Iorio et al., 2000; Gonzalez-Urzelai et al., 2003; Carey and Garrett, 1996; Freeborn et al., 1997). Studies measuring physician adherence to the recommendation of giving advice to stay active have also shown poor compliance (Frankel et al., 1999; Schers et al., 2000; Turner et al., 1998).

The lack of significant success in shifting doctors' management of back pain towards more evidence-based care highlights the fact that changing doctors' behaviour is complex and requires a comprehensive understanding of factors that may be influential; doctors' knowledge and beliefs, their training, and previous experiences, all strongly influence their management of back pain (Cherkin et al., 1994). Numerous studies have investigated why doctors do not adhere to back-pain guideline recommendations (Schers et al., 2001; Breen et al., 2004; Breen et al., 2006; Dahan et al., 2007; Espeland and Baerheim, 2003; McIntosh and Shaw, 2003; Rogers, 2002; Shye et al., 1998; Skelton et al., 1995; Schers et al., 2000; Little et al., 1998). Most commonly identified barriers have included the perception of the patient's preference for non-evidence-based care (e.g. their desire to have an X-ray imaging), insufficient knowledge about guideline recommendations, and a lack of diagnostic confidence leading to imaging requests. Similar factors have also been found to influence the management decisions of physiotherapists and chiropractors (Battie et al., 1994; Cherkin et al., 1988).

Several studies have found that clinicians treating back pain may hold alternative beliefs regarding the association of pain and activity that may influence their practice behaviour (Poiraudeau et al., 2006; Linton et al., 2002). In a recent study that we performed, general practitioners with a self-reported special interest in back pain were more likely to hold back pain-management beliefs and practices that are contrary to the best available evidence (Buchbinder et al., 2009). Compared to those without a special interest in back pain, these doctors were more likely to believe that complete bed rest and avoidance of work is appropriate for acute LBP, and lumbar spine X-rays are useful. Furthermore, the disparity between those with and without a special interest in back pain was still evident after adjusting for the presence of special interests in musculoskeletal and occupational medicine and recent post-graduate education in back pain, and, unlike the rest of the population, these beliefs were not modified by a mass media campaign specifically designed to educate the public about the best way to manage non-specific acute LBP. This raises concerns about potential vested financial and/or professional interests and the issue of the preparedness of clinicians to change (Bero et al., 1998) – another important barrier that has not been well studied to date.

The patient's presentation of their symptoms, and their knowledge, beliefs, and expectations from the consultation, patient satisfaction, provision of reassurance, relationship to work, and maintenance of doctor–patient relationship, are also important determinants of physician behaviour in managing back pain (Little et al., 1998; Chew-Graham and May, 1999). Societal factors, such as prevailing community views and existing legislation regarding sickness absence and compensation, may also affect medical behaviour and decisions (Dixon, 1990). For example, recent changes to legislation about whiplash in Australia have improved outcomes for neck-related disability (Cameron et al., 2008).

Workplace factors also play an important role. For example, efforts by employers to accommodate the LBP sufferer at work are important in reducing duration of disability due to back pain (Loisel et al., 1997). Appropriate modification of work duties, enabling either no lost time or early return to work, also reduces both the duration of back claims and the incidence of new back claims (Frank et al., 1998).

Systematic reviews of trials of interventions to improve physician practice have shown that passive strategies, such as providing access to medical education materials alone, are ineffective

(Bero et al., 1998; Overmeer et al., 2004; Love et al., 2005). Most other strategies are effective under some conditions, but none are effective in all situations, suggesting that the local setting is also an important consideration (Oxman et al., 1995; Grimshaw and Russell, 1993). Multifaceted approaches have also been shown to be more effective than single interventions (Grimshaw and Russell, 1993). Targeting health professionals alone may account for this relative lack of success, and provides further justification for a societal approach to significantly address the problem.

Mismatch of population perception of back pain with current evidence

The need to re-educate the public about back pain was identified over a decade ago (Deyo, 1996). Yet the results of recent studies performed in different countries continue to demonstrate mistaken population perceptions about back pain (Poiraudeau et al., 2006; Ihlebæk and Eriksen, 2003; Klaber Moffett et al., 2000; Gross et al., 2006). For example, a widely held belief in the UK is that back pain most often results from major pathology such as a 'slipped disc' or 'trapped nerve' (Klaber Moffett et al., 2000). In contrast, a recent study that investigated the beliefs of community pharmacists in the UK found they generally expressed positive attitudes about back pain, and were able to offer evidence-based advice, although there was some question about the representativeness of the sample (Silcock et al., 2007).

The Australian campaign and its evaluation

The Victorian WorkCover Authority (VWA) back-pain mass media campaign was developed based upon the messages delineated in *The Back Book*, an evidence-based patient-educational booklet produced in the UK by a multidisciplinary team of authors (Table 25.1; Roland et al., 1996). The messages were simple and in line with current evidence: back pain is not a serious medical problem; disability can be improved and even prevented by positive attitudes; and treatment should consist of continuing to perform usual activities, not resting for prolonged periods, exercising, and remaining at work (Burton et al., 1999). It counselled individuals with LBP, their doctors, and employers to avoid excessive medicalization of the problem, and unnecessary diagnostic testing and treatment. It emphasized that there is a lot that people with back pain can do to help themselves. A major emphasis was therefore on shifting the responsibility of control onto the individual and promoting self-management. It tackled fear-avoidance beliefs and promoted gradual exposure to painful activities, stressing that it was unlikely to be harmful. To ensure that the campaign did not discourage patients with serious pathology from seeking early medical assessment, advertisements highlighting 'red flag' symptoms were also shown.

The campaign included electronic, print, and outdoor media, and targeted both the community and treating doctors. The major medium of the campaign was television commercials that were aired in prime-time slots commencing in September 1997. The intensity of the campaign varied with a concentrated campaign for 3 months, initially followed by a low-key maintenance campaign until September 1998. A further 3-month concentrated television campaign was aired from September 1999, followed by a low-key maintenance campaign until February 2000.

The commercials included recognized international and national medical experts in orthopaedic surgery, rehabilitation, rheumatology, general practice, physiotherapy, chiropractic therapy, sports, and occupational medicine. There were also advertisements by well-known sporting and local television personalities, characters who had successfully managed their own back pain. All advertisements concluded with endorsements by the relevant national or state professional

Table 25.1 Key features, evaluation, and outcomes of the Australian, Scottish, Norwegian, and Canadian mass media back-pain campaigns (modified from Buchbinder et al., 2008, with permission.)

Title and years of campaign	Back pain – Don't take it lying down 1997–99	Working Backs Scotland 2000–03	Active back 2002–05	Back@lt 2005–08
Setting	State of Victoria in Australia	Scotland	Two counties (Vestfold and Aust-Agder) in Norway	Province of Alberta in Canada
Primary medium	Television commercials	Radio commercials	Combination of local television, radio, cinema, and commercials	Radio commercials
Intensity and frequency	Intense campaign for 12 months at beginning and final 3 months; 'top-up' low-intensity yearly ads were planned but never implemented	Intense campaign on all 15 commercial stations for 4 weeks; short 'booster' campaigns in February and October 2001, 2002 and February 2003	4 1-month campaigns	During peak listening months only
Overall cost	USD 7.6 million over 3 years	Not known	USD 531 000 specifically for media campaign	USD 930 000 over 3 years
Main messages	Back pain is not a serious problem; Continue usual activities, don't rest for prolonged periods, continue exercising and remain at work if possible; Positive attitudes are important and it is up to you; X-rays are not useful; Surgery may not be the answer; Keep employees at work	Stay active; Try simple pain relief; If you need it, get advice; Don't take back pain lying down; There's a lot you can do to help yourself; The prognosis should be good	Low back pain is not dangerous; X-ray is not useful; Activity helps improvement; Surgery is rarely necessary	Back pain: Don't take it lying down; The key to feeling better sooner is to stay active
Other media	Radio and printed advertisements, outdoor billboards, posters, seminars, workplace visits and publicity articles	Website (www.workingbacksscotland.com) Printed advertisements, outdoor billboards, posters, seminars, workplace visits, and publicity articles	Website (www.aktivrygg.no) Posters with the messages of the campaign at health care clinics	Website (www.wcb.ab.ca/back@it) Posters, pamphlets, billboard and bus advertisements, articles in public/industry news publications; TV public service announcements

Other interventions	The Back Book [39] translated into 16 languages; management guidelines for compensable back pain provided to all Victorian doctors	Leaflets and posters provided to employers, health professionals; 35 000 information packs to all health professionals; other materials developed and distributed during the campaign	Information paper delivered to all households, primary care physicians, physiotherapists, chiropractors, and social security officers	
Evaluation	Quasi-experimental design: Telephone surveys of the general population before, during, and after the campaign with the state of NSW as the control group; before–after postal surveys of general practitioners in both states; descriptive analysis of Victorian WorkCover Authority claims database	Before–after observational study: Monthly telephone surveys of the general population from before the campaign and over the following 3 years; before–after comparison of Royal Mail sickness absence rates and new awards of social security benefits for back pain in Scotland versus the rest of the United Kingdom	Quasi-experimental design: Telephone surveys of the general population before, during, and after the campaign with the county of Telemark as the control group; before-after postal surveys of health professionals; analysis of sickness absence, surgery rates for disc herniation, and imaging for low back pain	Quasi-experimental design: Telephone surveys of the general population before, during, and after the campaign with the province of Saskatchewan as the control group; interrupted time series of indicators of health care utilization and work-related disability from 5 years before the campaign until its conclusion
Outcomes	Significant and sustained shift in population beliefs and doctors' back-pain beliefs and stated behaviour in Victoria and no changes in NSW; significant reductions in total numbers of back-pain workers' compensation claims, medical and total payments for back claims, and rate of days compensated for back claims over the duration of the campaign in Victoria.	Significant and sustained shift in public beliefs regarding staying active and self-reported change in comparable advice to stay active provided by health professionals over 3 years; no change in advice about work or number who said they stayed off work; no effect on sickness absence or new awards of social security benefits for back pain.	Significant shift in public beliefs regarding staying active and at work, ability to self-manage, and better use of X-rays in Vestfold and Aust-Agder and no changes in Telemark; no changes in sickness behaviour or sickness listing and no important improvement in back-pain beliefs of health care providers.	Evaluation results not yet reported.

medical bodies. Virtually every professional body with a stake in back pain in Australia supported the campaign and had input into the wording and content of the advertisements.

Radio, billboard advertisements, posters, seminars, visits by personalities to workplaces, publicity articles, and publications supported the television campaign. *The Back Book* was sent to all treating practitioners in Victoria to be given to patients suffering from back pain and, in the latter stages of the campaign, to insurers to be passed on to claimants. Guidelines for the management of employees with compensable LBP, developed over a 3-year period with consultation from a wide variety of treating practitioners (Victorian WorkCover Authority, 1996), were also introduced simultaneously.

Evaluation of the Australian campaign showed dramatic improvements in both community and general practitioners' beliefs (Buchbinder et al., 2001a; Buchbinder et al., 2001b). Importantly, the campaign penetrated the wider community and uniformly shifted population beliefs irrespective of age, sex, education level, occupation, employment status, type of work (manual or not), income, country of birth (i.e. Australia or other), residence (i.e. metropolitan or rural), previous back-pain experience, and whether respondents reported awareness of back-pain advertising or not. In line with the population strategy of prevention, there was a favourable shift in the whole population distribution of prior beliefs – i.e. those with poorer prior beliefs improved by the same amount as those with intermediate and better prior beliefs. These belief changes were accompanied by a decline in number of workers' compensation claims for back pain and health care utilization over the duration of the campaign (Buchbinder et al., 2001a).

Follow-up studies have demonstrated that the improvements in both population and general practitioners' beliefs have been sustained over time (end of 2002 and mid-2004, respectively; Buchbinder and Jolley, 2004; Buchbinder and Jolley, 2005; Buchbinder and Jolley, 2007). However, there has been some decay in effect, likely due to an ill-informed lack of any reinforcement from ongoing small 'top-up' media reminders. These had been planned but were not implemented, coincident with the change in state government and senior Victorian WorkCover Authority staff that occurred at the end of 1999.

Other mass media campaigns for back pain

Similar public health campaigns have now been, or are currently being, carried out in other countries including Scotland, Norway, and Canada (Waddell et al., 2007; Alberta Back Pain Campaign, 2006; Werner et al., 2008a; Werner et al., 2008b; Werner et al., 2007). The observed effects have varied, most likely related to the major media that were used, the intensity of the campaigns and the available funding, as well as setting-specific contextual factors and the type of evaluation performed (Buchbinder et al., 2008).

The Scottish campaign, *The Working Backs Scotland Campaign*, was performed between 2000 and 2003 and used radio rather than television commercials (Table 25.1; Waddell et al., 2007). Its major messages were stay active, try simple pain relief and, if you need it, get advice. It resulted in a significant shift in public beliefs regarding staying active despite the pain, and it influenced the behaviour of health professionals to provide advice more in keeping with the campaign messages. There was little indication that the campaign had altered work-related LBP disability in terms of reduction in sickness absence or new awards of social security benefits for back pain. However, in contrast to the Victorian campaign, explicit recommendations about work had not been presented.

The Norwegian Back Pain Network *Active Back* Campaign was a small, low-budget intervention carried out in two counties, Vestfold and Aust-Agder, between 2002 and 2005 (Table 25.1; Werner et al., 2008a; Werner et al., 2008b). It comprised a low-budget mass media campaign directed towards the general public, as well as more targeted interventions, including an information campaign targeted to physicians, physiotherapists, and chiropractors in primary health care, an information campaign directed towards social security officers and a practical intervention in six co-operating workplaces. Similar to the Australian campaign, the main messages were that back pain is usually benign, X-rays rarely show the reason for back pain, recovery is aided by remaining active and returning to work as soon as possible even if pain is present, and surgery is needed infrequently.

Evaluation of the media campaign demonstrated a small but significant shift in population beliefs towards more optimistic, self-coping attitudes but no overall changes in sickness behaviour (Werner et al., 2008b), and no important improvements in the back-pain beliefs of health care providers exposed to the campaign (Werner et al., 2008a). The study authors concluded that a much larger investment with wider coverage would have been needed to effect changes comparable to those seen in Australia.

Similarly to the Scottish campaign, the Canadian campaign 'Back@It', which has been underway in the province of Alberta since 2005, is using radio as the major medium of the campaign due to the expense of television commercials (Table 25.1) (Alberta Back Pain Campaign, 2006). The messages and slogan are based upon the Australian campaign and an ongoing evaluation of the campaign is expected to be completed shortly.

Based upon empirical Australian data and results of similar campaigns performed elsewhere, there is now growing evidence that public policy initiatives designed to influence population attitudes and beliefs about back pain can achieve a sustained change in patient and clinician behaviour. While there has been variable demonstration of improvements in desirable economic and clinical outcomes, there is strong observational evidence that beliefs predict outcome (Woby et al., 2004).

Although each media campaign sought to promote positive beliefs about back pain, encourage self-coping strategies and continued activity, and reduce negative beliefs about the inevitable consequences of back pain, the nature of the campaigns varied widely. It appears that the more intensive and expensive television media campaign conducted in Australia was more effective than low-budget and limited campaigns. In addition, only those campaigns that made explicit recommendations regarding work changed work-related outcomes.

The advantages of public health approaches to influence population perceptions about pain

Disability related to back pain is a public health problem, since it affects a substantial proportion of the community and involves the use of substantial common resources. Therefore, public health approaches, such as the ones described above, may be much more cost effective than strategies targeted to the individual and/or individual health professionals (Rose, 1985). They may also be of use in priming the population in order to enhance the effects of more targeted strategies (Redman et al., 1990).

The advantages of using the mass media to deliver public health messages include the ability to reach large numbers of people simultaneously, including those difficult-to-identify high-risk groups and those who might be difficult to reach through traditional medical delivery (Redman et al., 1990). Psychosocial interventions that result in improved self-management skills and greater confidence to deal with the problem have been shown to be able to reduce disability associated with chronic disease and improve quality of life (Dixon et al., 2007). In the area of back pain, the available data suggest that informative interventions could be of even more value when initiated early, even prior to the onset of symptoms (Symonds et al., 1995).

If successful, this approach results in a favourable shift in the whole population distribution of prior beliefs in keeping with the 'population strategy' of prevention (Rose, 1985), which paradoxically, with a small shift in risk across the whole population, may provide more substantial public health benefit than a large shift in risk for a small subgroup (Rose, 1992). In addition, by influencing a large proportion of the community at the same time, there is societal support for sustained behavioural change and so less may be needed to maintain the message. Although use of the media is not cheap, it is less expensive than provision of similar messages via face-to-face services (Redman et al., 1990) and, depending upon the messages presented, cost savings, in terms of reductions in time lost from work, compensation costs, and/or health care utilization may be considerable.

Furthermore, the population approach may be an effective way of modifying doctor and other health professional behaviour, both through direct influences as well as through the change in attitudes of their patients. Finally, employer attitudes and beliefs and workplace philosophies may also be influenced through similar means.

Planning and evaluating social marketing campaigns which target population perceptions about pain

There is limited empirical understanding of the characteristics of effective (or ineffective) health campaigns based upon underlying general theories of health behaviour change. Several investigators who were involved in the planning and/or evaluation of mass media campaigns for back pain therefore recently reviewed the content and outcome of the campaigns conducted in Australia, Norway, and Canada, and their collective experience, in order to guide others who may be contemplating similar campaigns (Buchbinder et al., 2008). We used the Cochrane Effective Practice and Organisation of Care Review Group data collection checklist to summarize the relevant campaign and evaluation study characteristics (The Data Collection checklist, 2002; Table 25.1), and examined general theories of health behaviour change from the mass media literature to determine whether it is possible to develop a theoretical framework to explain the observed outcomes.

Based upon our findings, which were reviewed by a group of international back pain experts and participants at a workshop of the 2006 Low Back Pain Forum VIII: Primary Care Research on Low Back Pain conference, we identified five considerations relevant to the planning and evaluation of mass media interventions for back pain, together with specific items to consider for each one, based upon the theoretical framework of Hornick and Yanovitzky (Figure 25.1; Hornick and Yanovitzky, 2003). Consideration of these important issues may improve the outcome of mass media interventions for back pain.

Conclusion

Observational evidence exists indicating that beliefs predict outcome from LBP. While the results from quasi-experimental research on the Australian mass media campaign aimed at changing societal beliefs and attitudes about back pain appear to make a compelling evidence-based case for societal approaches to this problem, results of other similar campaigns have been mixed. Little is known about which communication strategies or media formats are most effective, but it appears that more intensive, explicit, and expensive media campaigns may be more effective than low-budget campaigns.

Mass media campaigns designed to alter population perceptions about pain may be a highly cost-effective method for reducing the overall burden of chronic painful conditions. In particular,

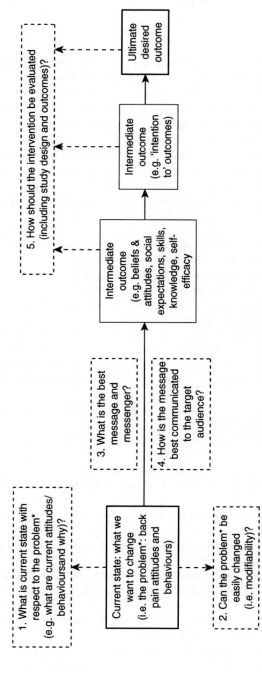

Fig. 25.1 Considerations relevant to the planning and evaluation of mass media interventions for low back pain based upon the theoretical framework of Hornick and Yanovitzky (2003) and modified from Buchbinder et al., 2008, with permission.

messages that emphasize that there is a lot you can do to help yourself and encourage a shift in the responsibility of control onto the individual may lead to behaviourally appropriate improvements in the self-management abilities of the general community. This could augment the effectiveness of more targeted strategies.

References

Agency for Health Care Policy Research. 1994: *Management guidelines for acute low back pain*. Agency for Health Care Policy and Research, US Department of Health and Human Services.

Alberta Back Pain Campaign. 2006. *Back Active*. Available from: www.backactive.ca.

Andreasen, A. 2006: *Social marketing in the 21st century*. Thousand Oaks, Calif: Sage Publications.

Australian Acute Musculoskeletal Pain Guidelines Group. 2003: *Evidence-based management of acute musculoskeletal pain*. Brisbane: Australian Academic Press.

Australian Bureau of Statistics. 2007: *Australian Social Trends, Work Related Injuries*. Canberra: ABS.

Australian Institute of Health & Welfare. 2006: *Australia's Health 2006: The tenth biennial health report of the Australian Institute of Health and Welfare*. Canberra: AIHW.

Battie, M., Cherkin, D., Dunn, R., Ciol, M. and Wheeler, K. 1994: Managing low back pain: attitudes and treatment preferences of physical therapists. *Physical Therapy* **74**, 219–26.

Bero, L., Grilli, R., Grimshaw, J., Harvey, E., Oxman, A. and Thomson, M. 1998: Closing the gap between research and practice: an overview of systematic reviews of interventions to promote the implementation of research findings. *British Medical Journal* **317**, 465–8.

Bishop, P. and Wing P.C. 2003: Compliance with clinical practice guidelines in family physicians managing worker's compensation board patients with acute lower back pain. *Spine J* **3**, 442–50.

Borkan, J., Reis, S., Ribak, J., Werner, S. and Porath, A. 1995: Guidelines for the treatment of low back pain in primary care: Israeli Low Back Pain Guideline Group.

Breen, A., Austin, H., Campion-Smith, C., Carr, E. and Mann, E. 2006: "You feel so hopeless": A qualitative study of GP management of acute back pain. *Eur J Pain* **11**, 21–9.

Breen, A., Carr, E., Mann, E. and Crossen-White, H. 2004: Acute back pain management in primary care: a qualitative pilot study of the feasibility of a nurse-led service in general practice. *J Nurs Manag* **12**, 201–9.

Britt, H., Miller, G., Charles, J., Pan, Y., Valenti, L., Henderson, J., et al. 2007: *General practice activity in Australia 2005-06*. Canberra: AIHW.

Britt, H., Miller, G. and Knox, S. 2001: *Imaging orders by general practitioners in Australia 1999-00*. Canberra: AIHW.

Buchbinder, R., Gross, D., Werner, E. and Hayden, J. 2008: Understanding the characteristics of effective public health interventions for back pain and methodological challenges in evaluating their effects. *Spine* **33**, 74–80.

Buchbinder, R. and Jolley, D. 2004: Population-based intervention to change back pain beliefs: a three-year follow up study. *BMJ* **328**, 321.

Buchbinder, R. and Jolley, D. 2005: Effects of a media campaign on back beliefs is sustained three years after its cessation. *Spine* **30**, 1323–30.

Buchbinder, R. and Jolley, D. 2007: Improvements in general practitioner beliefs and stated management of back pain persist four and a half years after the cessation of a public health media campaign. *Spine* **32**, E156–62.

Buchbinder, R., Jolley, D. and Wyatt, M. 2001: Population based intervention to change back pain beliefs and disability: three part evaluation. *BMJ* **322**, 1516–20.

Buchbinder, R., Jolley, D. and Wyatt, M. 2001: Volvo award winner in clinical studies: effects of a media campaign on back pain beliefs and its potential influence on management of low back pain in general practice. *Spine* **26**, 2535–42.

Buchbinder, R., Staples, M. and Jolley, D. 2009: Doctors with a special interest in back pain have poorer knowledge about how to treat back pain. *Spine* **34**, 1218–26.

Burton, A., Tillotson, K., Main, C. and Hollis, S. 1995: Psychosocial predictors of outcome in acute and subchronic low back trouble. *Spine* **20**, 722–8.

Burton, A., Waddell, G., Tillotston, K. and Summerton, N. 1999: Information and advice to patients with back pain can have a positive effect. A randomised controlled trial of a novel educational booklet in primary care. *Spine* **24**, 1–8.

Cameron, I.D., Rebbeck, T., Sindhusake, D., Rubin, G., Feyer, A.M., Walsh, J., et al. 2008: Legislative change is associated with improved health status in people with whiplash. *Spine* **33**, 250–4.

Carey, T. and Garrett, J. 1996: Patterns of ordering diagnostic tests for patients with acute low back pain. The North Carolina Back Pain Project. *Ann Intern Med* **125**, 807–14.

Cherkin, D., Deyo, R., Wheeler, K. and Ciol, M. 1994: Physician variation in diagnostic testing for low back pain. Who you see is what you get. *Arthritis & Rheumatism* **37**, 15–22.

Cherkin, D.C., MacCornack, F.A. and Berg, A.O. 1988: Managing low back pain-a comparison of the beliefs and behaviors of family physicians and chiropractors. *Western J Med* **149**, 475–80.

Chew-Graham, C. and May, C. 1999: Chronic low back pain in general practice: the challenge of the consultation. *Fam Pract* **16**, 46–9.

Dahan, R., Borkan, J., Brown, J., Reis, S., Hermoni, D. and Harris, S. 2007: The challenge of using the low back pain guidelines: a qualitative research. *J Eval Clin Pract* **13**, 616–20.

Deyo, R. 1996a: Acute low back pain: a new paradigm for management. *BMJ* **313**, 1343–4.

Deyo, R. 1996b: Drug therapy for back pain. Which drugs help which patients? *Spine* **21**, 2840–9.

Deyo, R., Diehl, A. and Rosenthal, M. 1987: Reducing roentgenography use. Can patient expectations be altered? *Arch Intern Med* **147**, 141–5.

Deyo, R. and Phillips, W. 1996: Low back pain. A primary care challenge. *Spine* **21**, 2826–32.

Di Iorio, D., Henley, E. and Doughty, A. 2000: A survey of primary care physician practice patterns and adherence to acute low back problem guidelines. *Arch Fam Med* **9**, 1015–21.

Dionne, C.E., Dunn, K.M. and Croft, P.R. 2006: Does back pain prevalence really decrease with increasing age? A systematic review. *Age and Ageing* **35**, 229–34.

Dixon, A. 1990: The evolution of clinical policies. *Medical Care* **28**, 201–20.

Dixon, K., Keefe, F., Scipio, C., Perri, L. and Abernethy, A. 2007: Psychological interventions for arthritis pain management in adults: a meta-analysis. *Health Psychol* **26**, 241–50.

Espeland, A., Albrektsen, G. and Larsen, J. 1999: Plain radiography of the lumbosacral spine. An audit of referrals from general practitioners. *Acta Radiologica* **40**, 52–9.

Espeland, A. and Baerheim, A. 2003: Factors affecting general practitioners' decisions about plain radiography for back pain: implications for classification of guideline barriers--a qualitative study. *BMC Health Serv Res* **3**, 8.

Frank, J., Sinclair, S., Hogg-Johnson, S., Shannon, H., Bombardier, C., Beaton, D., et al. 1998: Preventing disability from work-related low-back pain. New evidence gives new hope--if we can just get all the players onside. *CMAJ* **158**, 1625–31.

Frankel, B., Moffett, J., Keen, S. and Jackson, D. 1999: Guidelines for low back pain: changes in GP management. *Fam Pract* **16**, 16–22.

Freeborn, D., Shye, D., Mullooly, J., Eraker, S. and Romeo, J. 1997: Primary care physicians' use of lumbar spine imaging tests. Effects of guidelines and practice pattern feedback. *JGIM* **12**, 619–25.

Fullen, B., Maher, T., Bury, G., Tynan, A., Daly, L. and Hurley, D. 2007: Adherence of Irish general practitioners to European guidelines for acute low back pain: a prospective pilot study. *Eur J Pain* **11**, 614–23.

Gonzalez-Urzelai, V., Palacio-Elua, L. and Lopez-de-Munain, J. 2003: Routine primary care management of acute low back pain: adherence to clinical guidelines. *Eur Spine J* **12**, 589–94. Epub 2003 Nov 6.

Grimshaw, J. and Russell, I. 1993: Effect of clinical guidelines on medical practice: a systematic review of rigorous evaluations. *The Lancet* **342**, 1317–22.

Gross, D., Ferrari, R., Russell, A., Battié, M., Schopflocher, D., Hu, R., et al. 2006: A population-based survey of back pain beliefs in Alberta and Saskatchewan - Prelude to social marketing intervention. *Spine* **31**, 2142–5.

Hakala, P., Rimpela, A., Salminen, J.J., Virtanen, S.M. and Rimpela, M. 2002: Back, neck and shoulder pain in Finnish adolescents: National cross sectional surveys. *BMJ* **325**, 743–5.

Hartvigsen, J. and Christensen, K. 2008: Pain in the back and neck are with us until the end - A nationwide interview-based survey of Danish 100-year-olds. *Spine* **33**, 909–13.

Henschke, N., Maher, C.G., Refshauge, K.M., Herbert, R.D., Cumming, R.G., Bleasel, J., et al. 2008: Prognosis in patients with recent onset low back pain in Australian primary care: inception cohort study. *BMJ* **337**, a171.

Hornick, R. and Yanovitzky, I. 2003: Using theory to design evaluations of communication campaigns: The case of the National Youth Anti-Drug Media Campaign. *Communication Theory* **13**, 204–24.

Ihlebæk, C. and Eriksen, H. 2003: Are the "myths" of low back pain alive in the general Norwegian population? *Scand J Public Health* **31**, 395–8.

Indahl, A., Velund, L. and Reikeraas, O. 1995: Good prognosis for low back pain when left untampered. A randomized clinical trial. *Spine* **20**, 473–7.

Ireland, D.C.R. 1998: Australian repetition strain injury phenomenon. *Clin Orthop Rel Res* **351**, 63–73.

Jackson, J. and Browning, R. 2005: Impact of national low back pain guidelines on clinical practice. *South Med J* **98**, 139–43.

Jeffries, L.J., Milanese, S.F. and Grimmer-Somers, K.A. 2007: Epidemiology of adolescent spinal pain. A systematic overview of the research literature. *Spine* **32**, 2630–7.

Klaber Moffett, J., Newbronner, E., Waddell, G., Croucher, K. and Spear, S. 2000: Public perceptions about low back pain and its management: a gap between expectations and reality? *Health Expect* **3**, 161–8.

Kotler, P., Roberto, N. and Lee, N. 2002: *Social marketing: improving the quality of life.* 2nd ed. Thousand Oaks, Calif: Sage Publications.

Leboeuf-Yde, C. and Kyvik, K.O. 1998: At what age does low back pain become a common problem? A study of 29,424 individuals aged 12-41 years. *Spine* **23**, 228–34.

Linton, S., Vlaeyen, J. and Ostelo, R. 2002: The back pain beliefs of health care providers: are we fear-avoidant? *J Occup Rehabil* **12**, 223–32.

Little, P., Cantrell, T., Roberts, L., Chapman, J., Langridge, J. and Pickering, R. 1998: Why do GPs perform investigations?: the medical and social agendas in arranging back X-rays. *Family Practice* **15**, 264–5.

Little, P., Smith, L., Cantrell, T., Chapman, J., Langridge, J. and Pickering, R. 1996: General practitioners' mangement of acute back pain: a survey of reported practice compared with clinical guidelines. *BMJ* **312**, 485–8.

Loisel, P., Abenhaim, L., Durand, P., Esdaile, J.M., Suissa, S., Gosselin, L., et al. 1997: A population-based, randomized clinical trial on back pain management. *Spine* **22**, 2911–18.

Loisel, P., Buchbinder, R., Hazard, R., Keller, R., Pransky, G., Scheel, I., et al. 2005: Prevention of work disability due to musculoskeletal disorders: The challenge of implementing evidence. *J Occup Rehab* **15**, 507–24.

Love, T., Crampton, P., Salmond, C. and Dowell, A. 2005: Patterns of medical practice variation: variability in referral for back pain by New Zealand general practitioners. *New Zealand Med J* **118**, 1–9.

Malmivaara, A., Hakkinen, U., Aro, T., Heinrichs, M., Koskenniemi, L., Kuosma, E., et al. 1995: The treatment of acute low back pain - bed rest, exercises, or ordinary activity? *N Engl J Med* **332**, 351–5.

McIntosh, A. and Shaw, C. 2003: Barriers to patient information provision in primary care: patients' and general practitioners' experiences and expectations of information for low back pain. *Health Expect* **6**, 19–29.

Nachemson, A., Waddell, G. and Norlund, A. 2000: Epidemiology of neck and back pain. In: Nachemson A, Jonsson E, eds. *Neck and back pain. The scientific evidence of causes, diagnosis, and treatment.* Philadelphia: Lipppincott Williams & Wilkins p. 165–88.

Orchard, J., Read, J. and Anderson, I. 2005: The use of diagnostic imaging in sports medicine. *Med J Aust* **183**, 482–6.

Overmeer, T., Linton, S., Holmquist, L., Eriksson, M. and Engfeldt, P. 2004: Do evidence-based guidelines have an impact in primary care? A cross-sectional study of Swedish physicians and physiotherapists. *Spine* **30**, 146–51.

Oxman, A., Thomson, M., Davis, D. and Haynes, R. 1995: No magic bullets: a systematic review of 102 trials of interventions to improve professional practice. *Canadian Med Assoc J* **153**, 1423–31.

Pengel, L.H., Herbert, R.D., Maher, C.G. and Refshauge, K.M. 2003: Acute low back pain: systematic review of its prognosis. *BMJ* **327**, 9.

Poiraudeau, S., Rannou, F., Le Henanff, A., Coudeyre, E., Rozenberg, S., Huas, D., et al. 2006: Outcome of subacute low back pain: influence of patients' and rheumatologists' characteristics. *Rheumatol* **45**, 718–23.

Raspe, H., Hueppe, A. and Neuhauser, H. 2008: Back pain, a communicable disease? *Int J Epidemiol* **37**, 69–74.

Redman, S., Spencer, E. and Sanson-Fisher, R. 1990: The role of mass media in changing health-related behaviour: a critical appraisal of two methods. *Health Promo Intl* **5**, 85–101.

Rogers, W. 2002: Whose autonomy? Which choice? A study of GPs' attitudes towards patient autonomy in the management of low back pain. *Fam Pract* **19**, 140–5.

Roland, M., Waddell, G., Moffat, J., Burton, K., Main, C. and Cantrell, T. 1996: *The Back Book.* United Kingdom: The Stationary Office.

Rose, G. 1985: Sick individuals and sick populations. *Int J Epidemiol* **30**, 427–32.

Rose, G. 1992: *The Strategy of Preventive Medicine.* Oxford: Oxford University Press.

Rozenberg, S., Allaert, F., Savarieau, B., Perahia, M. and Valat, J. 2004: Compliance among general practitioners in France with recommendations not to prescribe bed rest for acute low back pain. *Joint Bone Spine* **71**, 56–9.

Schers, H., Braspenning, J., Drijver, R., Wensing, M. and Grol, R. 2000: Low back pain in general practice: reported management and reasons for not adhering to the guidelines in The Netherlands. *Br J Gen Pract* **50**, 640–4.

Schers, H., Wensing, M., Huijsmans, Z., van Tulder, M. and Grol, R. 2001: Implementation barriers for general practice guidelines on low back pain a qualitative study. *Spine* **26**, E348–53.

Schroth, W., Schectman, J., Elinsky, E. and Panagides, J. 1992: Utilization of medical services for the treatment of acute low back pain: conformance with clinical guidelines. *J Gen Intern Med* **7**, 486–91.

Shye, D., Freeborn, D., Romeo, J. and Eraker, S. 1998: Understanding physicians' imaging test use in low back pain care: the role of focus groups. *Int J Qual Health Care* **10**, 83–91.

Silcock, J., Klaber Moffett, J., Edmondson, H., Waddell, G. and Burton, A. 2007: Do community pharmacists have the attitudes and knowledge to support evidence based self-management of low back pain? *BMC Musculoskel Dis* **8**, 10.

Skelton, A., Murphy, E., Murphy, R. and O'Dowd, T. 1995: General practitioner perceptions of low back pain patients. *Fam Pract* **12**, 44–8.

Staal, J.B., Hlobil, H., van Tulder, M.W., Waddell, G., Burton, A.K., Koes, B.W., et al. 2003: Occupational health guidelines for the management of low back pain: an international comparison.[see comment]. *Occupational & Environmental Med* **60**, 618–26.

Symonds, T., Burton, A., Tillotston, K. and Main, C. 1995: Absence resulting from low back trouble can be reduced by psychosocial intervention at the work place. *Spine* **20**, 2738–44.

Symonds, T., Burton, A., Tillotston, K. and Main, C. 1996: Do attitudes and beliefs influence work loss due to low back trouble? *Occup Med* **46**, 25–32.

Taimela, S., Kujala, U.M., Salminen, J.J. and Viljanen, T. 1997: The prevalence of low back pain among children and adolescents - A nationwide, cohort-based questionnaire survey in Finland. *Spine* **22**, 1132–6.

The Data Collection checklist. 2002: Available from: http://www.epoc.uottawa.ca/checklist2002.doc.

Turner, J., LeResche, L., Von Korff, M. and Ehrlich, K. 1998: Back pain in primary care. Patient characteristics, content of initial visit, and short-term outcomes. *Spine* **23**, 463–9.

van der Weide, W., Verbeek, J. and van Tulder, M. 1997: Vocational outcome of intervention for low-back pain. *Scandinavian J Work, Environment & Health* **23**, 165–78.

van Tulder, M., Koes, B. and Bouter, L. 1997: Conservative treatment of acute and chronic nonspecific low back pain. A systematic review of randomized controlled trials of the most common interventions. *Spine* **22**, 2128–56.

van Tulder, M., Tuut, M., Pennick, V., Bombardier, C. and Assendelft, W. 2004: Quality of primary care guidelines for acute low back pain. *Spine* **29**, E357–62.

Victorian WorkCover Authority. 1995–1996: *Statistical report*, 485 LaTrobe St Melbourne.

Victorian WorkCover Authority. 1996: Guidelines for the management of employees with compensible low back pain.

Waddell, G. 1996: Low back pain: a twentieth century health care enigma [Keynote address for primary care forum]. *Spine* **21**, 2820–5.

Waddell, G., Feder, G. and Lewis, M. 1997: Systematic reviews of bed rest and advice to stay active for acute low back pain. *Br J Gen Pract* **47**, 647–52.

Waddell, G., O'Connor, M., Boorman, S. and Torsney, B. 2007: Working Backs Scotland. A Public and Professional Health Education Campaign for Back Pain. *Spine* **32**, 2139–43.

Watson, K.D., Papageorgiou, A.C., Jones, G.T., Taylor, S., Symmons, D.P.M., Silman, A.J., et al. 2002: Low back pain in schoolchildren: occurrence and characteristics. *Pain* **97**, 87–92.

Weinreich, N. 1999: *Hands on social marketing: A step by step guide*. Thousand Oaks, Calif: Sage Publications.

Werner, E.L., Gross, D.P., Lie, S.A. and Ihlebaek, C. 2008a: Healthcare provider back pain beliefs unaffected by a media campaign. *Scandinavian J Primary Health Care* **26**, 50–6.

Werner, E.L., Ihlebaek, C., Laerum, E., Wormgoor, M.E.A. and Indahl, A. 2008b: Low back pain media campaign: no effect on sickness behaviour. Patient Education & *Counseling* **71**, 198–203.

Werner, E., Ihlebaek, C., Skouen, J. and Laerum, E. 2005: Beliefs about low back pain in the Norwegian general population: are they related to pain experiences and health professionals? *Spine* **30**, 1770–6.

Werner, E., Lærum, E., Wormogoor, M., Lindh, E. and Indahl, A. 2007: Peer support in an occupational setting preventing LBP-related sick leave. *Occup Med* **57**, 590–5.

Woby, S., Watson, P., Roach, N.K., and Urmston, M. 2004: Are changes in fear-avoidance beliefs, catastrophizing, and appraisals of control, predictive of changes in chronic low back pain and disability? *Euro J Pain* **29**, 1818–22.

Chapter 26

The potential for prevention: overview

Peter Croft, Danielle van der Windt, Helen Boardman, and Fiona M. Blyth

This book has argued that, at a population level, the occurrence of chronic pain reflects a combination of the occurrence of

- diseases and injuries which trigger painful experiences and
- a propensity for those experiences to become amplified and chronic.

Such a propensity may have a long trajectory over the life-course or arise in the context of the disease or injury.

In this final chapter, some examples, mainly from prospective cohort studies, are added to the detailed picture provided in the earlier chapters in this section and elsewhere in the book, to illustrate the potential for prevention, even if there are, as yet, few examples (outside the occupational field and the back-pain media campaigns, described in Chapters 24 and 25, respectively) of evidence-based population interventions targeted at reducing chronic pain.

Primary prevention

Primary prevention of diseases or injuries that cause pain, such as cancer or road traffic accidents, is one approach to the prevention of chronic pain, although the fraction of all chronic pain in the general population attributable to such diseases or to neuropathic pain remains unclear.

The major group of conditions for which primary prevention might result in a substantial impact on population levels of chronic pain are the common chronic pain syndromes, such as musculoskeletal conditions (Bergman, 2007) and headaches. The disease model of prevention is relevant to some of these conditions – e.g. prevention of osteoarthritic change in the joints or prevention of migraine. However, the evidence so far suggests that, for people with back, neck, shoulder, joint, or head pain, the main determinants of who will go on to develop chronic symptoms relate to a broad biopsychosocial model of chronicity and to a general propensity for chronicity which appears or develops throughout the life-course.

The implication is that comprehensive primary prevention policies will need to target a range of biopsychosocial influences at all ages. Examples can be found throughout the book of potential areas for intervention, and earlier chapters in this section addressed occupation and public and professional beliefs about pain as two areas where population interventions may be plausible.

Tackling propensity

In addition to disease- and injury-based primary prevention approaches, targets for primary prevention also include risk factors for chronicity, or the 'propensity to chronic pain' discussed in Chapter 1. Evidence about these potential targets, ranging from risk factors for joint pain in older people to the origins of persistent low back pain in children or of chronic widespread pain in adults, points consistently to a number of potentially modifiable risks. These include physical inactivity, overweight, low social status as measured by education or occupational class, psychological distress (e.g. anxiety and depression; cognitions, beliefs, and concerns about pain), physical and emotional stress in childhood, social inequality, and the cultural environment concerning pain and pain-related disability. Such a list is selective – there may be other environmental or health-related primary prevention targets. Translating the evidence of association and risk into targets for prevention is also a simplification of research that is often concerned with unravelling complex pathways of causality and which is as yet still evolving.

Risk factors for pain onset and chronicity which are general public health targets

A crucial component of the evidence, in the absence of public health intervention studies, is provided by incidence studies. These can provide estimates of what predicts future onset of chronic pain. Some examples of evidence relating to chronic pain generally, or to common syndromes of pain, are considered below.

It is likely that these general public health targets will have benefits in reducing population risks of chronic pain.

Obesity

Guh et al. (2009) searched and reviewed systematically all prospective studies with sufficient numbers to estimate incidence rates of each co-morbid disease combination with obesity. They identified studies relating to 18 co-morbidities which provided good evidence of links to pre-existing obesity, including many cancers, osteoarthritis (OA), and chronic back pain. Heim and colleagues (2008) studied 55- to 85-year olds in a Dutch population sample and showed an increased incidence of all pain (2.3 times in men and 2.8 times in women) for persons in the highest compared to the lowest quartile of body mass index (BMI). Life-course influences have been studied and Lake et al. (2000), for example, showed that obesity in young women at age 23 years predicted onset of back pain at age 33. One of the most studied associations is that of BMI and chronic knee pain or clinical OA of the knee in older people, for which both mechanical and metabolic mechanisms have been proposed. Blagojevic et al. (2010) confirmed, in a systematic review of risks for the onset of knee OA, consistent evidence for a role of obesity. Jinks et al. (2006) used cohort data to calculate that 19% of new cases of severe knee pain, over a 3-year period in a UK population aged >50, would be prevented if there were a one-category shift in BMI in this age group in the general population.

Physical activity

Although recent systematic reviews and guidelines have favoured exercise as being beneficial for OA and back pain, the potential role of physical activity generally in reducing the incidence of chronic pain is more controversial. This relates to the lack of evidence that moderate levels of physical activity affect disease processes in OA, for example, and to concerns that strenuous physical activity might cause some musculoskeletal problems as well as preventing others. However, on balance, there is an emerging and consistent body of evidence that modest levels of regular physical activity at all ages can have beneficial effects on reducing the onset and persistence of pain and on improving pain-related function, possibly via mechanisms linked to weight control and mental health as well as to fitness and musculoskeletal health.

Evidence about the close association between pain and physical function in older and middle-aged persons has been discussed elsewhere in this book. Buchner et al. some years ago (1992) pointed to the general beneficial potential of physical activity on musculoskeletal function, and Conn et al. (2008), in a meta-analysis of physical activity and arthritis, estimated small but consistent beneficial effects on pain and physical function. Dugan et al. (2009) followed up 2400 community-dwelling middle-aged women from a national sample in America; they found that increasing physical activity score at baseline was associated with a lower bodily pain score on the Short Form-36 (SF-36) at 3-year follow-up, after adjusting, among other things, for baseline co-morbidity, education level, and BMI. They also showed that the link between physical activity and reduced mobility at follow-up was mediated almost entirely by chronic pain. Wedderkopp et al. (2009) identified that high physical activity in childhood protected against later development of back pain; Thomas et al. (1999) found that pre-existing low levels of physical activity were a risk factor for the development of chronicity in adults consulting with a new episode of back pain in primary care; and Hartvigsen and Christensen (2007) found that, even in a group of 70–100-year olds, active lifestyle protected against back pain.

Psychological health

Promotion of mental health is another public health target relevant to the population burden of chronic pain. Depression predicts the onset of new episodes of pain and is a risk factor for persistence of pain (Leino and Magni, 1993). Major depressive illness in a Canadian cohort predicted the development of chronic pain over an 8-year period (Patten et al., 2008). There is clear evidence that the association also works in the other direction, chronic pain often preceding the development of psychological distress (McBeth et al., 2002); the potential for gains in health from prevention of chronic pain is heightened by this interaction of psychological distress and pain.

Less severe degrees of emotional distress, which are more common and therefore potentially more important in terms of population-level prevention, also predict onset and persistence of pain, e.g. new episodes of low back pain (Croft et al., 1995; Thomas et al., 1999); this even occurs among persons with no prior recalled history of previous episodes of pain, and has been observed for musculoskeletal pain more generally (Leino and Magni, 1993). In systematic reviews of the transition from acute to chronic pain, psychological factors have been identified as contributing to the likelihood of subsequent chronic back pain (Pincus et al., 2002), and somatization and poor sleep as contributing to the onset of chronic widespread pain (Gupta et al., 2007). In research reviewed in detail in other chapters, such propensities have been shown to be traceable back to early childhood experiences and potentially to biological mechanisms related to stress pathways. From this perspective, primary prevention of pain becomes inextricably linked with promotion of mental health.

The combination of physical and mental abuse is emerging as a population risk factor for chronic pain, although much of the evidence relies on recall. In one systematic review (Paras et al., 2009), physical and emotional abuse predicted chronic non-specific pain (odds ratio (OR) for association with prior sexual abuse: 2.2), and fibromyalgia and pelvic pain (OR for association with prior episode of rape: 3.4 and 3.3, respectively). The population-attributable proportion, however, remains uncertain, since the frequency of exposure is not firmly established.

Some of the beneficial effects of physical activity referred to above may act via effects on psychological health. Evidence is emerging, for example, that factors such as 'neighbourhood walkability' is linked to lower depression levels in older men (Berke et al., 2007), whilst increasing physical activity was linked with decreasing depressive symptoms in middle-aged women, independent of pre-existing physical and psychological health, in a 5-year follow-up study in Australia (Brown et al., 2005). Seavey et al. (2003) followed up 1149 men and 964 women, who were free of arthritis in 1974, for 20 years in a Canadian cohort study; BMI, gender, and depression predicted arthritis at follow-up, and leisure-time physical activity was protective. In another cohort study of older persons, depression increased incident disability, partly in relation to decreased physical activity and reduced social interaction (Penninx et al., 1999).

The account in Chapter 25 by Buchbinder highlights another component of psychological status relevant to pain, namely cognitions about pain and about its capacity to interfere with life. Poor self-rated health, e.g. in a population sample free of arm pain (Palmer et al., 2008), was associated with onset and persistence of this musculoskeletal syndrome 18 months later. However, it is unclear to what extent beliefs and attitudes may pre-date the onset of pain overall – Severeijns et al. (2005) suggest, for example, that catastrophizing ideas about pain are generally low in prevalence in the community and only weakly predictive for future development of chronic pain in that setting, and so have limited potential for screening or as a target for primary prevention. Most prospective studies of ideas, beliefs, and perceptions about pain have been carried out in persons who already have pain, where there is more evidence of the strength of the association with outcome (e.g. Foster et al., 2008), and it may be that they are more important as targets for secondary prevention in the context of current pain experience. On the other hand, Buchbinder in Chapter 25 demonstrates the potential for tackling perceptions about back pain at a population level. In population and public health terms it might be more appropriate to see these as representing cultural attitudes rather than individual psychological attributes.

Social factors

As pointed out in Chapter 3, social factors present major potential targets for population-level interventions to reduce chronic pain. Hestbaek et al. (2008) found a protective effect of more favourable socioeconomic circumstances in adolescence on future chronic low back pain. Macfarlane and colleagues have demonstrated that social factors act across the life-course in influencing the onset of chronic widespread pain (e.g. Macfarlane et al., 2009), and other studies have identified adverse socioeconomic factors, such as low income, to be predictors of declining function in persons with pain (e.g. Mackenbach et al., 2001). Population-level studies are suggesting small but distinct effects of area-level factors (e.g. the level of deprivation in an area) in addition to individual social characteristics (see Chapter 3; e.g. Jordan et al., 2008).

Education level

Education level provides an example of a specific social factor that is a potential population-level target. It is set relatively early in life, and is thus a measure of long-term influence. In an 11-year follow-up of Norwegian adults from the general population (Hagen et al., 2006), low educational level was a risk factor for future onset of back-pain disability in a population cohort, and the authors summarized that the likelihood of reporting disability in adults falls by 14% for each additional year of formal education reported. In a prospective population-based study (the Ontario Children's Study), Mustard et al. (2005) showed that low parental education had an independent effect on future low back-pain occurrence in adult life. In a systematic review of evidence for educational status as a causal factor, Dionne and colleagues identified evidence that less well-educated groups had higher rates of disabling back pain (Dionne et al., 2001). By contrast, Kempen and colleagues (1999) called into question the extent of the contribution of education level to chronic pain experience, suggesting that there was evidence of a specific but rather limited moderating effect of education on the dominant role of the medical diagnosis. However, such small but distinctive effects may have large consequences for the common conditions that are the major public health targets for chronic pain prevention.

On balance, increasing the proportion of young persons continuing into higher education seems to offer one possible population-level intervention, which might be desirable for many other reasons. However, it is far from clear what mechanisms are mediating the effect of education level on chronic pain incidence. Furthermore, there is an unanswered ecological question about why the historical rise in higher education numbers, e.g. in the UK from 1945 onwards, has been accompanied by a seeming rise in chronic pain rather than a decline in response to the improved education levels.

Social influences

Social influences on the phenotype of chronic illness in the population offers a second example and a different perspective. The idea of an amplified 'chronic pain syndrome' was introduced in Section 1 and has reappeared throughout this book. There is evidence for such a phenotype from general analyses of population health. Schur et al. (2007), for example, investigated clusters of symptom syndromes in 3912 twins. The biggest proportion was generally healthy, but the commonest illness cluster (17% of the sample) was depression, low back pain, and headache. In an analysis of 30 years of an American cohort study, low household income and low levels of physical activity predicted an unremitting decline in future general health (Kaplan et al., 2007). In a long-term UK follow-up of a cohort of schoolchildren, children who were noted as 'often complaining of aches and pains' were more likely to be permanently sick and disabled at ages 45–50 years (Henderson et al., 2009). It seems likely that, although individual characteristics will vary substantially, part of the population picture of chronic pain is that it clusters with other aspects of ill-health, and part of this clustering represents a trajectory over time and through life. Social disadvantage plays an influential population-level role in shaping this trajectory.

Secondary and tertiary prevention of chronic pain

We are mainly concerned in this book with the possibility that there could be population-level interventions to prevent chronic pain.

However, Chapter 2 pointed out that people with chronic pain so commonly present to primary care in developed countries that effective treatment could have population effects. Whether this is secondary or tertiary prevention depends on one's perspective – tackling prognostic factors for chronicity in people presenting with pain can be viewed as either tertiary prevention of the consequences of chronic pain or secondary prevention of chronic disabling pain. For simplicity we consider attempts to control, reduce, or remove pain as secondary prevention, accepting that any successful reduction of pain may represent clinically important tertiary prevention of pain and disability. The issue for public health is whether these approaches also count as reasonable efforts at secondary long-term prevention of chronic pain syndrome in the population.

Many areas of primary prevention are equally relevant to secondary prevention (e.g. physical activity or behavioural change) and examples have been considered above. Indeed, much of the evidence about the benefits of physical activity and psychological interventions comes from secondary and tertiary prevention studies (e.g. Karmisholt and Gotzsche, 2005). However, the most widely used intervention in primary care is analgesic medication. We have considered one detailed example in this book – Zhang and Doherty's comprehensive systematic review of the evidence for effectiveness of pharmacological treatments for OA in Chapter 23.

We know the following about OA:

1 The clinical syndrome of joint pain in older people is more common than the radiographic disease.

2 It is the dominant cause of disability in older people.

3 Self-reported pain in older people is considered predominantly to refer to clinical OA.

4 Drug treatments are provided for two-thirds of people attending primary care with clinical OA.

Zhang and Doherty identify modest effect sizes for a range of pharmacological interventions. These interventions could potentially be applied to the large number of people with joint pain for the many years they survive with the condition, although some sufferers will also receive other interventions such as joint replacements. This is potentially a large population exposure to drugs. The authors also highlight some of the potential side effects of drug use which, although estimates of the incidence of these may be low, would involve significant numbers of people, again because of the high numbers exposed. The authors provide a clear basis for useful clinical decision-making, on the basis of the current evidence. However, a broader question to address is whether medication is a sensible public health intervention for the prevention of chronic pain in populations.

Population patterns of medicines use

Using medicines to relieve pain is common. Most people who experience pain report that they use medicines to ease pain, either prescribed or over-the-counter. Population surveys of the use of medicines in Europe, USA, and Canada have shown consistent figures between countries and between studies for analgesic use, depending on the precise definitions used, and there has been a significant rise in the proportion of people in the general population using analgesics from 1980 onwards. Table 26.1 illustrates some examples from this evidence base.

There is general agreement between such surveys on the demographic associations of analgesic use – women are more likely to report using both prescription analgesia and over-the-counter medication, and persons from less well-off sectors of society tend to report higher levels of use, although this varies with study setting and with type of analgesic use. Opioids for chronic pain in the USA, for example, are more frequently used by non-Hispanic whites than by other groups (Parsells Kelly et al., 2008), whilst the Tromsø studies (Eggen, 1994) reported higher analgesic use in persons with higher education levels. Other characteristics linked with higher analgesic use, noted in the studies in Table 26.1, include persons who report lower general health, poor sleep, less physical activity, depression, and overweight.

The demographics of analgesic use in persons with chronic pain tend then to be the same demographics as those of persons more likely to have chronic pain in the first place. However, in most of these studies, it is not clear whether the demographic picture of analgesic use arises only from the higher prevalence of chronic pain in these groups or from higher recourse to analgesics by people with chronic pain in these groups.

Whether these rates of use are, in general, reasonable or not is less a public health issue than a moral and clinical one of the right-to-pain-relief. Regardless of any long-term benefits or costs of using medication for acute or episodic or end-of-life pain, the humane requirements of pain relief are a crucial component of these figures. Appropriate and equal access to strong and effectively used analgesia in acute pain and emergency medicine continues, for example, to be an important global concern. In America, despite evidence that the proportion of patients with pain in emergency medicine departments receiving appropriate opioid analgesia increased following government initiatives in the 1990s, this form of analgesia still remains unequally available to different social groups (Pletcher et al., 2008).

The short-term pain relief provided by analgesia may, in practice, provide one public health approach to the population burden of common acute or episodic pains such as headache or minor musculoskeletal pain. This may also be true of short-term pain relief in chronic pain. Systematic reviews of the efficacy of chronic pain treatments, such as Zhang and Doherty in Chapter 23 or Keller et al.'s 2007 review of non-surgical treatments for back pain, have consistently reported modest but definite effects of analgesia in providing short-term relief of chronic pain.

Table 26.1 Prevalence studies of analgesic use

Ref	Country	Design	Group	Drug	Prevalence
Pitkala, 2002 (relates to 1989)	Finland	Population	Adults	Analgesic use	29%
Eggen, 1994	Tromso	Population 21–61	Men	Recent analgesic	13%
			Women	Recent analgesia	28%
Furu et al., 1997	Finnmark	Population 20–62	Men	Recent analgesic	17%
			Women	Recent analgesic	33%
Antonov 1998	Sweden	Population 18–84	Men	Prescription analgesic	7.2%
			Women		12.2 %
Antonov 1998	Sweden	Population 18–84	Men	Over the counter(OTC)	20.0%
			Women		30.4%
Andersson 1999	Sweden	Population 25–74		Analgesics for chronic pain	14%
Pitkala, 2002 (relates to 1999)	Finland	Population	Adults	Analgesic use	41%
Curhan 2002	US	Nurses 33–77	Women	Regular acetaminophen	20%
Curhan 2002	US	Nurses 33–77	Women ≤51	Regular NSAIDs	42%
			Women >51	Regular aspirin	25%
Motola 2004	Italy	Population	Adults	Regular NSAIDs	23%
Turunen 2005	Finland	Population	Adults	Prescription analgesic	27%
Turunen 2005	Finland	Population	Adults	OTC	41%
Blyth 2005	Australia	Population, 18-plus	Chronic pain	Medication	47%
Hargreave 2010	Denmark	Population 18–45	Men	Continuous regular analgesics	18%
			Women		27%
Brefel-Courbon 2009	France	Population	Adults	Chronic analgesic prescriptions	20%
Brefel-Courbon 2009	France	Population	Osteoarthritis	Chronic analgesia	33%
			Parkinsons	Chronic analgesia	33%
Sadowski 2009	Canada	Population	65-plus	Analgesia use during 1 year	34%

The public health issue surrounding long-term analgesic use for chronic pain however is different, and concerns the following question:

Are medicines of value in the long-term prevention of chronic pain and its consequences?

As Zhang and Doherty show for the common long-term problem of OA, and as others have shown, e.g. for opioid therapy for chronic non-cancer pain (Trescot et al., 2008), there is very little evidence regarding long-term benefits of analgesic medication for the prevention of chronic pain. This is not to argue against using analgesia for chronic pain, but for setting such use in the context of the potential for harm and the lack of effectiveness of long-term analgesic use as a public health approach to preventing the common problem of chronic pain and its consequences.

Just as the assumption that pain relief is universally available for those who need it is incorrect and remains a suitable target for global policy-making, so also is the assumption incorrect and unproven that universal availability of potent analgesics will result in the reduction of chronic pain in the population alongside a positive cost–benefit profile. We should be concerned from a public health point-of-view with the escalating use of analgesics, especially opioid medications, for the long-term public health control and prevention of chronic pain.

The example of opioids Zhang and Doherty review the efficacy of opioids for OA pain, estimating the evidence as showing a definite effect but identifying the evidence base as restricted exclusively to short-term studies. The literature on the use of opioids in chronic pain more generally also points to little clear evidence of effectiveness beyond 6 months (Trescot et al., 2008). Ballantyne, in one of a series of reasoned articles, highlights the value of opioids for short-term pain relief in chronic pain (i.e. some months), but points out that their benefits in improving function are less clear (Ballantyne and Shin, 2008). In a meta-analysis of trials of opioids for chronic back pain, no evidence for significant pain reduction was found compared with placebo or controls taking non-opioids; no trials were longer than 16 weeks (Martell et al., 2007). This latter paper also estimated a figure for lifetime substance misuse of 43% in persons taking opioids for back pain. As with other investigations of the risk of misuse, these authors emphasize the influence of prior misuse or mental health problems on misuse rates, but also highlight that the attributable risk in relation to these predictors is high because they are so common in back-pain sufferers.

There is consistent evidence of increasingly frequent use of strong opioids in the management of chronic non-cancer pain in the USA, Europe, and elsewhere. Parsells Kelly and colleagues (2008) presented results from the telephone-based Slone Surveys of a representative sample of US adults ($n = 19 150$ over a 10-year period): 4.9% of this sample reported using opioids, 2% regularly and 2.9% less regularly. The authors estimated that 4 million US adults use opioids regularly, and this increases with age and among females and people with lower education levels. In a subset of persons with back pain, 11–13% were using opioids. In Northern Europe, 3% of the population are estimated to be using opioids regularly, and this again is linked to increased age, reduced education, and negative perceived health (Eriksen et al., 2006).

Caudill-Slosberg and colleagues (2004), among others, have shown that these figures represent a clear increase from earlier years: use of potent opioids increased in a US health care organization from 2% to 9% between 1980 and 2000, despite no parallel increase in consultations for musculoskeletal pain (the latter was responsible for 28% of adult visits in both years). There is evidence of parallel increases elsewhere in the world, although not all of the observed patterns are consistent with each other. For example, in a comparison of the Nordic countries from 2002 to 2006

(Hamunen et al., 2009), total use of opioids increased in all countries except Sweden; increase according to type of opioid (strong or mild) varied between the countries, although oxycodone use increased in all except Iceland. The authors of this comparison related the patterns of change primarily to the marketing of the drugs, but noted that the general trend was towards increased use.

Confirmation that most of this opioid use is among persons with common chronic pain syndromes can be found in a study in which 2% of survey responders had used opioids for at least 1 month, with 63% of regular users reporting arthritis and 59% back pain (Hudson et al., 2008). This study illustrates another consistent finding – use of long-term opioids rises with the number of pain complaints; in this study there was an average of two pain conditions reported by each opioid user.

Perhaps the most striking finding from the surveys of analgesic use in the general population is that if a person is using one medication, they are very likely to be using another. Users of treatments tend to have high rates of use of multiple medications. Parsells Kelly et al.'s analysis of the Slone Surveys in America (2008) found that 32% of regular opioid users were using >5 other prescription drugs, including 12% who were using non-steroidal anti-inflammatory drugs (NSAIDs) and 31% who were using antidepressants, compared with 7.5%, 2%, and 7%, respectively, of individuals not on opioids.

Non-pharmacological interventions for chronic pain will also be used alongside opioid medications. Nicholas and colleagues have raised an important issue about this: the potentially negative effect of the use of strong analgesia such as opioids on these other approaches to the management of persistent non-cancer pain, notably on techniques designed to facilitate long-term behavioural change (Nicholas et al., 2006). They highlight that the use of opioids may directly contradict the principles of behavioural approaches to pain management – e.g. by reinforcing 'avoidance responses' (e.g. sickness absence) which promote disability.

There is also continuing debate on the long-term safety of opioids for chronic non-cancer pain, relating to issues such as misuse, poisoning and overdose on the one hand versus the problem of under-prescribing for pain on the other. The reality is that long-term studies of effectiveness and safety are not available in the context of dramatically rising rates of prescribing of these medicines (e.g. Ballantyne and Shin, 2008; Von Korff and Deyo, 2004). What does seem clear is that opioid use will not solve the population problem of chronic pain. Many persons on opioid treatment continue to experience significant pain and activity limitations (Eriksen et al., 2006). The public health concern, once the issue of optimal global availability of opioids for humane and effective treatment of acute, traumatic, and end-of-life pain has been addressed (Ballantyne, 2007), is that the widespread use of opioids for the long-term management of chronic pain might prove to be ineffective, costly and counterproductive.

Conclusion

This last example summarizes the dilemma posed so elegantly by Geoffrey Rose in his writings. Clinicians must always be concerned with the sick individual, and the individual person in pain represents perhaps par excellence the requirement for the clinician to provide the best treatment available. Humane and effective approaches to immediate pain relief may not, however, be the best approaches to the different problem of managing chronic pain over time and preventing its adverse consequences on daily activity and social life. Sick populations may require completely different perspectives on prevention, involving interventions designed to shift the risk of chronic pain and its consequences in the population as a whole, regardless of what is done for the individual at high risk. Public health policy and practice, directed at primary prevention of chronic pain in populations, offers the potential to reduce the frequency of chronic pain and the impact which it has on societies. The universality of pain as part of the human experience however means that the scientific, clinical, and policy pursuit of the optimal treatment for the sick individual in pain needs to continue in tandem with the scientific, public health, and policy pursuit of the optimal approach to the population in pain.

References

Andersson HI, Ejlertsson G, Leden I, Scherstén B. 1999: Impact of chronic pain on health care seeking, self care, and medication. Results from a population-based Swedish study. *J Epidemiol Community Health* **53**, 503–9.

Antonov KIM, Isacson DGL. 1998: Prescription and non-prescription analgesic use in Sweden. *Ann Pharmacother* **32**, 485–94.

Ballantyne JC. 2007: Opioid analgesia: perspectives on right use and utility. *Pain Physician* **10**, 479–91.

Ballantyne JC, Shin NS. 2008: Efficacy of opioids for chronic pain: a review of the evidence. *Clin J Pain* **24**, 469–78.

Bergman S. 2007: Public health perspective – how to improve the musculoskeletal health of the population. *Best Pract Res Clin Rheumatol* **21**, 191–204.

Berke EM, Gottlieb LM, Moudon AV, Larson EB. 2007: Protective association between neighbourhood walkability and depression in older men. *J Am Geriatr Soc* **55**, 526–33.

Blagojevic M, Jinks C, Jeffery A, Jordan KP. 2010: Risk factors for onset of osteoarthritis of the knee in older adults: a systematic review and meta-analysis. *Osteoarthritis Cartilage* **18**, 24–33.

Blyth FM, March LM, Brnabic AJ, Cousins MJ. 2004: Chronic pain and frequent use of health care. *Pain* **111**, 51–8.

Brefel-Courbon C, Grolleau S, Thalamas C, Bourrel R, Allaria-Lapierre V, Loï R, et al. 2009: Comparison of chronic analgesic drugs prevalence in Parkinson's disease, other chronic diseases and the general population. *Pain* **141**, 14–8.

Brown WJ, Ford JH, Burton NW, Marshall AL, Dobson AJ. 2005: Prospective study of physical activity and depressive symptoms in middle-aged women. *Am J Prev Med* **29**, 265–72.

Buchner DM, Beresford SA, Larson EB, LaCroix AZ, Wagner EH. 1992: Effects of physical activity on health status in older adults. II. Intervention studies. *Annu Rev Public Health* **13**, 469–88.

Caudill-Slosberg MA, Schwartz LM, Woloshin S. 2004: Office visits and analgesic prescriptions for musculoskeletal pain in US: 1980 vs 2000. *Pain* **109**, 514–19.

Conn VS, Hafdahl AR, Minor MA, Nielsen PJ. 2008: Physical activity interventions among adults with arthritis: meta-analysis of outcomes. *Semin Arthritis Rheum* **37**, 307–16.

Croft PR, Papageorgiou AC, Ferry S, Thomas E, Jayson MI, Silman AJ. 1995: Psychologic distress and low back pain. Evidence from a prospective study in the general population. *Spine* **20**, 2731–7.

Curhan GC, Bullock AJ, Hankinson SE, Willett WC, Speizer FE, Stampfer MJ. 2002: Frequency of use of acetaminophen, nonsteroidal anti-inflammatory drugs, and aspirin in US women. *Pharmacoepidemiol Drug Saf.* **11**, 687–93.

Dionne CE, Von Korff M, Koepsell TD, Deyo RA, Barlow WE, Checkoway H. 2001: Formal education and back pain: a review. *J Epidemiol Community Health* **55**, 455–68.

Dugan SA, Everson-Rose SA, Karavolos K, Sternfeld B, Wesley D, Powell LH. 2009: The impact of physical activity level on SF-36 role-physical and bodily pain indices in midlife women. *J Phys Act Health* **6**, 33–42.

Eggen AE. 1994: Pattern of drug use in a general population – prevalence and predicting factors: the Tromsø study. *Int J Epidemiol* **23**, 1262–72.

Foster NE, Bishop A, Thomas E, Main C, Horne R, Weinman J, et al. 2008: Illness perceptions of low back pain patients in primary care: what are they, do they change and are they associated with outcome? *Pain* **136**, 177–87.

Eriksen J, Sjøgren P, Bruera E, Ekholm O, Rasmussen NK. 2006: Critical issues on opioids in chronic non-cancer pain: an epidemiological study. *Pain* **125**, 172–9.

Furu K, Straume B, Theile DS. 1997: Legal drug use in a general population: association with gender, mortality, health care utilisation, and lifestyle characteristics. *J Clin Epidemiol* **50**, 341–9.

Guh DP, Zhang W, Bansback N, Amarsi Z, Birmingham CL, Anis AH. 2009: The incidence of co-morbidities related to obesity and overweight: a systematic review and meta-analysis. *BMC Public Health* **9**, 88.

Gupta A, Silman AJ, Ray D, Morriss R, Dickens C, MacFarlane GJ, et al. 2007: The role of psychosocial factors in predicting the onset of chronic widespread pain: results from a prospective population-based study. *Rheumatology* **46**, 666–71.

Hagen KB, Tambs K, Bjerkedal T. 2006: What mediates the inverse association between education and occupational disability from back pain? A prospective cohort study from the Nord-Trøndelag health study in Norway. *Soc Sci Med* **63**, 1267–75.

Hamunen K, Paakkari P, Kalso E. 2009: Trends in opioid consumption in the Nordic countries 2002-2006. *Eur J Pain* **13**, 954–62.

Hargreave M, Andersen TV, Nielsen A, Munk C, Liaw KL, Kjaer SK. 2010: Factors associated with a continuous regular analgesic use – a population-based study of more than 45 000 Danish women and men 18-45 years of age. *Pharmacoepidemiol Drug Saf* **19**, 65–74.

Hartvigsen J, Christensen K. 2007: Active lifestyle protects against incident low back pain in seniors: a population-based 2-year prospective study of 1387 Danish twins aged 70-100 years. *Spine* **32**, 76–81.

Heim N, Snijder MB, Deeg DJ, Seidell JC, Visser M. 2008: Obesity in older adults is associated with an increased prevalence and incidence of pain. *Obesity* **16**, 2510–17.

Henderson M, Hotopf M, Leon DA. 2009: Childhood temperament and long-term sickness absence in adult life. *Br J Psychiatry* **194**, 220–3.

Hestbaek L, Korsholm L, Leboeuf-Yde C, Kyvik KO. 2008: Does socioeconomic status in adolescence predict low back pain in adulthood? A repeated cross-sectional study of 4,771 Danish adolescents. *Eur Spine J* **17**, 1727–34.

Hudson TJ, Edlund MJ, Steffick DE, Tripathi SP, Sullivan MD. 2008: Epidemiology of regular prescribed opioid use: results from a national, population-based survey. *J Pain Symptom Manage* **36**, 280–8.

Jinks C, Jordan K, Croft P. 2006: Disabling knee pain – another consequence of obesity: results from a prospective cohort study. *BMC Public Health* **6**, 258.

Jordan KP, Thomas E, Peat G, Wilkie R, Croft P. 2008: Social risks for disabling pain in older people: a prospective study of individual and area characteristics. *Pain* **137**, 652–61.

Kaplan GA, Baltrus PT, Raghunathan TE. 2007: The shape of health to come: prospective study of the determinants of 30-year health trajectories in the Alameda County Study. *Int J Epidemiol* **36**, 542–8.

Karmisholt K, Gøtzsche PC. 2005: Physical activity for secondary prevention of disease. Systematic reviews of randomised clinical trials. *Dan Med Bull* **52**, 90–4.

Keller A, Hayden J, Bombardier C, van Tulder M. 2007: Effect sizes of non-surgical treatments of non-specific low-back pain. *Eur Spine J* **16**, 1776–88.

Kempen GI, Brilman EI, Ranchor AV, Ormel J. 1999: Morbidity and quality of life and the moderating effects of level of education in the elderly. *Soc Sci Med* **49**, 143–9.

Lake JK, Power C, Cole TJ. 2000: Back pain and obesity in the 1958 British birth cohort: cause or effect? *J Clin Epidemiol* **53**, 245–50.

Leino P, Magni G. 1993: Depressive and distress symptoms as predictors of low back pain, neck-shoulder pain, and other musculoskeletal morbidity: a 10-year follow-up of metal industry employees. *Pain* **53**, 89–94.

Macfarlane GJ, Norrie G, Atherton K, Power C, Jones GT. 2009: The influence of socioeconomic status on the reporting of regional and widespread musculoskeletal pain: results from the 1958 British Birth Cohort Study. *Ann Rheum Dis* **68**, 1591–5.

Mackenbach JP, Borsboom GJ, Nusselder WJ, Looman CW, Schrijvers CT. 2001: Determinants of levels and changes of physical functioning in chronically ill persons: results from the GLOBE Study. *J Epidemiol Community Health* **55**, 631–8.

Martell BA, O'Connor PG, Kerns RD, Becker WC, Morales KH, Kosten TR, et al. 2007: Systematic review: opioid treatment for chronic back pain: prevalence, efficacy, and association with addiction. *Ann Intern Med* **146**, 116–27.

McBeth J, Macfarlane GJ, Silman AJ. 2002: Does chronic pain predict future psychological distress? *Pain* **96**, 239–45.

Motola D, Vaccheri A, Silvani MC, Poluzzi E, Bottoni A, De Ponti F, et al. 2004: Patterns of NSAID use in the Italian general population: a questionnaire-based survey. *Eur J Clin Pharmacol.* **60**, 731–8.

Mustard CA, Kalcevich C, Frank JW, Boyle M. 2005: Childhood and early adult predictors of risk of incident back pain: Ontario Child Health Study 2001 follow-up. *Am J Epidemiol* **162**, 779–86.

Nicholas MK, Molloy AR, Brooker C. 2006: Using opioids with persisting noncancer pain: a biopsychosocial perspective. *Clin J Pain* **22**, 137–46.

Palmer KT, Reading I, Linaker C, Calnan M, Coggon D. 2008: Population-based cohort study of incident and persistent arm pain: role of mental health, self-rated health and health beliefs. *Pain* **136**, 30–7.

Paras ML, Murad MH, Chen LP, Goranson EN, Sattler AL, Colbenson KM, et al. 2009: Sexual abuse and lifetime diagnosis of somatic disorders: a systematic review and meta-analysis. *JAMA* **302**, 550–61.

Parsells Kelly J, Cook SF, Kaufman DW, Anderson T, Rosenberg L, Mitchell AA. 2008: Prevalence and characteristics of opioid use in the US adult population. *Pain* **138**, 507–13.

Patten SB, Williams JV, Lavorato DH, Modgill G, Jetté N, Eliasziw M. 2008: Major depression as a risk factor for chronic disease incidence: longitudinal analyses in a general population cohort. *Gen Hosp Psychiatry* **30**, 407–13.

Penninx BW, Leveille S, Ferrucci L, van Eijk JT, Guralnik JM. 1999: Exploring the effect of depression on physical disability: longitudinal evidence from the established populations for epidemiologic studies of the elderly. *Am J Public Health* **89**, 1346–52.

Pincus T, Burton K, Vogel S, Field AP. 2002: A systematic review of psychological factors as predictors of chronicity/disability in prospective cohorts of low back pain. *Spine* **27**, E109–20.

Pitkala KH, Strandberg TE, Tilvis RS. 2002: Management of nonmalignant pain in home-dwelling older people: a population-based survey. *J Am Geriatr Soc.* **50**, 1861–5.

Pletcher MJ, Kertesz SG, Kohn MA, Gonzales R. 2008: Trends in opioid prescribing by race/ethnicity for patients seeking care in US emergency departments. *JAMA* **299**, 70–8.

Sadowski CA, Carrie AG, Grymonpre RE, Metge CJ, St John P. 2009: Medication use among children <12 years of age in the United States: results from the Slone Survey. *Pediatrics.* **124**, 446–54.

Schur EA, Afari N, Furberg H, Olarte M, Goldberg J, Sullivan PF, et al. 2007: Feeling bad in more ways than one: comorbidity patterns of medically unexplained and psychiatric conditions. *J Gen Intern Med* **22**, 818–21.

Seavey WG, Kurata JH, Cohen RD. 2003: Risk factors for incident self-reported arthritis in a 20 year followup of the Alameda County Study Cohort. *J Rheumatol* **30**, 2103–11.

Severeijns R, Vlaeyen JW, van den Hout MA, Picavet HS. 2005: Pain catastrophising and consequences of musculoskeletal pain: a prospective study in the Dutch community. *J Pain* **6**, 125–32.

Thomas E, Silman AJ, Croft PR, Papageorgiou AC, Jayson MI, Macfarlane GJ. 1999: Predicting who develops chronic low back pain in primary care: a prospective study. *BMJ* **318**, 1662–7.

Trescot AM, Helm S, Hansen H, Benyamin R, Glaser SE, Adlaka R, et al. 2008: Opioids in the management of chronic non-cancer pain: an update of the American Society of Interventional Pain Physicians' (ASIPP) guidelines. *Pain Physician* **11** (Suppl 2), S5–S62.

Turunen JH, Mantyselka PT, Kumpusalo EA, Ahonen RS. 2005: Frequent analgesic use at population level: prevalence and patterns of use. *Pain* **115**, 374–81.

Von Korff M, Deyo RA. 2004: Potent opioids for chronic musculoskeletal pain: flying blind? *Pain* **109**, 207–9.

Wedderkopp N, Kjaer P, Hestbaek L, Korsholm L, Leboeuf-Yde C. 2009: High-level physical activity in childhood seems to protect against low back pain in early adolescence. *Spine J* **9**, 134–41.

Index